T0342092

The False Discovery Rate

STATISTICS IN PRACTICE

Series Editor
Geert Molenberghs

Statistics in Practice is an important international series of texts which provide detailed coverage of statistical concepts, methods and worked case studies in specific fields of investigation and study.

With sound motivation and many worked practical examples, the books show in down-to-earth terms how to select and use an appropriate range of statistical techniques in a particular practical field within each title's special topic area.

The books provide statistical support for professionals and research workers across a range of employment fields and research environments. Subject areas covered include medicine and pharmaceutics; industry, finance and commerce; public services; the earth and environmental sciences, and so on.

The books also provide support to students studying statistical courses applied to the above areas. The demand for graduates to be equipped for the work environment has led to such courses becoming increasingly prevalent at universities and colleges.

It is our aim to present judiciously chosen and well-written workbooks to meet everyday practical needs. Feedback of views from readers will be most valuable to monitor the success of this aim.

The False Discovery Rate

Its Meaning, Interpretation and Application in Data Science

N.W. Galwey
GlaxoSmithKline Research and Development
Stevenage
UK

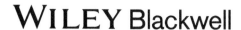

Registered Office(s)
John Wiley & Sons, Inc., 111 River Street, Hoboken, NJ 07030, USA
John Wiley & Sons Ltd, The Atrium, Southern Gate, Chichester, West Sussex, PO19 8SQ, UK

For details of our global editorial offices, customer services, and more information about Wiley products visit us at www.wiley.com.

Library of Congress Cataloging-in-Publication Data
Names: Galwey, N.W., author. | John Wiley & Sons, publisher.
Title: The false discovery rate : its meaning, interpretation and
    application in data science / N.W. Galwey.
Description: Hoboken, NJ : Wiley-Blackwell, 2025. | Includes
    bibliographical references and index.
Identifiers: LCCN 2024034645 (print) | LCCN 2024034646 (ebook) | ISBN
    9781119889779 (hardback) | ISBN 9781119889786 (adobe pdf) | ISBN
    9781119889793 (epub)
Subjects: LCSH: Statistical hypothesis testing. | Mathematical statistics.
Classification: LCC QA277 .G25 2025 (print) | LCC QA277 (ebook) | DDC
    519.5/6–dc23/eng20241010
LC record available at https://lccn.loc.gov/2024034645
LC ebook record available at https://lccn.loc.gov/2024034646

Cover Design: Wiley

Cover Images: Courtesy of N.W. Galwey

Set in 9.5/12.5pt STIXTwoText by Straive, Pondicherry, India
Printed and bound by CPI Group (UK) Ltd, Croydon, CR0 4YY
C9781119889779_251024

Contents

Preface and Acknowledgement

The motivation to write this book came from an occasion when members of GlaxoSmithKline's (GSK's) Research Statistics Group invited me to talk about the False Discovery Rate (FDR) for twice as long as we had originally planned. I concluded that if this group of very able, highly educated statisticians felt that they did not know as much about the FDR as they wanted to, there must be many other statisticians and researchers in the same situation. This book is intended to enable such people to use the FDR with practical proficiency, and with a full understanding of its meaning.

I am grateful to members of the Research Statistics Group and other GSK colleagues, in particular G.Q. Cai, Tanja Högg, Anna Hutchinson, Tasos Papanikos and Paul Wilson, for comments on drafts of various parts of the book. Further afield, I am grateful to Jane Hutton, Julia Mortera and Amy Wilson for similar help; and closer to home, to my wife, Caroline Galwey. I am particularly grateful to Stephen Senn, for endorsing the project at the commissioning stage, and for reviewing the entire draft manuscript. Any errors of fact or interpretation that remain are the sole responsibility of the author.

Computer code relating to the numerical and graphical examples, and other supplementary material, is available from the book's website, at www.wiley.com/go/falsediscoveryrate.

About the Companion Website

This book is complemented by a companion website.

www.wiley.com/go/falsediscoveryrate

The companion website provides computer code (R scripts) to reproduce the numerical and graphical examples in the book.

1

Introduction

1.1   A Brief History of Multiple Testing

In the beginning was the significance threshold. By the early twentieth century, researchers with an awareness of random variation became concerned that the interesting results that they wished to report might have occurred by chance. Mathematicians worked to develop methods for quantifying this risk, and in 1926, R.A. Fisher wrote,

> ...it is convenient to draw the line at about the level at which we can say: 'Either there is something in the treatment, or a coincidence has occurred such as does not occur more than once in twenty trials'.

That is, he suggested a threshold of $\alpha = 0.05$, adding,

> If one in twenty does not seem high enough odds, we may, if we prefer it, draw the line at one in fifty (the 2 per cent. point) or one in a hundred (the 1 per cent. point). (Fisher, 1926, p. 504)

Fisher's suggestion was taken up by researchers, but for the next few decades they did not usually calculate the probability of obtaining, by coincidence, the observed result of each particular study. Such a calculation required a substantial amount of work by a trained mathematician. Instead, the researcher calculated a test statistic – z, t, F, χ^2 or r (the correlation coefficient), depending on the design of the study and the question asked – and compared the value obtained with a published table of values corresponding to particular thresholds, typically $\alpha = 0.05$, 0.01 and 0.001. For example, suppose that a researcher analysing data from an experiment obtained the result $t = -3.1$, with 8 degrees of freedom (d.f. $= 8$). If they were interested in large effects either positive or negative, they would consult a table of values of the t statistic for a two-sided test, and find that $P(|T_8| > 2.306) = 0.05$ and $P(|T_8| > 3.355) = 0.01$. Hence, they would conclude that their result was significant at the 5% ($\alpha = 0.05$) level, but not at the 1% ($\alpha = 0.01$) level. Though no probability had been calculated, such a conclusion could be reported in terms of a p-value – in this case, $p < 0.05$.

The False Discovery Rate: Its Meaning, Interpretation and Application in Data Science, First Edition.
N.W. Galwey.
© 2025 John Wiley & Sons Ltd. Published 2025 by John Wiley & Sons Ltd.
Companion website: www.wiley.com/go/falsediscoveryrate

By the late 1970s, many researchers had desktop or pocket calculators offering statistical functions, or even had access to programmable computers. This enabled them to present the actual p-value associated with their result, rather than comparing the result to pre-specified thresholds. In the present case, they would report $p = 0.015$. However, the preoccupation with thresholds that had its origin in arithmetical convenience persisted, and a value of $p > 0.05$ was (and is) typically presented as 'non-significant' ('NS'), whereas $p < 0.05$ is 'significant' (often indicated by '*'); $p < 0.01$ is 'highly significant' ('**'); and $p < 0.001$ is 'very highly significant' ('***').

By this time, such significance tests had become the mainstay of statistical data analysis in the biological and social sciences – a status that they still retain. However, it was apparent from the outset that there are conceptual problems associated with such tests. Firstly, the test does not address precisely the question that the researcher most wants to answer. The researcher is not primarily interested in the probability of their dataset – in a sense its probability is irrelevant, as it is an event that has actually happened. What they really want to know is the probability of the hypothesis that the experiment was designed to test. This is the problem of 'inverse' or 'Bayesian' probability, the probability of things that are not – and cannot be – observed. Secondly, although the probability that a single experiment will give a significant result by coincidence is low, if more tests are conducted, the probability that at least one of them will do so increases.

Initially, these difficulties were dealt with by an informal understanding that if results were unlikely to be obtained by coincidence, then the probability that they were indeed produced by coincidence was low, and hence the hypothesis that this had occurred – the null hypothesis, H_0 – could be rejected. It followed that among all the 'discoveries' announced by many researchers working over many years, it would not often turn out that the null hypothesis had, after all, been correct. As long as every study and every statistical analysis conducted required a considerable effort on the part of the researcher, there was some reason for confidence in this argument: researchers would not usually waste their time and other resources striving to detect effects that were unlikely to exist.

However, in the last decades of the twentieth century, technological developments changed the situation. There were several aspects to this expansion of the scope for statistical analysis, namely:

- Increased capacity for statistical calculations, initially by centralised mainframe computers, and later by personal computers and other devices that could be under the control of a small research group or an individual.
- Increased capacity for electronic data storage. 'The world's technological per-capita capacity to store information has roughly doubled every 40 months since the 1980s' (Hilbert and López 2011, quoted by https://en.wikipedia.org/wiki/Big_data, accessed 15 April 2024).
- Development of electronic automated measuring devices, electronic data loggers for capturing the measurements from traditional devices such as thermometers, and high-throughput laboratory technologies for obtaining experimental data (the latter particularly in genetics and genomics).
- Development of user-friendly software, usually with a 'point-and-click' interface, enabling researchers to perform their own routine statistical analyses and ending their dependence on specialist programmers or statisticians for this service.

By the 1990s, the term 'big data' started to be used to refer to such developments. The management, manipulation and exploration of these huge datasets were characterised as a discipline called 'data science', distinct from classical statistics:

> While the term data science is not new, the meanings and connotations have changed over time. The word first appeared in the '60s as an alternative name for statistics. In the late '90s, computer science professionals formalized the term. A proposed definition for data science saw it as a separate field with three aspects: data design, collection, and analysis. It still took another decade for the term to be used outside of academia. (Amazon Web Services, https://aws.amazon.com/what-is/data-science/, accessed 15 April 2024)

When thousands of statistical hypothesis tests could be performed with negligible effort either in the collection or the analysis of the data, the prospect that multiple testing would lead to significant results in cases where H_0 was true – false positives – became effectively a certainty.

The problem of false-positive results is exacerbated if the multiple testing that has caused it is not apparent when the results are reported. This can occur, inadvertently or deliberately, due to several distinct mechanisms, for example, as follows:

1) Repeatedly testing the same null hypothesis. Specifically,
   - repeated testing of the same hypothesis by the same method, stopping when a significant result is obtained and reporting only the last test: a flagrant abuse of statistical significance testing;
   - less obviously, testing of the same null hypothesis in unconnected studies, reporting only the one or a few that give significant results, perhaps with no awareness that the other studies existed.
2) Testing a number of related null hypotheses, and reporting only those that give a significant result. Specifically,
   - simple failure to report the number of hypotheses, directly comparable with each other, that have been considered (e.g., the number of candidate genes that have been tested for association with a heritable disease);
   - testing each of several types of event (e.g., adverse health outcomes) for association with each of several exposures (e.g., potential environmental risk factors) resulting in a large number of pair-wise combinations;
   - in clinical trials, testing the effect of the medical intervention on secondary outcomes in addition to the pre-specified primary end-point;
   - also in clinical trials, testing the effect of the intervention on subsets of the patients recruited (e.g., older males, a particular ethnic group, patients with a particular comorbidity...).
3) Testing the same hypothesis by a number of different statistical methods. Specifically,
   - selection of different variables for inclusion as covariates in a multivariable regression model;
   - inclusion versus deletion of outliers;

- application of different analysis methods to the same data (logarithmic transformation, square root transformation, choice of a value for a 'tuning parameter' or the number of spline knot-points in advanced regression-analysis methods), and reporting only the one that gives the most satisfactory results.

If such concealment of multiplicity is practised deliberately, it is known as 'data dredging' or '*p*-hacking', and is a form of scientific malpractice. But even if multiplicity is not concealed from the reader, it may not be properly taken into account. In 1995, Benjamini and Hochberg reported that:

> In medical research, for example, [three published papers] examined samples of reports of comparative studies from major medical journals. They found that researchers overlook various kinds of multiplicity, and as a result reporting tends to exaggerate treatment differences (Pocock et al. 1987).

Simple recognition of the multiplicity that is present may be enough to prevent such exaggeration: before embarking on a more formal method for taking account of multiplicity, a researcher should consider the requirements, assumptions, and difficulties that this would entail. Nevertheless, often such a formal approach is called for. In this case, the appropriate method depends on the type of multiplicity present. Always assuming that the multiple testing has occurred in good faith (e.g., because the same hypothesis has been tested in several independent studies, all of which have been reported), and not as a result of an attempt to mislead, the methods required are as follows.

In the first broad category, when the same hypothesis has been tested in several separate studies, it is often appropriate to combine the results of these in a single analysis, known as a 'meta-analysis'. This approach is now commonly applied to clinical trials data: an introduction to the methods used is given by Ortiz et al. (2022).

In the third category, when the same hypothesis is tested by different methods in the same dataset, the appropriate remedy is to divide the dataset (if it is sufficiently large) into a training set, used to choose the most appropriate statistical model specifications, and a test set, 'used for assessment of the generalization error of the final chosen model. Ideally, the test set should be kept in a "vault," and be brought out only at the end of the data analysis' (Hastie et al. 2001, Section 7.2).

It is the second of the broad categories of multiplicity outlined in the preceding numbered list, in which a clearly specified set of distinct but related hypotheses are tested, that is addressed by Benjamini and Hochberg's paper, and is the focus of this book.

The problem of multiplicity continued to grow in the years following the publication of Benjamini and Hochberg's paper. In 2005, Ioannidis noted a 'high rate of non-replication (lack of confirmation) of research discoveries', and drew attention to an 'increasing concern that in modern research, false findings may be the majority or even the vast majority of published research claims'. He argued, on methodological grounds, that this must indeed be the case: his paper is entitled 'Why most published research findings are false'. The probability that a research claim is true, he stated, may depend on study power and bias, the number of other studies on the same question, and, importantly, the ratio of true to no relationships among the relationships probed in each scientific field. In this framework, a research finding is less likely to be true when the studies conducted in a field are smaller; when effect sizes are smaller; when there is a greater number and lesser preselection of tested relationships; where there is greater flexibility in designs, definitions, outcomes, and analytical modes; when there is greater financial and other interest and prejudice; and when more teams are involved in a scientific field in chase of statistical significance.

By the early 2010s, the problem of multiplicity (combined with the other factors noted by Ioannidis) was being referred to as a 'replication crisis':

> The replication crisis is frequently discussed in relation to psychology and medicine, where considerable efforts have been undertaken to reinvestigate classic results, to determine whether they are reliable, and if they turn out not to be, the reasons for the failure. Data strongly indicate that other natural and social sciences are affected as well. (https://en.wikipedia.org/wiki/Replication_crisis, accessed 15 April 2024)

In the subsequent years, awareness of the problem, and of the difficulty of getting negative evidence published when reported discoveries cannot be replicated, has spread to the non-scientific press (e.g., Ridley 2023).

In response to such concerns, the journal *Basic and Applied Social Psychology* took a decision to ban the presentation of p-values (Trafimow and Marks 2015). This radical step attracted close attention from researchers in a wide range of disciplines and also from statisticians, and the American Statistical Association (ASA) responded by convening a board of more than 20 experts to develop a policy statement on p-values and statistical significance. The resulting document was published, with an accompanying editorial, in *The American Statistician* in 2016 (Wasserstein and Lazar 2016). It comprised a set of six principles, set out in some detail, that sought to defend against the improper use and interpretation of p-values, while giving due recognition to their value when used properly. The accompanying editorial concluded,

> Though there was disagreement on exactly what the statement should say, there was high agreement that the ASA should be speaking out about these matters.
> Let us be clear. Nothing in the ASA statement is new. Statisticians and others have been sounding the alarm about these matters for decades, to little avail. We hoped that a statement from the world's largest professional association of statisticians would open a fresh discussion and draw renewed and vigorous attention to changing the practice of science with regards to the use of statistical inference.

Has the ASA succeeded in this ambition? p-values continue to be widely reported as a key result of a statistical data analysis, though they are now accompanied by a formal consideration of multiplicity much more often than was the case in the early days of significance testing. Still, the ASA statement was perhaps too detailed and nuanced to give practitioners the clear steer they desired, and significance tests continue to be viewed with unease. One response has been a steady increase in enthusiasm for Bayesian statistical methods, which address the null hypothesis and its alternative, H_1 (that the effect in question is real), directly, and seek to quantify and compare the probabilities of these alternatives, in the light of the data from the study. But this very attractive goal is approached at a price: to apply Bayesian methods, the researcher must be able and willing to quantify their relative degree of belief in each hypothesis (expressed as a probability) *before* the results of the study are known, and the reasonableness of such a 'prior probability distribution' is always open to challenge.

Within the 'frequentist' (i.e., non-Bayesian) statistical tradition, which considers the probability of data rather than of hypotheses, formal approaches to the problem of multiplicity go back a long way: they began with a proposed method of compensation published by Bonferroni in 1936. His approach was a contribution to probability theory in general; however, it can be expressed in the language of significance testing by noting that if m significance tests are conducted using a significance threshold α, then

$$P(p < \alpha \text{ for at least one test} | H_0 \text{ true for all tests}) \leq m\alpha.$$

Hence, one can compensate for the multiple testing either

- by specifying a more stringent significance threshold, $\alpha' = \alpha/m$, testing each p-value against this new threshold, and declaring a significant result only if $p < \alpha'$; or, equivalently,
- by multiplying each p-value by m, and comparing it to the original threshold, declaring significance only if $mp < \alpha$.

This 'Bonferroni correction' or 'Bonferroni adjustment' has long been applied in contexts where multiplicity is recognised to be an issue and where there is a clearly specified 'family' of tests under consideration, to provide the appropriate value of m. Control of the false-positive rate (also known as the family-wise error rate, FWER) is duly achieved at level α. However, like the proposed Bayesian solution, this achievement comes at a price, this time paid in 'statistical power': even when a real effect is present (i.e., when H_1 is true), the probability of obtaining a significant result in each individual test is reduced. That is, the false-negative rate (β) is increased, and equivalently the 'power' of the test $(1 - \beta)$ is reduced. (This is referred to as the 'disjunctive power' of the test. However, note that the power of a set of m tests to give *at least one* significant result, referred to as the 'conjunctive power', is not necessarily reduced below the single-test value by a multiple testing adjustment. The distinction between disjunctive and conjunctive power has been discussed by Senn and Bretz (2007).)

The reduction in statistical power due to adjustment for multiplicity can be severe. One of the most spectacular examples comes from human genetics. The sequencing of the 23 pairs of chromosomes in the human genome was completed by the Human Genome Project in 2003, and the high-throughput genotyping technologies developed during the project then made possible the identification of variants between individuals at millions of genetic loci (locations on the chromosomes). The association of each of a set of variants, distributed over the genome, with a heritable disease could then be tested in a genome-wide association study (GWAS). It has become conventional to account for the multiple testing in such a study by setting the significance threshold for the test at each locus to $\alpha' = 5 \times 10^{-8}$ (https://en.wikipedia.org/wiki/Genome-wide_association_study#Methods, accessed 15 April 2024). If the overall significance threshold is $\alpha = 0.05$, this is equivalent to adjusting for $m = \alpha/\alpha' = 0.05/(5 \times 10^{-8}) = 1,000,000$ tests. The number of loci considered may be much larger than this – up to several million – but many of the variant loci are rare (technically, have a low minor allele frequency) and/or are close to other variant loci, both of which reduce their effective contribution to multiplicity (Xu et al. 2014). But $m = 1$ million is quite enough to present difficulties: the resulting stringent significance threshold is only likely to be achieved in a study of a very large number of individuals.

The research community rose to the challenge. The first successful attempt at such an approach was the Wellcome Trust Case Control Consortium's (WTCCC's) publication in 2007 of its 'Genome-wide association study of 14 000 cases of seven common diseases and 3000 shared controls,' which reported 24 genetic association signals significant at a threshold (generous by today's standards) of $\alpha' = 5 \times 10^{-7}$. The Consortium noted that 'On the basis of prior findings and replication studies thus-far completed, almost all of these signals reflect genuine susceptibility effects,' thereby addressing the poor replication track record of previous molecular-genetic association studies (Ioannidis and Trikalinos 2005).

Within two years, Manolio et al. (2009) reported that 'Genome-wide association studies have identified hundreds of genetic variants associated with complex human diseases and traits'. However, they also noted that 'Most variants identified so far confer relatively small increments in risk, and explain only a small proportion of familial clustering, leading many to question how the remaining, "missing" heritability can be explained'. They referred to this 'missing heritability' as the '"dark matter" of genome-wide association', and noted that many explanations had been suggested for it, 'including much larger numbers of variants of smaller effect yet to be found' – that is, that the stringent significance threshold, required to take account of multiplicity, had exacted its price in loss of statistical power.

An approach to mitigating this loss of power, while still taking account of multiplicity, was offered in the paper by Benjamini and Hochberg (1995) quoted earlier. In a retrospective account of the genesis and reception of this paper, 'Discovering the false discovery rate' (2010), Benjamini emphasised the pivotal role of a paper by Soriç (1989), 'who argued forcefully against the use of uncontrolled single-hypothesis testing when many are tested, and used the expected number of false discoveries divided by the number of discoveries as a warning that "a large part of statistical discoveries may be wrong"'. This warning shifted the focus from:

- the number of false positives considered as a proportion of the cases in which H_0 *is true* (the false-positive rate), to
- the number of false positives considered as a proportion of the cases in which H_0 *is rejected* (the false discovery rate).

Benjamini and Hochberg realised that this shift in focus offered 'a very appealing error rate, that rather than being merely a warning can serve as a worthy goal to control'. If the cases in which H_0 was rejected and H_1 accepted were to be announced as 'discoveries', the researcher could decide what proportion of false discoveries they were willing to tolerate, taking account of all the circumstances: the resources available for confirmatory studies, the reputational cost of a false discovery, and so on. They could then select a significance threshold that controlled the proportion of false positives among the discoveries at this acceptable level, for example, the level $q^* = 0.1$. Benjamini and Hochberg named this control level the false discovery rate (FDR). The prospect of controlling the FDR was 'appealing' because in many circumstances the resulting significance threshold is much more generous than that required to control the FWER, resulting in a much smaller loss of statistical power.

When the FDR is used as a criterion for reporting research results, the researcher is no longer required to choose between using a Bonferroni-corrected *p*-value, necessitating very large studies that result in frustratingly few significant discoveries, or a Bayesian approach with a questionable prior distribution. If the FDR is controlled by the method of Benjamini and Hochberg (the 'BH-FDR' criterion), the multiplicity and the need for confirmatory research can be openly acknowledged, and this research can be planned, and budgeted for, based on a realistic prediction of the proportion of 'discoveries' that will be replicated.

Recognition of the merit of this approach was by no means instantaneous. Benjamini (2010) reminisced that following their initial submission of a paper on the topic in 1989, it was only '5 years and three journals later [that] the paper was accepted for publication' – admittedly with some key additional insights on the most useful way to estimate the FDR. But,

> Acceptance of the FDR idea remained slow even after Benjamini and Hochberg (1995) was published...The dramatic change in attitude came when genetic research took a new dimension, in quantitative trait loci and microarrays analyses, where the number of hypotheses tested in an experiment reached thousands. This seemed unthinkable 10 years earlier: for example, our simulations...had been criticized for considering 4–64 hypotheses, as 'no one uses multiple comparisons for problems with 50 or 100 tested hypotheses'. Alas, facing the new challenges, tools that balance multiplicity control and power were needed, and FDR methodology could yield useful answers.

There was no need for Benjamini to say 'alas'. The FDR is now routinely used and proving its worth in a wide range of disciplines, from geography (de Castro and Singer 2006) to medical statistics (Jager and Leek 2014) to genomics (the study of differential gene expression) (Chen et al. 2021) – though researchers in genetic association still prefer to use stringent significance thresholds that control the false-positive rate.

The aim of this book is to take the reader beyond an operational understanding of the FDR, to a conceptual understanding that considers its relationship to other measures of the strength of statistical evidence – the *p*-values, FWERs, Bayesian posterior probabilities and confidence intervals produced in the analysis of research data, and the power, precision and sample size calculations used in study design. The hope is that this will enable the reader to use FDR values with greater confidence, and to discuss them with greater insight into their meaning.

To achieve this aim, some use of mathematical tools is essential. It is assumed that the reader has previously encountered basic notation of statistics and probability theory, such as that used in this introduction. If not, they are recommended to consult introductory texts

such as Moore and McCabe (1999) and Hacking (2001). More advanced or elaborate notation, when unavoidable, is defined and explained when it is introduced.

1.2 Outline of the Book

Following this introductory chapter, the book starts by introducing the concept of a statistical significance test of a null hypothesis (H_0). H_0 may be true or false, and the test may lead
to acceptance or rejection of the H_0 (rejection being a positive result); hence, there are four
possible outcomes (true positive, false positive, true negative and false negative), which can
be represented in a 2×2 'confusion matrix'. Two further foundational concepts for multiple
testing are introduced:

- the false-positive rate, which relates the frequency of undesirable false-positive results to
  the proportion of tests in which H_0 is true, and is represented by the p-value conventionally used to present significance-test results; and
- the false discovery rate (FDR), relating the frequency of false positives to the proportion of
  tests in which H_0 is rejected.

Clearly, it is desirable that the FDR should be controlled in a way that minimises the
consequent false-negative rate, and the Benjamini–Hochberg (BH) criterion is introduced
as a means of achieving this.

The BH criterion makes the assumption that in the cases in which H_0 is true, the hypotheses tested are independent of each other. However, in practice there are likely to be correlations among the hypotheses, and the consequences of this are next explored. The
exploration leads to the reassuring conclusion that when such correlations are positive,
the BH criterion is conservative.

Methods for graphical presentation of the FDR are then explored, first on the probability
(p) scale, and then on the $-\log_{10}(p)$ scale. Graphical presentation aids understanding of the
BH criterion, and transformation to the $-\log_{10}(p)$ scale further facilitates interpretation of
the results. Graphical presentation is also valuable as a diagnostic tool, for detection of correlations among the hypotheses tested, and consequent adjustment of the interpretation.

The concepts and methods presented so far are then applied to real data, obtained from an
experimental study of *Arabidopsis thaliana*, a species widely used as a model organism in
plant genetics and genomics. Such a study can produce many response variables (in the
present case gene expression levels) with complex groupings and interrelationships, and
the experimental design typically leads to several hypotheses to be tested in relation to each
response variable. These relationships lead to several sets of multiple tests, to each of which
the methods can be applied. The resulting patterns of FDRs can then be interpreted and
compared, to make inferences about the biological processes occurring and to identify
hypotheses that merit further investigation.

As noted in the preceding 'brief history' (Section 1.1), the BH-FDR criterion is a relatively
recent development in dealing with multiple hypothesis-testing situations. It is next compared with longer-established methods based more directly on the p-value, starting with the
Šidák and Bonferroni 'corrections'. These methods replace the original p-value with a more

stringent value, based simply on the number of hypotheses tested, that can then be interpreted in the same way as the original value – a goal known as conservation of the 'family-wise error rate' (FWER). Developments of these methods that take account of known relationships among the hypotheses tested (e.g., that they test the $g(g-1)/2$ possible pair-wise comparisons among g groups) are then reviewed.

These methods that control the FWER and the BH criterion that controls the FDR are then compared, generally to the advantage of the BH criterion. However, the distinction between 'exploratory' and 'confirmatory' objectives in relation to hypothesis testing is noted, and the value of control of the FWER in a confirmatory study is acknowledged. In this context, it is noted that when a single hypothesis is tested in a single study, the p-value and the FDR are equivalent. This leads on to a generalisation of the Bonferroni correction, Holm's method, that identifies a subset of the hypotheses tested in which both the FDR and the FWER are controlled. To conclude this comparison of the attributes of the FDR and the p-value (the false-positive rate), it is noted that the distinction between them is not confined to statistical significance testing, but is present also in simple diagnostic tests, and in the prosecutor's fallacy.

Another relatively recent development in the application of statistics is the increasing popularity of Bayesian methods, and the FDR is next considered in this context, first noting that it can be given a Bayesian interpretation. It is shown that in some circumstances a conventional p-value can be interpreted as a Bayesian posterior probability, and the idea that this may offer a solution to the multiplicity problem is considered. It is shown that any such solution depends critically on the specification of an appropriate prior probability distribution, and the attempt to do so is connected back to the FDR.

The FDR, as defined up to this point, strictly speaking relates to a subset of the multiple hypotheses tested, not to any individual hypothesis, and it has been objected that this makes it too generous, as it assesses each hypothesis on the basis of all hypotheses for which evidence against H_0 is stronger. This leads to the concept of the local FDR, that is, the FDR specific to each hypothesis. Methods for attempting to estimate this, without becoming excessively vulnerable to the stochastic variation associated with each hypothesis test, are considered. These include the ingenious idea of re-ranking the individual-test FDRs, to take account of the under-estimation of each one.

So far it has been assumed that the significance test from which the p-values are obtained is valid in the cases in which H_0 is true. However, this will not be the case if the statistical model on which the test is based has been mis-specified: for example, if sampling units are assumed to be independent, but in reality there is a correlation between the observations made on them. Such mis-specification, even if slight, becomes important in the multiple-testing context: if the probability of a significant result departs slightly from that indicated by H_0, this may cause a substantial excess or deficit in the number of discoveries reported. A method has been proposed to overcome this problem by estimating the FDR in relation to an empirically identified 'uninteresting' distribution of test statistics, rather than the distribution on a purely mathematically defined null hypothesis. The defence provided by this approach in the context of an experiment with unrecognised pseudoreplication, and an experiment with unrecognised block effects, is explored.

A set of p-values from a multiple-testing study is often not the only information available concerning the set of hypotheses: there is typically other information, which can be expressed in the form of one or more auxiliary covariates. A method has been developed for adapting the FDR to take account of such a covariate, and this is next described. The output of the method is a new set of p-values, and if more than one auxiliary covariate is available, these output p-values can be used as input for repeated application of the method.

If researchers are persuaded to move from approaches based directly on the p-value to an approach based on the BH-FDR for the interpretation of multiple-testing results, they will want to be able to connect the BH-FDR to their standard practices as closely as possible. One of these standard practices is the calculation of confidence intervals (CIs) around reported effect sizes, and these CIs have a well-defined relationship to p-values. CIs that have an analogous relationship to the BH-FDR are therefore required. A criterion that enables the calculation of such CIs, the false coverage rate (FCR), is next described.

Up to this point, the focus has been on the application of the FDR to the data-analysis and reporting phases of an investigation. However, the concept of the p-value is routinely used at the planning stage to guide statistical power and sample size calculations, and another point on which researchers will want to be confident is the appropriateness of such calculations if control of the FDR is the goal. The book concludes with a presentation of tools for achieving this, first in relation to the sample size required to achieve a specified FDR, then in relation to the significance threshold required to achieve the same goal when the sample size is fixed.

1.3 Summary

The history of statistical significance testing is reviewed. The first formal steps were taken early in the twentieth century, and quantified the probability of obtaining an extreme result by coincidence alone.

The values of standard test statistics (z, t, F, χ^2, r, etc.) observed from trials were compared with tabulated values corresponding to particular probability thresholds, typically $\alpha = 0.05$, 0.01 and 0.001. The results were expressed in terms of p-values, for example, '$p < 0.05$', but the actual p-value was not calculated.

By the late 1970s, many researchers had access to electronic calculators or even computers, and could report their actual p-values. However, the preoccupation with thresholds that had its origin in arithmetical convenience has persisted. Thus, typically:

- $p > 0.05$ is interpreted as 'non-significant' ('NS'),
- $p < 0.05$ is 'significant', indicated by '*',
- $p < 0.01$ is 'highly significant', indicated by '**',
- $p < 0.001$ is 'very highly significant', indicated by '***'.

Such significance tests became, and remain, the mainstay of statistical data analysis in the biological and social sciences. However, it was always apparent that there are conceptual problems associated with them, namely:

- the test indicates the probability of the data conditional on a hypothesis, whereas the researcher is primarily interested in the probability of a hypothesis conditional on the data (the 'inverse' or 'Bayesian' probability), and

- the probability that a single experiment will give a significant result by coincidence is low, but if more tests are conducted, the probability that at least one of them will do so increases.

These problems were initially dealt with informally by assuming that:

- researchers would not spend time and resources seeking to refute a null hypothesis, H_0, that was likely to be true, and
- the cost in time and resources would limit the number of hypotheses that researchers were able to test.

Hence, among the 'discoveries' announced by many researchers over many years, it would rarely turn out that H_0 had, after all, been correct.

In the late twentieth century, technological developments changed the situation: the capacity for statistical calculation and data storage increased immensely. The term 'big data' began to be used, and a discipline called 'data science' for the management, manipulation and exploration of huge datasets, distinct from classical statistics, began to be recognised.

The problem of false-positive results is exacerbated if the multiple testing is not apparent when the results are reported, or if its implications are not recognised. Several mechanisms that can cause this to occur, inadvertently or deliberately, are identified.

The problem of multiplicity continued to grow in the early twenty-first century. It was argued that 'false findings may be...the vast majority of published research claims' (Ioannidis 2005: 'Why most published research findings are false').

In 2015, the journal *Basic and Applied Social Psychology* sought to address the 'replication crisis' by banning the presentation of *p*-values.

In response, the ASA convened a board of experts to develop a policy on the subject. The resulting document sought to defend against the improper use and interpretation of *p*-values, while giving due recognition to their value when used properly.

Significance tests continue to be viewed with unease, leading to an increase in enthusiasm for Bayesian statistical methods. However, to use these, the researcher must specify the probabilities of H_0 and the alternative H_1 that are assumed before the results of the study are known. Such a 'prior probability distribution' is always open to challenge.

In the alternative, 'frequentist' statistical tradition, formal approaches to the problem of multiplicity begin with the method of Bonferroni (1936), in which the threshold α is replaced by α/m, where m is the number of tests in the 'family' under consideration. This 'Bonferroni correction' or 'Bonferroni adjustment' controls the false-positive rate (the family-wise error rate (FWER)) at level α.

However, the Bonferroni adjustment also increases the false-negative rate (β), and reduces the 'statistical power' of each test ($1 - \beta$). This reduction in power can be severe, requiring very large sample sizes to overcome it. This approach is discussed in the context of genome-wide association studies (GWAS) of heritable human disease.

In the first decade of the twenty-first century, GWAS rapidly identified hundreds of genetic variants associated with complex diseases and traits, but these explained only a small proportion of familial clustering. The 'missing' heritability might be explained by much larger numbers of variants of smaller, unrecognised effect. If so, the Bonferroni-type adjustment had exacted its price in loss of statistical power.

Benjamini and Hochberg (1995) proposed mitigating this loss of power, by shifting the focus:

- from the proportion of false positives in the cases in which H_0 *is true* (the false-positive rate)
- to the proportion in the cases in which H_0 *is rejected*. They named this the false discovery rate (FDR).

The researcher can select a significance threshold that controls the FDR at an acceptable level, for example, $q^* = 0.1$.

The resulting significance threshold is often much more generous than that required to control the FWER, resulting in a much smaller loss of statistical power.

Recognition of the merit of this approach was by no means instantaneous. However, the introduction of genetic microarray analyses, testing thousands of hypotheses, led to a dramatic change in attitude. The FDR is now routinely used and proving its worth in a wide range of disciplines.

The aim of this book is to take the reader beyond an operational understanding of the FDR, to a conceptual understanding that considers its relationship to the other measures of the strength of statistical evidence mentioned in the earlier text. The hope is that this conceptual understanding will enable the reader to use FDR values with greater confidence, and to discuss them with greater insight into their meaning.

This introductory chapter ends with an outline of the book, showing the reader the material to be covered, how it is structured, and how it will assist the reader both to understand and to apply the FDR.

References

Benjamini, Y. (2010). Discovering the false discovery rate. *Journal of the Royal Statistical Society B* 72: 405–416.

Benjamini, Y. and Hochberg, Y. (1995). Controlling the false discovery rate: a practical and powerful approach to multiple testing. *Journal of the Royal Statistical Society B* 57: 289–300.

Bonferroni, C.E. (1936). *Teoria statistica delle classi e calcolo delle probabilità. Pubblicazioni del R Istituto Superiore di Scienze Economiche e Commerciali di Firenze.*

de Castro, M.C. and Singer, B.H. (2006). Controlling the false discovery rate: a new application to account for multiple and dependent tests in local statistics of spatial association. *Geographical Analysis* 38: 180–208.

Chen, X., Robinson, D.G., and Storey, J.D. (2021). The functional false discovery rate with applications to genomics. *Biostatistics* 22: 68–81. https://doi.org/10.1093/biostatistics/kxz010.

Fisher, R.A. (1926). The arrangement of field experiments. *Journal of the Ministry of Agriculture of Great Britain* 33: 503–513.

Hacking, I. (2001). *An Introduction to Probability and Logic.* Cambridge: Cambridge University Press 302 pp.

Hastie, T., Tibshirai, R., and Friedman, J. (2001). *The Elements of Statistical Learning. Data Mining, Inference and Prediction.* New York: Springer 533 pp.

Hilbert, M. and López, P. (2011). The world's technological capacity to store, communicate, and compute information. *Science* 332: 60–65. https://doi.org/10.1126/science.1200970.

Ioannidis, J.P.A. (2005). Why most published research findings are false. *PLoS Medicine* 19: e1004085. https://doi.org/10.1371/journal.pmed.0020124.

Ioannidis, J.P. and Trikalinos, T.A. (2005). Early extreme contradictory estimates may appear in published research: the Proteus phenomenon in molecular genetics research and randomized trials. *Journal of Clinical Epidemiology* 58: 543–549.

Jager, L.R. and Leek, J.T. (2014). An estimate of the science-wise false discovery rate and application to the top medical literature. *Biostatistics* 15: 1–12. https://doi.org/10.1093/biostatistics/kxt007.

Manolio, T.A., Collins, F.S., Cox, N.J. et al. (2009). Finding the missing heritability of complex diseases. *Nature* 461: 747–753. https://doi.org/10.1038/nature08494, PMID: 19812666; PMCID: PMC2831613.

Moore, D.S. and McCabe, G.P. (1999). *Introduction to the Practice of Statistics*, 3e. New York: W.H. Freeman and Company 825 pp.

Ortiz, A.F.H., Camacho, E.C., Rojas, J.C. et al. (2022). A practical guide to perform a systematic literature review and meta-analysis. *Principles and Practice of Clinical Research* 7 (4): 47–57. https://doi.org/10.21801/ppcrj.2021.74.6.

Pocock, S.J., Hughes, M.D., and Lee, R.J. (1987). Statistical problems in reporting clinical trials. *Journal of the American Statistical Association* 84: 381–392.

Ridley, M. (2023). Science Fiction: the crisis in research. *Spectator*, issue of 12 August 2023.

Senn, S. and Bretz, F. (2007). Power and sample size when multiple endpoints are considered. *Pharmaceutical Statistics* 6: 161–170.

Soriç, B. (1989). Statistical "discoveries" and effect size estimation. *Journal of the American Statistical Association* 84: 608–610.

The Wellcome Trust Case Control Consortium (2007). Genome-wide association study of 14,000 cases of seven common diseases and 3,000 shared controls. *Nature* 447: 661–678. https://doi.org/10.1038/nature05911.

Trafimow, D. and Marks, M. (2015). Editorial. *Basic and Applied Social Psychology* 37: 1–2.

Wasserstein, R.L. and Lazar, N.A. (2016). The ASA statement on *p*-values: context, process, and purpose. *The American Statistician* 70: 129–133. https://doi.org/10.1080/00031305.2016.1154108.

Xu, C., Tachmazidou, I., Walter, K. et al. (2014). Estimating genome-wide significance for whole-genome sequencing studies. *Genetic Epidemiology* 38: 281–290. https://doi.org/10.1002/gepi.21797. Epub 2014 Feb 14. PMID: 24676807; PMCID: PMC4489336.

2

The Meaning of the False Discovery Rate (FDR)

2.1 True Hypothesis Versus Conclusion from Evidence: The Confusion Matrix

A false discovery rate (FDR), like a p-value, is based on consideration of two hypotheses, a *null hypothesis* (H_0) and an *alternative hypothesis* (H_1). The null hypothesis is usually that some phenomenon of interest is absent: it is some statement like 'There is no real difference between the effect of Treatment A and Treatment B', or 'There is no real association between the explanatory variable X and the response variable Y'. The alternative hypothesis is that the phenomenon is present: that there *is* such an effect or such an association. If the experimental or observational evidence strongly favours H_1, that is,

- if the observed difference between the effects of Treatments A and B is large on average, relative to the variation (considered to be random) between observations on the same treatment, or
- if the observed association between X and Y is strong, relative to the random variation between observations of Y at the same value of X,

then H_0 is rejected and H_1 is accepted. But when random variation is present, there is a possibility that a large observed difference or a strong observed association will occur by chance, and H_0 will be wrongly rejected. Conversely, random variation may obscure a real difference or association, causing H_0 to be wrongly accepted. These possible outcomes can be organised in a *confusion matrix*, as shown in Table 2.1.

H_0 and H_1 can be specified for each of a set of statistical tests, conducted on data from different experiments or observational studies, or on different hypotheses within the same experiment or observational study. The conclusion drawn from each test must then belong in one of the four positions in this matrix – though we can never know in which row a particular test-conclusion belongs, as we can never know with certainty which hypothesis is true. Still, we can assign symbols to represent the number of tests in each position, as shown in Table 2.2. That is,

U = number of true negative conclusions.

V = number of false positive conclusions.

The False Discovery Rate: Its Meaning, Interpretation and Application in Data Science, First Edition.
N.W. Galwey.
© 2025 John Wiley & Sons Ltd. Published 2025 by John Wiley & Sons Ltd.
Companion website: www.wiley.com/go/falsediscoveryrate

Table 2.1 The confusion matrix relating the four possible outcomes of a hypothesis test.

True hypothesis	Conclusion from evidence	
	H_0	H_1
H_0	True negative	False positive (Type I error)
H_1	False negative (Type II error)	True positive

Table 2.2 Symbols for the counts in the confusion matrix.

True hypothesis	Conclusion from evidence	
	H_0	H_1
H_0	U	V
H_1	T	S

T = number of false negative conclusions.

S = number of true positive conclusions.

The confusion matrix shows that there are two types of error that can be made when drawing a conclusion from a test:

- a false-positive conclusion, also known as a Type I error, and
- a false-negative conclusion, also known as a Type II error.

Although we cannot know how many tests belong in each position in the matrix, we can deduce the relationships expected between U, V, T and S in a specified scenario. In particular, we can connect them to the p-value and the FDR.

2.2 The Meaning of the p-Value

The relationship between the confusion matrix and the p-value will be presented briefly here: for a fuller account of the conceptual basis of the p-value, see, for example, Moore and McCabe (1999, Section 6.2, Tests of significance, and Section 6.3, Use and abuse of tests, pp. 453–483). Or, for a more philosophical approach with less emphasis on guidance for conventional practice, see Hacking (2001, Chapter 18, Significance and power, pp. 209–228). The familiar statistical tests of significance – the Z test, t test, χ^2 test and others – give a value of a test statistic from a set of experimental or observational data. The p-value is then the probability (p) of obtaining a value of the test statistic as extreme as, or more extreme than, that observed, if:

- H_0 is true, and
- the assumptions on which the test is based are satisfied: that is, the statistical model specified is precisely correct in relation to the data on which the test was performed.

A probability threshold α is specified for the announcement of a significant result, typically $\alpha = 0.05$, and H_0 is rejected if the p-value is below this value: that is, if $p < \alpha$.

If we envisage performing the same significance test repeatedly on independent samples of observations, then each p is itself a realisation of a random variable P, and if H_0 is true and the assumptions of the significance test are satisfied, then

$$P \sim \text{Uniform}(0, 1), \tag{2.1}$$

from which it follows that

$$P(P < \alpha \mid H_0) = \alpha. \tag{2.2}$$

The vertical-bar symbol '|' in this formula means 'conditional on' or 'given that'. It then follows that, as $U + V \to \infty$,

$$\frac{V}{U + V} \to \alpha. \tag{2.3}$$

That is, if we confine our attention to the part of the confusion matrix in which H_0 is true (the upper row), then when a large number of tests are performed, the proportion of them in which H_0 is rejected will tend towards α. For example, if we specify $\alpha = 0.05$, we will obtain a significant result in a proportion 0.05 of our tests by chance alone. This is known as the *false-positive rate*, and we can also express it as a percentage, in this case 5%.

2.3   The Meaning of the FDR: Its Relationship to the Confusion Matrix and the *p*-Value

A similar argument relates the FDR to the confusion matrix, but now we focus on the part of the confusion matrix in which H_0 is rejected and H_1 is our conclusion from the evidence (the right-hand column). We can then state that

$$\text{FDR} = \frac{V}{V + S}. \tag{2.4}$$

Because we cannot know for certainty whether H_0 is true for any test, we cannot know the exact value of V, nor therefore the exact value of $\frac{V}{V + S}$, but we can make some theoretical statements about this quantity. We can consider the situation in which there is an effectively infinite population of hypotheses potentially available for testing – for example:

- a study of many chemical compounds, each of which may have an activity indicating potential medical value (H_1), or may not (H_0);
- a study of the many genes within a particular species of organism, in which the expression of each gene may be influenced by an environmental stimulus (H_1), or may not (H_0).

If the hypotheses that we test are a random sample from this population, then the 'expected' (i.e., average) value of the FDR in such a sample, $E\left(\dfrac{V}{V+S}\right)$, is the value that would be obtained if the whole population of hypotheses could be tested. Moreover, the larger the sample, the more closely the value in the sample will approach the population value: that is, as $V + S \to \infty$,

$$\text{FDR} \to E\left(\frac{V}{V+S}\right). \tag{2.5}$$

The meaning of the ratios in Displays (2.3) and (2.4) is compared graphically in Figure 2.1. The areas in the confusion matrices in this figure represent the relative frequencies of the different outcomes. (Note that the hatched area in the ratio at the bottom of the figure, coloured red in the electronic version of this book, represents a different row and column within the confusion matrix, depending on whether the p-value or the FDR is being calculated.) Comparison of Panels (a) and (b) of Figure 2.1 shows that

$$p = P(\text{significant test result} \mid H_0 \text{ is true}),$$

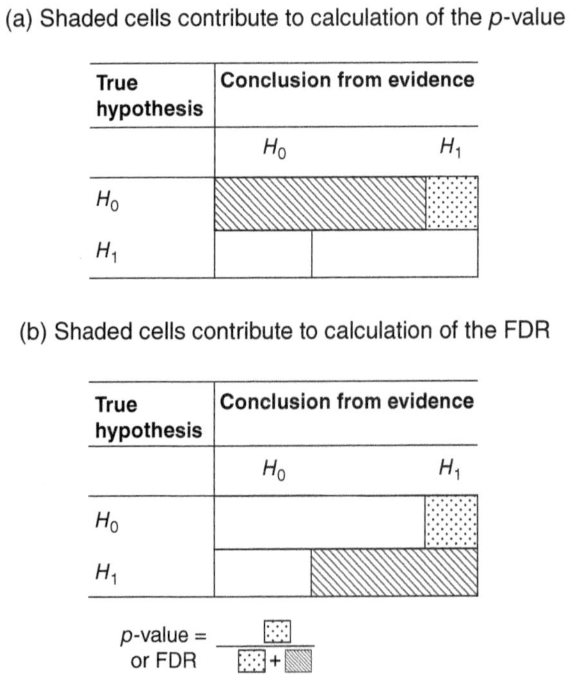

(a) Shaded cells contribute to calculation of the p-value

(b) Shaded cells contribute to calculation of the FDR

Figure 2.1 (a) and (b) The relationship between the p-value and the FDR, in terms of the confusion matrix.

whereas

$$\text{FDR} = P(H_0 \text{ is true } | \text{ significant test result}).$$

2.4 Control of the FDR While Minimising False-Negative Results: The Benjamini–Hochberg (BH) Criterion

In order to put these ideas to use, we must confront the fact that for any individual significance test, we can never know for certain which hypothesis is true, H_0 or H_1. This is not a problem in relation to the p-value, as all the reasoning in connection with p is *conditional on* H_0 being true. However, when considering the FDR, though we know with certainty the number of tests for which we rejected H_0 and accepted H_1, namely $(V + S)$, we can never know V or S, nor hence the proportion $\dfrac{V}{V + S}$, with certainty. But an ingenious method has been found for *controlling* this proportion at a chosen level, as follows (Benjamini and Hochberg 1995).

Suppose that m significance tests are performed, and give the p-values $p_1, p_2... p_m$. Note that:

- each of these observed p-values, p_i, $i = 1...m$, represented by a lower-case 'p', is considered to be a realisation of a random variable, P_i, represented by a capital 'P', which could take any value in the range $[0, 1]$. The observed p-value, p_i in the case of the ith hypothesis, is a realisation of P_i.
- for the moment we assume that the p-values are mutually independent: that is, $P(P_i < p_i)$ does not depend on the p-value for any other hypothesis, $p_{i'}$, $i' \neq i$. Relaxation of this assumption will be considered later (Section 2.8).

Rank these p-values in ascending order, $p_{(1)} \leq p_{(2)} \leq ... \leq p_{(m)}$. (Note the use of brackets in the subscript to distinguish the labelling of the ranked p-values from that of the p-values in their original order. The observed value $p_{(i)}$ is considered to be a realisation of the random variable $P_{(i)}$.) Then specify a rate q^* at which we wish to control the FDR. For example, if we specify $q^* = 0.1$, we indicate that we want on average no more than 10% of our significant test results to be false discoveries. Then find the largest p-value for which

$$p_{(i)} \leq \frac{i}{m}q^*. \tag{2.6}$$

This is done by a *step-down procedure*. Starting with the largest p-value, $p_{(m)}$, determine whether it satisfies Inequality (2.6). If not, proceed to the next-largest p-value, $p_{(m-1)}$. Continue in this way until a p-value is encountered that satisfies Inequality (2.6). Specify this as the kth ordered p-value, $p_{(k)}$, and interpret it as the largest significant p-value: that is, reject H_0 for this test and for all tests giving smaller p-values, namely the tests giving $p_{(i)}$ for $i = 1...k$.

Now suppose that for m_0 of the significance tests H_0 is true, and for the other m_1 tests H_1 is true, that is, $m_0 + m_1 = m$. It can then be proved that the expected (i.e., average) proportion of false discoveries among the test results declared significant is

$$E\left(\frac{V}{V+S}\right) \le \frac{m_0}{m}q^* \le q^*. \tag{2.7}$$

The expected FDR is less than q^*, and we express this by saying that the FDR is *controlled* at rate q^*.

The full proof of this result is given by Benjamini and Hochberg: an outline of it is as follows. If $p_{(k)}$ is specified as the largest significant p-value, the number of discoveries announced is

$$V + S = k.$$

Also, in this case, for an individual test for which the null hypothesis is true, the probability that a significant result will be obtained is

$$P\left(P_i \le P_{(k)} \mid H_0\right) = p_{(k)}.$$

Therefore, if the m_0 tests for which H_0 is true are independent – a crucial condition – the expected number of false-positive tests is

$$E(V) = m_0 P\left(P_i \le P_{(k)} \mid H_0\right) = m_0 p_{(k)}.$$

Hence, the expected FDR is

$$E\left(\frac{V}{V+S}\right) = \frac{E(V)}{V+S} = \frac{m_0 p_{(k)}}{k}. \tag{2.8}$$

We wish to achieve

$$E\left(\frac{V}{V+S}\right) = E\left(\frac{V}{k}\right) \le q^*, \tag{2.9}$$

that is,

$$\frac{m_0 p_{(k)}}{k} \le q^*. \tag{2.10}$$

Now m_0 is unknown, so we cannot substitute values that will meet this criterion directly. However, we can note that

$$m_0 \le m,$$

so

$$\frac{m_0 p_{(k)}}{k} \le \frac{m p_{(k)}}{k}. \tag{2.11}$$

Hence, if we specify values that meet the criterion

$$\frac{m p_{(k)}}{k} \le q^*, \tag{2.12}$$

we can combine Inequalities (2.11) and (2.12) to give

$$\frac{m_0 p_{(k)}}{k} \le \frac{m p_{(k)}}{k} \le q^*, \tag{2.13}$$

and our required criterion (2.10) is satisfied. Rearranging Inequality (2.13), we obtain

$$p_{(k)} \leq \frac{k}{m} q^*, \tag{2.14}$$

and this tells us the largest p-value that we can consider significant, $p_{(k)}$, while controlling the FDR at rate q^*.

For example, suppose that significance tests are conducted for $m = 50$ hypotheses, giving the p-values shown in Table 2.3 (simulated data). Now suppose that we wish to select some of these hypotheses for further investigation, while ensuring that on average our selection procedure will give us not more than 30% of false discoveries: that is, while controlling the FDR at $q^* = 0.3$. We first sort the p-values into ascending order, as shown in Table 2.4. Then for each ordered value $p_{(i)}$, we calculate i/m, as also shown. For each of the new values of i (the ordered hypothesis numbers), we then determine whether it is true that

$$p_{(i)} \leq \frac{i}{m} q^*. \tag{2.15}$$

We then find the largest p-value for which this is the case. If the number of hypotheses is large enough for an algorithm to be needed for this purpose, we start from the largest p-value, $p_{(m)}$, and examine each successive smaller value in turn until we reach the first one for which Inequality (2.15) is true: this is the *step-down procedure*. In the present set of p-values, we find that this is $p_{(16)} = 0.07900$, and we therefore specify that $k = 16$, and $p_{(k)} = p_{(16)}$ is the largest p-value to be considered significant. A proportion $k/m = 16/50 = 0.32$, that is, 32% of our hypotheses, those with strongest support for H_1 from the data, will go forward for further investigation.

Table 2.3 Unordered p-values. i = unordered hypothesis number.

i	p_i	i	p_i	i	p_i	i	p_i	i	p_i
1	0.44156	11	0.13081	21	0.23433	31	0.98225	41	0.00029
2	0.79081	12	0.14529	22	0.32222	32	0.07895	42	0.02138
3	0.95563	13	0.03513	23	0.72925	33	0.99766	43	0.00790
4	0.07900	14	0.11818	24	0.71578	34	0.66271	44	0.00284
5	0.96820	15	0.19151	25	0.22049	35	0.86558	45	0.00616
6	0.93158	16	0.10690	26	0.49395	36	0.00083	46	0.00233
7	0.46724	17	0.31911	27	0.17801	37	0.00309	47	0.02990
8	0.54795	18	0.69420	28	0.86287	38	0.00033	48	0.00258
9	0.34050	19	0.95185	29	0.26797	39	0.11475	49	0.07595
10	0.51841	20	0.71867	30	0.27948	40	0.12869	50	0.00197

Table 2.4 Ordered p-values with calculations for the BH procedure, with q^* specified as 0.3. i = ordered hypothesis number.

i	Unordered hypothesis number	$p_{(i)}$	i/m	$(i/m)q^*$	$p_{(i)} \leq (i/m)q^*$	i	Unordered hypothesis number	$p_{(i)}$	i/m	$(i/m)q^*$	$p_{(i)} \leq (i/m)q^*$
1	41	0.00029	0.02	0.006	TRUE	26	21	0.23433	0.52	0.156	FALSE
2	38	0.00033	0.04	0.012	TRUE	27	29	0.26797	0.54	0.162	FALSE
3	36	0.00083	0.06	0.018	TRUE	28	30	0.27948	0.56	0.168	FALSE
4	50	0.00197	0.08	0.024	TRUE	29	17	0.31911	0.58	0.174	FALSE
5	46	0.00233	0.10	0.030	TRUE	30	22	0.32222	0.60	0.180	FALSE
6	48	0.00258	0.12	0.036	TRUE	31	9	0.34050	0.62	0.186	FALSE
7	44	0.00284	0.14	0.042	TRUE	32	1	0.44156	0.64	0.192	FALSE
8	37	0.00309	0.16	0.048	TRUE	33	7	0.46724	0.66	0.198	FALSE
9	45	0.00616	0.18	0.054	TRUE	34	26	0.49395	0.68	0.204	FALSE
10	43	0.00790	0.20	0.060	TRUE	35	10	0.51841	0.70	0.210	FALSE
11	42	0.02138	0.22	0.066	TRUE	36	8	0.54795	0.72	0.216	FALSE
12	47	0.02990	0.24	0.072	TRUE	37	34	0.66271	0.74	0.222	FALSE
13	13	0.03513	0.26	0.078	TRUE	38	18	0.69420	0.76	0.228	FALSE
14	49	0.07595	0.28	0.084	TRUE	39	24	0.71578	0.78	0.234	FALSE
15	32	0.07895	0.30	0.090	TRUE	40	20	0.71867	0.80	0.240	FALSE
16	4	0.07900	0.32	0.096	TRUE	41	23	0.72925	0.82	0.246	FALSE
17	16	0.10690	0.34	0.102	FALSE	42	2	0.79081	0.84	0.252	FALSE
18	39	0.11475	0.36	0.108	FALSE	43	28	0.86287	0.86	0.258	FALSE
19	14	0.11818	0.38	0.114	FALSE	44	35	0.86558	0.88	0.264	FALSE
20	40	0.12869	0.40	0.120	FALSE	45	6	0.93158	0.90	0.270	FALSE
21	11	0.13081	0.42	0.126	FALSE	46	19	0.95185	0.92	0.276	FALSE
22	12	0.14529	0.44	0.132	FALSE	47	3	0.95563	0.94	0.282	FALSE
23	27	0.17801	0.46	0.138	FALSE	48	5	0.96820	0.96	0.288	FALSE
24	15	0.19151	0.48	0.144	FALSE	49	31	0.98225	0.98	0.294	FALSE
25	25	0.22049	0.50	0.150	FALSE	50	33	0.99766	1.00	0.300	FALSE

2.5 Graphical Illustration of the Benjamini–Hochberg FDR Criterion

A graphical presentation helps to show that the Benjamini–Hochberg step-down FDR criterion is consistent with intuition. Consider the case where H_0 is true for all the significance tests conducted, and the tests are mutually independent. For example, suppose that the hypotheses are tested using the Z statistic

$$Z \sim N(0, 1),$$

and the observed values z_i, $i = 1...m$ are independent realisations of this variable. The
p-values from a one-sided test will then be a random sample from the distribution

$$P \sim \text{Uniform}(0, 1).$$

Figure 2.2 shows a histogram of $m = 50$ such values (i.e., simulated data): all values between
0 and 1 occur about equally often, though with some irregularity because the sample is
finite. Figure 2.3 shows the scatter plot obtained when the p-values in this sample are sorted
into ascending order and plotted against their ranks divided by the number of p-values, that
is, when $p_{(i)}$ is plotted against i/m. i/m is the *expected* proportion of the p-values that are less
than or equal to $p_{(i)}$,

$$P(P_{(i)} \leq p_{(i)}|H_0) = i/m,$$

the mean proportion that would be obtained in an infinite population of such sets of p-
values, each set comprising m values. That is, the ordered observed p-values, $p_{(i)}$, are plotted
against the expected proportions on H_0. The points in this scatter plot lie approximately
along the diagonal line of unit slope passing through the origin: that is, each ordered p-value
is approximately equal to its expected value. When H_0 is true for all tests, the p-value is simply an approximate statement of its own proportional position in the ranking.

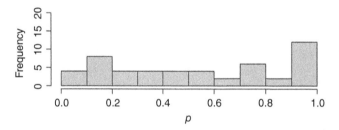

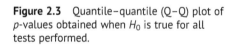

Figure 2.2 Histogram of p-values obtained when H_0 is true for all tests performed.

Figure 2.3 Quantile–quantile (Q–Q) plot of
p-values obtained when H_0 is true for all
tests performed.

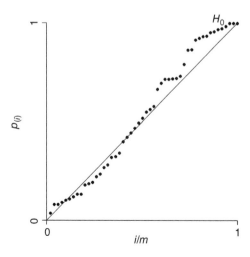

When m is large, this expected proportion is almost, but not quite, the same thing as the expected value of $p_{(i)}$, which is $i/(m+1)$. For an intuitive illustration of the difference between the two, consider the limiting case $m = 1$, in which the average value of a single p-value, on H_0, is $1/(1+1) = \frac{1}{2}$.

Now consider an example where H_0 is true for a proportion $m_0/m = 0.7$ (70%) of the p-values, but H_0 is false and H_1 is true for the remaining $m_1/m = 0.3$ (30%). The null hypothesis

$$H_0: \mu = 0$$

is again tested using a one-sided Z-test. The alternative hypothesis is specified as

$$H_1: \mu > 0,$$

that is, $\mu < 0$ is not considered to be a possibility. We specify that in the cases where H_0 is true,

$$Z \sim N(\mu = 0, \sigma = 1),$$

and when H_0 is true and a one-sided test is specified, the p-values are then drawn from a

$$P \sim \text{Uniform}(0, 1)$$

distribution as before. However, in the cases where H_1 is true,

$$Z \sim N(\mu = 2.5, \sigma = 1),$$

and there are consequently a relatively large number of p-values close to zero.

The histogram of the distribution of p-values resulting from the mixture of these two Z-distributions is presented in Figure 2.4, and the scatter plot of $p_{(i)}$ versus i/m in Figure 2.5. Both representations of the data show the impact of the tests for which H_0 is false: in the histogram, the bars close to $P = 0$ are taller, representing more p-values; in the scatter plot, nearly all the points lie below the diagonal line $p_{(i)} = i/m$, the H_0 line.

A plot such as that in Figure 2.3 or Figure 2.5, comparing the quantiles of a distribution of observed values with the quantiles of a standard mathematical distribution expected on some hypothesis, is known as a quantile–quantile (Q–Q) plot. When a Q–Q plot is obtained from a set of p-values, since these observed values are themselves probabilities, their distribution is compared directly with

$$P \sim \text{Uniform}(0, 1), \tag{2.16}$$

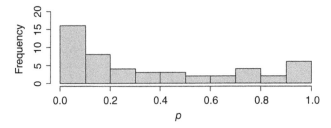

Figure 2.4 Histogram of p-values obtained when H_1 is true for a proportion $m_1/m = 0.3$ of tests.

Figure 2.5 Q–Q plot of p-values obtained when H_1 is true for a proportion $m_1/m = 0.3$ of tests.

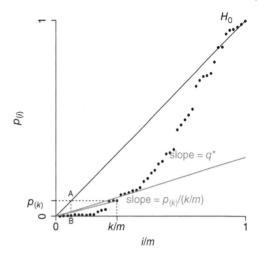

and not with a more mathematically elaborate distribution such as that of Z (as will be illustrated in Section 2.6). If the p-values are sampled from Distribution (2.16), then

$$P(P \le i/m) = i/m,$$

that is, the quantile of i/m is i/m itself, as also indicated by Equation (2.2).

The Q–Q plot obtained from the present set of p-values (Figure 2.5) can be used to illustrate how the Benjamini–Hochberg step-down procedure (BH procedure) controls the FDR. The rate q^* at which the FDR is to be controlled is represented on the Q–Q plot by a diagonal line with slope q^*, passing through the origin. In the present case, we choose to specify $q^* = 0.3$. The BH procedure specifies that the largest p-value to be considered significant, $p_{(k)}$, is the largest one that lies below this line. The horizontal coordinate of the point representing this p-value is k/m, the proportion of the test results declared significant. Its vertical coordinate, $p_{(k)}$, is the proportion *expected* to be declared significant if H_0 is true for all tests. We now drop a perpendicular from this point to the vertical axis, find the intersection between this perpendicular and the H_0 line (labelled A), then drop a perpendicular from A to the coordinate $p_{(k)}$ on the horizontal axis (labelled B). The vertical line AB divides the significant test results into two sets: the number to the left is an estimate of the number of false-positive results that we will have obtained by chance – term V in the confusion matrix – and the number to the right is an estimate of the additional number of true-positive results that we have obtained – term S. Thus, $\dfrac{p_{(k)}}{k/m}$ is an estimate of $\dfrac{V}{V+S}$, the FDR. The areas of the dotted-line-enclosed rectangles to the left and right of the line AB correspond to V and S, respectively, and to the stippled (blue in the e-version of the book) and hatched (red) rectangles in Figure 2.1b. Inspection of the slopes of the lines on the plot confirms that

$$\frac{p_{(k)}}{k/m} \le q^*,$$

and rearranging this inequality we obtain Inequality (2.14), as required.

It should be noted that in most applications the values $m_1/m = 0.3$ and $\mu = 2.5$ would be considered excessively optimistic, and the value $q^* = 0.3$ excessively generous. They are chosen here to enable clear illustration of concepts.

2.6 Use of the Q–Q Plot in Other Contexts

The Q–Q plot is central to the approach to the interpretation of the FDR taken in this book, so its use for the interpretation of p-values will here be briefly compared with its most common use, as a diagnostic tool to examine the distribution of residual values when a statistical model is fitted to data. In this context, the expected quantiles on the horizontal axis are usually not simply those of the Uniform(0, 1) distribution. For example, suppose that $n = 100$ observations are made of two continuous variables, X and Y, and the regression model

$$Y = \beta_0 + \beta_1 X + E, \tag{2.17}$$

where

$$E \sim N(0, \sigma)$$

is fitted to these data, as illustrated in Figure 2.6. The residual value for the ith pair of observations, (x_i, y_i), is calculated as

$$e_i = y_i - \left(\hat{\beta}_0 + \hat{\beta}_1 x_i\right), \tag{2.18}$$

where $\hat{\beta}_0$ and $\hat{\beta}_1$ are the estimates of β_0 and β_1, respectively.

If the fit of this model to the data is good, these residuals may be expected to be approximately normally distributed, and their agreement with this expectation can be judged visually by ordering them, and plotting them against the corresponding quantiles of the standard normal distribution,

$$Z \sim N(0, 1),$$

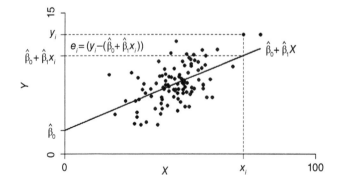

Figure 2.6   The line of best fit to $n = 100$ pairs of observations of variables X and Y.

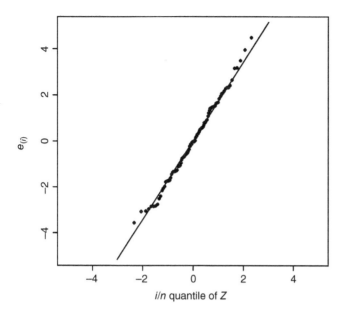

Figure 2.7 Quantile–quantile (Q–Q) plot of the ordered residuals from the fitted relationship between X and Y in Equation (2.17), against the corresponding quantiles of the standard normal distribution.

as shown in Figure 2.7. For example, the 5th-ranked observation out of $n = 100$ is plotted against $Z = -1.640$, because

$$P(Z \leq -1.640) = 5/100.$$

The points in this Q–Q plot lie approximately on a straight diagonal line, indicating that the agreement between the model and the data is good.

2.7 Alternatives to the BH Criterion

The Benjamini–Hochberg criterion is not the only possible approach to controlling the FDR: besides specifying a desired FDR and finding the largest significance threshold $p_{(k)}$ that is expected to achieve it in a particular set of tests, one can turn the argument around, specifying a significance threshold $p_{(k)}$ on some other basis and finding the FDR that it is expected to achieve, namely,

$$E\left(\frac{V}{V + S}\right) \leq \frac{p_{(k)}}{k/m}. \tag{2.19}$$

For example, one could specify the conventional significance threshold $\alpha = 0.05$ to the data-set presented in Table 2.3, as illustrated in Figure 2.8. On this basis, when it is determined from Table 2.4 that the largest p-value smaller than α is $p_{(k)} = p_{(13)} = 0.03513$, substitution of these values into Inequality (2.19) gives

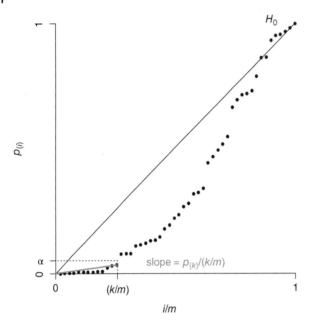

Figure 2.8 Q–Q plot showing the control of the FDR achieved by a pre-specified conventional significance threshold α.

$$E\left(\frac{V}{V+S}\right) \le \frac{0.03513}{13/50} = 0.135.$$

Conversely, one might decide that one's resources extended to further investigation of 30% of one's hypotheses, and accordingly specify the significance threshold at the p-value corresponding to the quantile $k/m = k/50 = 0.3$, as illustrated in Figure 2.9, whence $k = 15$. The largest p-value considered as significant would then be $p_{(15)} = 0.07895$, and this would be the effective significance threshold, $\alpha_{effective} = 0.07895$. The expected FDR would then be controlled at $\alpha_{effective}/(k/m) = 0.07895/(15/50) = 0.263$.

More generally, one can specify an arbitrary significance threshold from among the observed ordered p-values, $p_{(k)}$, and find the FDR that it is expected to achieve. (Note that in this context, the result $p_{(k)} = \alpha$ is considered significant: that is, the significance criterion is $p \le \alpha$, not $p < \alpha$.) This is not a conventional procedure, but it gives a useful illustration of the concepts and reasoning related to the FDR. Figure 2.10 shows an enlargement of the region close to the origin (i.e., the region containing the small values of $p_{(i)}$) from Figures 2.7–2.9, with two possible significance thresholds applied to the set of tests, $p_{(16)} = 0.07900$ and $p_{(14)} = 0.07595$. $p_{(16)}$ is the threshold given by the BH step-down procedure when the criterion $q^* = 0.3$ is applied, and the level at which the expected FDR is controlled by this threshold is indeed below 0.3, namely, $\dfrac{p_{(k)}}{k/m} = \dfrac{0.07900}{16/50} = 0.2469$. The threshold $p_{(14)}$, though more stringent, gives $\dfrac{0.07595}{14/50} = 0.2712$, a slightly higher

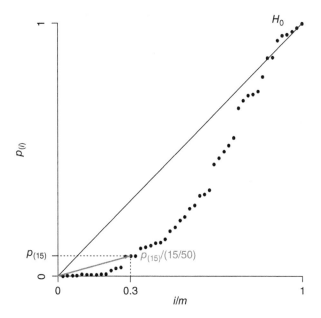

Figure 2.9 Q–Q plot showing the control of the FDR achieved by a pre-specified quantile threshold k/m.

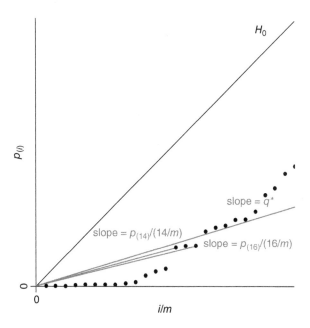

Figure 2.10 Q–Q plot showing the control of the FDR achieved by two different quantile thresholds, $14/m$ and $16/m$.

control-boundary for the FDR. Moreover, it gives a smaller set of test results announced as significant, a subset of those announced for $p_{(16)}$, and hence less statistical power. Thus, perhaps counterintuitively, the less stringent significance threshold is preferable in terms of both FDR and statistical power.

These alternative procedures control the FDR at a level that can be determined, but they are not specified in terms of this level: they are specified on other criteria – a significance threshold a, a quantile k/m, or a p-value $p_{(k)}$. The special feature of the Benjamini–Hochberg step-down False Discovery Rate criterion (the BH-FDR procedure) is that it specifies the subset of p-values selected in terms of level at which the FDR is controlled, q^*. Its special merit is that by identifying the largest value $p_{(k)}$ consistent with this criterion (as noted in Section 2.4), it defines the largest possible set of significant test results ('discoveries') consistent with the criterion. This in turn maximises the expected number of true-positive results S, and hence maximises the expected value of

$$\frac{S}{S+T} = P(H_0 \text{ rejected} \mid H_1 \text{ is true}).$$

That is, the BH-FDR criterion maximises the *statistical power* of the tests – the proportion of real effects that they discover. Equivalently, the BH-FDR criterion minimises the false-negative rate, which is the expected value of

$$\frac{T}{S+T} = P(H_0 \text{ accepted} \mid H_1 \text{ is true}) = 1 - P(H_0 \text{ rejected} \mid H_1 \text{ is true}).$$

2.8 Consequences of Correlations Among the Hypotheses Tested

An illustration will demonstrate the importance of the condition that the m_0 tests for which H_0 is true are independent. Consider a single normally distributed explanatory variable,

$$X \sim N(\mu_X, \sigma_X).$$

Then consider a large number, $m_{0.H}$, of normally distributed response variables,

$$Y_i \sim N(\mu_Y, \sigma_Y), i = 1...m_{0.H}.$$

For each of these response variables, the null hypothesis H_0 that Y_i is not associated with X is to be tested, with the one-sided alternative hypothesis H_1 that there is a positive association between Y_i and X. All the variables are measured on each of a very large number, n, of experimental units (e.g., subjects or patients). Now suppose that the n units are divided into a large number, $m_{0.S}$, of small samples, each of size n_S, so that $n = m_{0.S} n_S$, and that each of the $m_{0.H}$ null hypotheses is to be tested in each of the $m_{0.S}$ samples. Thus, $m_{0.S} m_{0.H}$ tests are to be conducted in total. The test of the ith null hypothesis on the jth sample gives rise to the p-value p_{ij}. The structure of the data is illustrated in Table 2.5, and that of the p-values in Table 2.6. (It is not suggested that this division of n experimental units into $m_{0.S}$ small samples would be sensible in practice: the purpose is to illustrate the concepts of independent and correlated p-values.)

Table 2.5 Structure of the data for tests of association between an explanatory variable X and $m_{0.H}$ response variables Y_i, $i = 1...m_{0.H}$, to be conducted on $n = m_{0.S}n_S$ experimental units divided into $m_{0.S}$ small samples of size n_S.

Sample	Unit	X	Y_1	...	Y_i	...	$Y_{m_{0.H}}$
1	1	x_{11}	y_{111}		y_{i11}		$y_{m_{0.H}11}$
	$\vdots$						$\vdots$
	k	x_{1k}	y_{11k}		y_{i1k}		$y_{m_{0.H}1k}$
	$\vdots$						$\vdots$
	n_S	x_{1n_S}	y_{11n_S}		y_{i1n_S}		$y_{m_{0.H}1n_S}$
	$\vdots$						$\vdots$
j	1	x_{j1}	y_{1j1}		y_{ij1}		$y_{m_{0.H}j1}$
	$\vdots$						$\vdots$
	k	x_{jk}	y_{1jk}		y_{ijk}		$y_{m_{0.H}jk}$
	$\vdots$						$\vdots$
	n_S	x_{jn_S}	y_{1jn_S}		y_{ijn_S}		$y_{m_{0.H}jn_S}$
	$\vdots$						$\vdots$
$m_{0.S}$	1	$x_{m_{0.S}1}$	$y_{1m_{0.S}1}$		$y_{im_{0.S}1}$		$y_{m_{0.H}m_{0.S}1}$
	$\vdots$						$\vdots$
	k	$x_{m_{0.S}k}$	$y_{1m_{0.S}k}$		$y_{im_{0.S}k}$		$y_{m_{0.H}m_{0.S}k}$
	$\vdots$						$\vdots$
	n_S	$x_{m_{0.S}n_S}$	$y_{1m_{0.S}n_S}$	...	$y_{im_{0.S}n_S}$	...	$y_{m_{0.H}m_{0.S}n_S}$

Table 2.6 Structure of p-values from the data-structure illustrated in Table 2.5.

Sample	Y_1	...	Y_i	...	$Y_{m_{0.H}}$	Variance over hypotheses[b]
1	p_{11}		p_{i1}		$p_{m_{0.H}1}$	
$\vdots$			$\vdots$			
j	p_{1j}		p_{ij}		$p_{m_{0.H}j}$	$\mathrm{var}(p_{.j})$
$\vdots$			$\vdots$			
$m_{0.S}$	$p_{1m_{0.S}}$	...	$p_{im_{0.S}}$	...	$p_{m_{0.H}m_{0.S}}$	
Variance over samples[a]			$\mathrm{var}(p_{i.})$			

[a] $\mathrm{var}(p_{i.})$ = variance of p_{ij} for the ith hypothesis over all $j = 1...m_{0.S}$ samples.
[b] $\mathrm{var}(p_{.j})$ = variance of p_{ij} for the jth sample over all $i = 1...m_{0.H}$ hypotheses.

Now suppose that there is no association between X and any of the Y variables, so that H_0 is true for every test, but that there are positive correlations between the Y variables. A dataset that meets these criteria can be produced as follows. We first produce n independent realisations of a variable distributed as X. We then specify

$$Y_i = \mu_Y + Z + E_i, \tag{2.20}$$

that is, the variation in each Y variable is the sum of two components, namely, Z, which is common to all the Y variables, and E_i, which is unique to the Y variable in question. To obtain the values of these Y variables, we then proceed as follows. We first produce n realisations of a latent (i.e., unobservable) variable Z, sampled from the distribution

$$Z \sim N(0, \sigma_Z). \tag{2.21}$$

These n realisations are independent of each other and of the realisations of X. We then produce n realisations of each of $m_{0.H}$ variables E_i, $i = 1...m_{0.H}$, sampled from the distribution

$$E_i \sim N(0, \sigma_E). \tag{2.22}$$

These $m_{0.H}n$ realisations are likewise independent of each other and of the realisations of X and Z. The realisations of Z and E_i are then substituted into Equation (2.20), to obtain the values of Y_i, $i = 1...m_{0.H}$.

The consequences of this data structure will be explored using simulated data with the specifications shown in Table 2.7.

The pattern in the simulated data obtained from these specifications is illustrated for $i = 1$ and 2 in Figures 2.11 and 2.12. The distributions of the observations of Y_1 and X, and the relationship between these variables, are presented in Figure 2.11a, and the corresponding patterns for Y_2 and X in Figure 2.11b. As expected, the observations of all three variables are approximately normally distributed, and there is little evidence of a relationship between either Y variable and X: in both cases, the line of best fit is nearly horizontal, and the p-value for the one-sided test for a positive slope is large – indeed, greater than 0.5, as in both cases the estimated slope is slightly negative. Though neither Y_1 nor Y_2 is related to X, these two response variables are clearly related to each other (Figure 2.12). The population correlation

Table 2.7 Specifications for a dataset with the structure indicated by Equation (2.20), Distributions (2.21) and (2.22), and Table 2.5.

Specification	Symbol	Value
Number of response variables, Y_i, $i = 1...m_{0.H}$	$m_{0.H}$	1,000
Number of small samples	$m_{0.S}$	1,000
Number of experimental units per small sample	n_S	10
Total number of experimental units	$n = m_{0.S}n_S$	10,000
Mean of single explanatory variable X	μ_X	4
Standard deviation of X	σ_X	1
Mean of response variables Y_i, $i = 1...m_{0.H}$	μ_Y	3
Standard deviation of latent variable Z, contributing to all Y_i, $i = 1...m_{0.H}$	σ_Z	$\sqrt{0.7}$
Standard deviation of residual variables E_i, $i = 1...m_{0.H}$, unique to each Y_i	σ_E	$\sqrt{0.3}$

coefficient between any two Y variables constructed on the basis of Equation (2.20) and Distributions (2.21) and (2.22) is

$$\rho = \sigma_Z^2/(\sigma_Z^2 + \sigma_E^2). \tag{2.23}$$

In the present case, $\rho = 0.7/(0.7 + 0.3) = 0.7$, and the observed value, $r = 0.707$, is close to this. The quantiles of the distribution of the observed r-values, over the $\frac{1}{2} \times 1000 \times (1000 - 1) = 499\,500$ pairwise combinations among the 1000 Y variables, are presented in Table 2.8. They show that the distribution is tightly focused around the population value: only $5\% + 5\% = 10\%$ of the r-values lie above 0.7138 or below 0.7006. This is because the number of observations contributing to each r-value is large ($n = 10,000$).

a) Y_1 versus X
b) Y_2 versus X

(a)

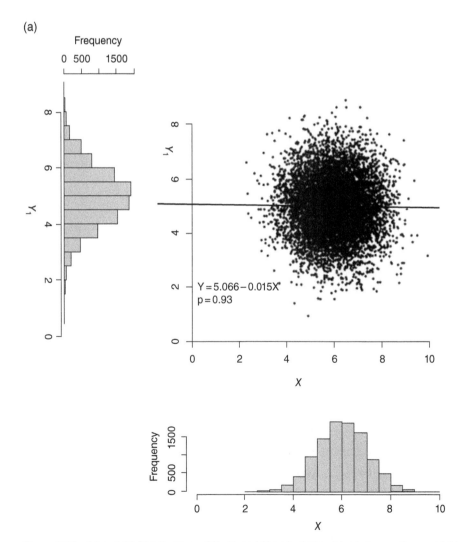

Figure 2.11 (a) and (b) Distributions of Y_1, Y_2 and X, and relationships between these variables.

(b)

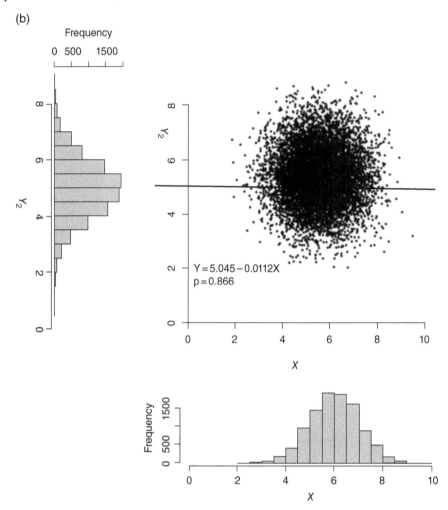

Figure 2.11 (Continued)

Now consider what happens when the *i*th null hypothesis H_0: 'Y_i is not associated with X' is tested repeatedly in each of the $m_{0.S}$ small samples. H_0 is true, so the *p*-value for each sample is an observation from a Uniform(0, 1) distribution. The samples are independent of each other, so the $m_{0.S}$ observed *p*-values are expected approximately to follow this distribution. The distributions obtained for $i = 1$ and 2, that is, in the case of Y_1 and Y_2, are presented in Figure 2.13, together with a scatter plot showing the relationship between the two sets of *p*-values – their bivariate distribution. Each set of *p*-values has an approximately Uniform(0, 1) distribution, as expected. The variance of the Uniform(0, 1) distribution is $\frac{1}{12} = 0.0833$, and the variance of the observed distribution of the *p*-values for the *i*th null hypothesis, over the $m_{0.S} = 1000$ small samples (i.e., the variance of the *p*-values in the *i*th column of Table 2.6), can be compared with this value. When this variance is calculated for each of the $m_{0.H} = 1000$ null hypotheses (i.e., for each column of Table 2.6), and the distribution of these variance estimates is considered, the percentiles are as presented in Table 2.9, in the column headed 'Percentile over hypotheses $i = 1...m_{0.H}$, of var($p_{i.}$)'. They show that the distribution is tightly focused around the population value.

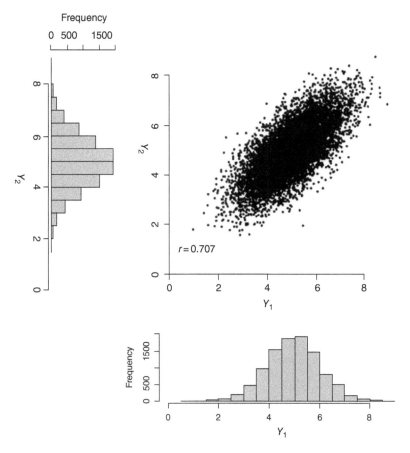

Figure 2.12 Distributions of, and relationship between, Y_1 and Y_2.

Table 2.8 Percentage points of the distribution of the observed correlation coefficient r over pairwise combinations of Y variables.

Percentage point	Percentile
0%	0.6873
5%	0.7006
50%	0.7073
95%	0.7138
100%	0.7247

However, the scatter plot in Figure 2.13 shows that the sets of p values obtained from $i = 1$ and 2 are not independent: if the p-value for the first null hypothesis is small in a particular sample, that for the second null hypothesis is usually also small. Conversely, if the first is large, the second is usually also large. Samples in which the first p-value is large and the second small, or *vice versa*, are rare. This pattern is due to the positive correlation between

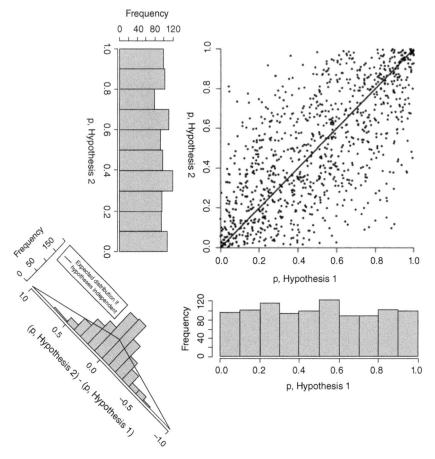

Figure 2.13 Univariate distributions, over the $m_{0.S}$ small samples, of p-values for Y_1 versus X and Y_2 versus X, and the corresponding bivariate distribution, when Y_1 and Y_2 are positively correlated.

Table 2.9 Distribution of the observed variance of the p-values obtained from hypothesis tests in small samples, over hypotheses and over samples.

	Percentile	
Percentage point	Over hypotheses $i = 1...m_{0.H}$, of var($p_{i.}$)	Over samples $j = 1...m_{0.S}$, of var($p_{.j}$)
0%	0.0771	0.0004
5%	0.0797	0.0060
50%	0.0827	0.0268
95%	0.0855	0.0491
100%	0.0893	0.0700

Y_1 and Y_2: if the correlation were perfect ($\rho = 1$), then the two significance tests would effectively be testing the same hypothesis, the two p-values from each small sample would be the same, and the points in the scatter plot would all lie exactly on the diagonal line. This pattern can be explored further by considering the distribution of the differences between the two p-values in each pair, shown in the histogram displayed diagonally at the bottom left of Figure 2.13. The values are concentrated in a narrow range, relative to the distribution expected if the two sets of p-values are independent.

The corresponding plots when the hypotheses are independent (i.e., obtained with the specification $\sigma_Z = 0$, $\sigma_E = 1$) are shown in Figure 2.14. The two univariate distributions

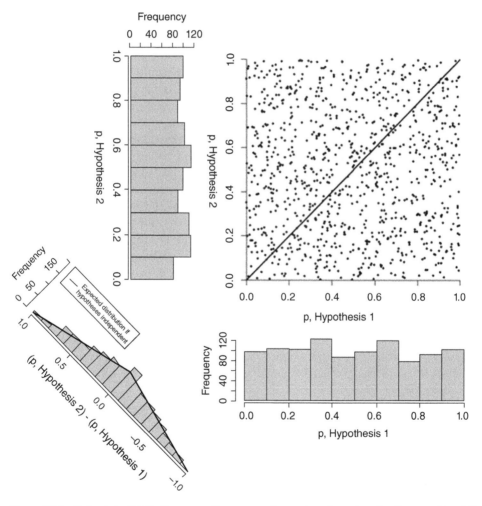

Figure 2.14 Univariate distributions, over the $m_{0.5}$ small samples, of p-values for Y_1 versus X and Y_2 versus X, and the corresponding bivariate distribution, when Y_1 and Y_2 are uncorrelated.

of *p*-values are almost unchanged, but the bivariate distribution and the distribution of the difference between the *p*-values are different. The points representing combinations of the two *p*-values are now fairly evenly distributed over the scatter plot: if one *p*-value is large, this gives no indication of the size of the other *p*-value. Consequently, the histogram of differences displayed diagonally conforms closely to the theoretical distribution of the differences between two independent observations from the Uniform(0, 1) distribution.

Returning to the simulated data obtained with the specification $\sigma_Z = \sqrt{0.7}$, $\sigma_E = \sqrt{0.3}$, we can consider the consequences of the pattern observed in Figure 2.13 for the distribution of *p*-values over hypotheses that are *not* independent, rather than over small samples that *are* independent. The corresponding histograms and scatter plot are presented in Figure 2.15. The histograms show that these *p*-values do not have an approximately Uniform(0, 1) distribution: because of the correlations between the *Y* variables, induced by the latent variable *Z* that makes a common contribution to all of them, the *p*-values tend to be similar to each other, as was seen in the bivariate plot and the histogram of differences for hypotheses 1 and 2 in Figure 2.13. Consequently, there is a deficiency of *p*-values close to 0, or close to 1, or at both ends of the distribution. The particular distribution of *p*-values varies considerably from sample to sample, depending on the small set of *Z*-values that contribute in common to all the *Y*-values for the sample, but in every case the *p*-values cluster, to a greater or lesser extent, around some central value. The bivariate plot confirms that the pairs of *p*-values are not uniformly distributed over the two-dimensional range, but also confirms that there is almost no correlation between the *p*-values for the two samples. The distribution of the difference between the *p*-values in each pair, shown in the histogram displayed diagonally at the bottom left of the figure, has a visibly narrower spread than the expected distribution if the *p*-values are uncorrelated, and is asymmetric because it is strongly influenced by the 20 random values of *Z* that contribute to the calculation of every *p*-value from these two samples. If the *p*-values for the $m_{0.\mathrm{H}} = 1000$ hypotheses were uncorrelated, the patterns in the plots in Figure 2.15 would be very similar to those in Figure 2.14. The tightness of the clustering of *p*-values in each sample can be quantified by the variance of the *p*-values over the $m_{0.\mathrm{H}} = 1000$ hypotheses for each of the $m_{0.\mathrm{S}} = 1000$ samples (i.e., for each row of Table 2.6): the variance is a summary statistic reflecting the differences between the values that contribute to it, so it extends the exploration of differences between *p*-values from hypotheses 1 and 2 to all the hypotheses. The percentiles of the distribution of these variance estimates are also presented in Table 2.9, in the column headed 'Percentile over samples $j = 1...m_{0.\mathrm{S}}$, of var(p_j)': they show that these variances are consistently smaller than that of the Uniform(0, 1) distribution.

Therefore, if H_0 is true for each of m_0 tests, but the *p*-values from these tests are not mutually independent but are positively correlated with each other, then if the significance threshold is set at $P_{(k)}$, it is no longer true that the expected number of false-positive tests is

$$\mathrm{E}(V) = m_0 \mathrm{P}\left(P_i \leq P_{(k)} \mid H_0\right) = m_0 P_{(k)}.$$

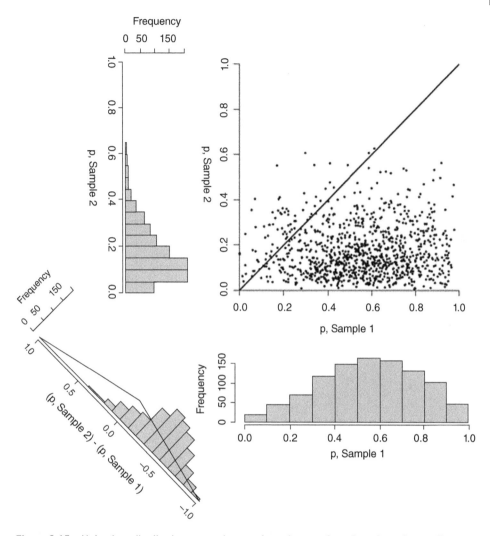

Figure 2.15 Univariate distributions, over the $m_{0.H}$ hypotheses, of p-values from the small samples for $j = 1$ and $j = 2$, and the corresponding bivariate distribution, when the Y_i variables are positively correlated.

There will be a deficiency of p-values close to 0 and close to 1, so that if a significance threshold below one-half is specified ($P_{(k)} < \frac{1}{2}$) – which in practice will always be the case – then

$$E(V) < m_0 p_{(k)},$$

that is, fewer false-positives are to be expected than the value of m_0 would suggest. One can say that in the presence of positive correlations, the *nominal* number of tests for which H_0 is true, m_0, is equivalent to a smaller *effective* number of tests – though in general it is not possible to specify this smaller number precisely. Thus, in the presence of positive correlations, the BH criterion is conservative: it anticipates more false-positive results than are actually expected to occur. (As noted, positive correlations also cause a deficiency of very large p-values, but as significance thresholds specified in practice are always close to 0, these large values do not affect the argument.)

In certain special cases it is possible to specify the smaller number of independent hypotheses to which the m_0 nominal hypotheses are equivalent, and in this case the deficiency of extreme p-values can be understood in terms of the expected values of $P_{(i)}$, $i = 1...m_0$. For example, suppose that $m_0 = 20$ hypotheses are tested. If they are all mutually independent, the expected values of $P_{(1)}...P_{(20)}$ on H_0 are then $i/(m_0 + 1)$, $i = 1...20$, that is, $1/21$, $2/21...$ $20/21$. However, suppose that the variables Y_i, $i = 1...20$, comprise ten pairs (Y_1 and Y_2, Y_3 and $Y_4 ... Y_{19}$ and Y_{20}) that are effectively duplicate measurements of the same response. The two p-values for the tests within each pair will then be identical. This approach is connected to the correlation-based view of the situation by the correlation matrix among the 20 Y variables:

	Y_1	Y_2	Y_3	Y_4	Y_5	Y_6	Y_7	Y_8	Y_9	Y_{10}	Y_{11}	Y_{12}	Y_{13}	Y_{14}	Y_{15}	Y_{16}	Y_{17}	Y_{18}	Y_{19}	Y_{20}
Y_1	1	1	0	0	0	0	0	0	0	0	0	0	0	0	0	0	0	0	0	0
Y_2	1	1	0	0	0	0	0	0	0	0	0	0	0	0	0	0	0	0	0	0
Y_3	0	0	1	1	0	0	0	0	0	0	0	0	0	0	0	0	0	0	0	0
Y_4	0	0	1	1	0	0	0	0	0	0	0	0	0	0	0	0	0	0	0	0
Y_5	0	0	0	0	1	1	0	0	0	0	0	0	0	0	0	0	0	0	0	0
Y_6	0	0	0	0	1	1	0	0	0	0	0	0	0	0	0	0	0	0	0	0
Y_7	0	0	0	0	0	0	1	1	0	0	0	0	0	0	0	0	0	0	0	0
Y_8	0	0	0	0	0	0	1	1	0	0	0	0	0	0	0	0	0	0	0	0
Y_9	0	0	0	0	0	0	0	0	1	1	0	0	0	0	0	0	0	0	0	0
Y_{10}	0	0	0	0	0	0	0	0	1	1	0	0	0	0	0	0	0	0	0	0
Y_{11}	0	0	0	0	0	0	0	0	0	0	1	1	0	0	0	0	0	0	0	0
Y_{12}	0	0	0	0	0	0	0	0	0	0	1	1	0	0	0	0	0	0	0	0
Y_{13}	0	0	0	0	0	0	0	0	0	0	0	0	1	1	0	0	0	0	0	0
Y_{14}	0	0	0	0	0	0	0	0	0	0	0	0	1	1	0	0	0	0	0	0
Y_{15}	0	0	0	0	0	0	0	0	0	0	0	0	0	0	1	1	0	0	0	0
Y_{16}	0	0	0	0	0	0	0	0	0	0	0	0	0	0	1	1	0	0	0	0
Y_{17}	0	0	0	0	0	0	0	0	0	0	0	0	0	0	0	0	1	1	0	0
Y_{18}	0	0	0	0	0	0	0	0	0	0	0	0	0	0	0	0	1	1	0	0
Y_{19}	0	0	0	0	0	0	0	0	0	0	0	0	0	0	0	0	0	0	1	1
Y_{20}	0	0	0	0	0	0	0	0	0	0	0	0	0	0	0	0	0	0	1	1

For hypotheses in the same pair, the correlation coefficient between the Y variables (highlighted in the matrix) is 1, for hypotheses in different pairs (not highlighted), it is 0. The

20 nominal hypotheses are then equivalent to only ten independent hypotheses, and the expected values of $P_{(1)}...P_{(20)}$ on H_0 are then 1/11, 1/11, 2/11, 2/11, ...10/11, 10/11. Next, suppose that the variables comprise five groups of four (Y_1 to Y_4, Y_5 to Y_8, Y_9 to Y_{12}, Y_{13} to Y_{16}, Y_{17} to Y_{20}), the variables within each group being effectively duplicate measurements of the same response. The correlation matrix among the Y variables is then as follows:

	Y_1	Y_2	Y_3	Y_4	Y_5	Y_6	Y_7	Y_8	Y_9	Y_{10}	Y_{11}	Y_{12}	Y_{13}	Y_{14}	Y_{15}	Y_{16}	Y_{17}	Y_{18}	Y_{19}	Y_{20}
Y_1	1	1	1	1	0	0	0	0	0	0	0	0	0	0	0	0	0	0	0	0
Y_2	1	1	1	1	0	0	0	0	0	0	0	0	0	0	0	0	0	0	0	0
Y_3	1	1	1	1	0	0	0	0	0	0	0	0	0	0	0	0	0	0	0	0
Y_4	1	1	1	1	0	0	0	0	0	0	0	0	0	0	0	0	0	0	0	0
Y_5	0	0	0	0	1	1	1	1	0	0	0	0	0	0	0	0	0	0	0	0
Y_6	0	0	0	0	1	1	1	1	0	0	0	0	0	0	0	0	0	0	0	0
Y_7	0	0	0	0	1	1	1	1	0	0	0	0	0	0	0	0	0	0	0	0
Y_8	0	0	0	0	1	1	1	1	0	0	0	0	0	0	0	0	0	0	0	0
Y_9	0	0	0	0	0	0	0	0	1	1	1	1	0	0	0	0	0	0	0	0
Y_{10}	0	0	0	0	0	0	0	0	1	1	1	1	0	0	0	0	0	0	0	0
Y_{11}	0	0	0	0	0	0	0	0	1	1	1	1	0	0	0	0	0	0	0	0
Y_{12}	0	0	0	0	0	0	0	0	1	1	1	1	0	0	0	0	0	0	0	0
Y_{13}	0	0	0	0	0	0	0	0	0	0	0	0	1	1	1	1	0	0	0	0
Y_{14}	0	0	0	0	0	0	0	0	0	0	0	0	1	1	1	1	0	0	0	0
Y_{15}	0	0	0	0	0	0	0	0	0	0	0	0	1	1	1	1	0	0	0	0
Y_{16}	0	0	0	0	0	0	0	0	0	0	0	0	1	1	1	1	0	0	0	0
Y_{17}	0	0	0	0	0	0	0	0	0	0	0	0	0	0	0	0	1	1	1	1
Y_{18}	0	0	0	0	0	0	0	0	0	0	0	0	0	0	0	0	1	1	1	1
Y_{19}	0	0	0	0	0	0	0	0	0	0	0	0	0	0	0	0	1	1	1	1
Y_{20}	0	0	0	0	0	0	0	0	0	0	0	0	0	0	0	0	1	1	1	1

The 20 nominal hypotheses are now equivalent to only five independent hypotheses, and the expected values of $p_{(1)}...p_{(20)}$ on H_0 are now 1/6, 1/6, 1/6, 1/6, 2/6, 2/6, 2/6, 2/6,...5/6, 5/6, 5/6, 5/6. Finally, suppose that the 20 Y variables are all effectively duplicate measurements of the same response. The 20 nominal hypotheses are now equivalent to a single hypothesis, all tests will give the same p-value and the expected values of $P_{(1)}...P_{(20)}$ on H_0 are all ½. This relationship between the effective number of independent tests and the expected values of $p_{(i)}, i = 1...m_0$, is presented graphically in Figure 2.16. As the effective number of hypotheses decreases, the expected values of $p_{(i)}$ shrink towards the centre of the Uniform(0, 1) distribution, the extreme values being shrunk most strongly.

Note that although the BH criterion depends on Equation (2.8) and hence on the independence of the m_0 tests for which H_0 is true, there is no such requirement for independence among the m_1 tests for which H_0 is false (Benjamini and Hochberg, 1995, Section 3.1): these may be positively or negatively correlated with each other.

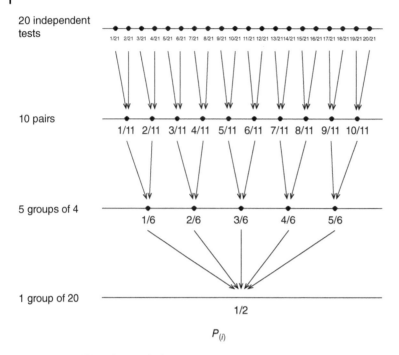

Figure 2.16 The relationship between the effective number of independent tests and the expected values of $P_{(i)}$.

2.9 The FDR in a Non-Statistical Context: A Diagnostic Test

The distinction between the false-positive rate and the FDR is relevant not just to statistical significance testing of null hypotheses, but to any type of test that can give either a false-positive or a false-negative result, such as a medical diagnostic test. For example, the faecal immunochemical test (FIT), used by the UK's National Health Service in routine screening of the older adult population for colorectal cancer (CRC), is estimated to have a specificity of 85.8%: that is, among individuals who do not have CRC, the false-positive rate (the statistician's Type I error rate – see Section 2.1) is $(100 - 85.8)/100 = 0.142$. The test is also estimated to have a sensitivity of 92.1%: that is, among individuals who *do* have CRC, the false-negative rate (the statistician's Type II error rate) is $(100 - 92.1)/100 = 0.079$ (D'Souza 2019). We can combine this information with information on the prevalence of the disease (American Cancer Society 2020) and demographic information (https://www.statista.com/statistics/270000/age-distribution-in-the-united-states/, accessed 15 April 2024) from a roughly comparable population in the US, in order to obtain a tentative estimate of the proportions in the confusion matrix for this test. In 2019, the number of individuals alive with a history of CRC in the US was 776,120 men + 768,650 women = 1,544,770. Of these, 56% were aged 65–84 years: that is, about $56/100 \times 1{,}544{,}770 = 865{,}071$ individuals. The total population of the US was 320 million, of whom 17.04% were aged ≥ 65 years, that is, $17.04/100 \times 320{,}000{,}000 = 54{,}528{,}000$ individuals. Hence, the percentage of those aged

Table 2.10 The confusion matrix for a medical diagnostic test.

	Test result		
True status	**Negative**	**Positive**	**Total**
Negative	$0.984135 \times 0.858 = 0.844389$	$0.984135 \times 0.142 = 0.139747$	0.984135
Positive	$0.015865 \times 0.079 = 0.001253$	$0.015865 \times 0.921 = 0.014612$	0.015865
Total	0.845642	0.154359	1

The proportions of outcomes in each cell are presented. Highlighted values are obtained directly from external sources.

≥65 years with a history of CRC was approximately $865,071/54,528,000 = 1.5865\%$. On the basis of these figures, the proportions in the cells of the confusion matrix are as shown in Table 2.10. The false-positive rate of the FIT test is then estimated to be $0.139747/(0.844389 + 0.139747) = 0.142$. However, the FDR is very different: $0.139747/(0.139747 + 0.014611) = 0.905$. The test has a low false-positive rate, but because CRC is fairly rare, the FDR is nevertheless high. For this reason, individuals who take the test as part of a routine screening programme are reassured that even if they are called back for an endoscopy because of a positive test result, they do not necessarily have bowel cancer.

These calculations should not be taken as a reliable indication of the FDR of the FIT test: they are based on readily available information from a population only roughly comparable with that being screened. In particular, in the UK at the time of writing, bowel cancer screening is available to everyone aged 60–74 years, but is not offered routinely to those aged 75 or older (https://www.nhs.uk/conditions/bowel-cancer-screening/, accessed 15 April 2024). Moreover, the proportion of individuals *known to have* a history of CRC in one population is very questionable as an estimate of the proportion with *as-yet undiagnosed* CRC in another. However, this analysis does show clearly the difference between the meaning of the false-positive rate and the FDR. (N.B. Changing the assumed ratio from 1:1 to, for example, '1 known history:5 undiagnosed' does not greatly change the false-positive–FDR relationship.)

The great difference between the false-positive rate and the FDR in this case shows the care that must be taken in interpreting the values in a confusion matrix. An example of potentially deliberate failure to do so, for a dishonest purpose, is the Prosecutor's Fallacy, in which a small probability of obtaining certain incriminating evidence if the accused person is innocent (the false-positive rate) is misrepresented as the probability that the accused is innocent given that the evidence has indeed been obtained (the FDR):

> The use of *p*-values [as legal evidence] can...lead to the prosecutor's fallacy because a *p*-value (which says something about the probability of observing the evidence [or more extreme evidence] given a hypothesis) is often wrongly interpreted as being the same as the probability of the hypothesis given the evidence. (Fenton, Neil and Berger, 2016)

The false-positive rate and the FDR are not the only ways of interpreting a confusion matrix. A Wikipedia article (https://en.wikipedia.org/wiki/Confusion_matrix, accessed 15 April 2024) shows no less than 21 ways of interpreting combinations of the four values U, V, T and S in Table 2.2, and even more names for these combinations. For example,

$$\frac{V}{V+U} = \text{false-positive rate,}$$

$$\frac{T}{T+S} = \text{false-negative rate,}$$

$$\frac{V}{V+S} = \text{false discovery rate (FDR),}$$

$$\frac{T}{T+U} = \text{false omission rate,}$$

$$\frac{U}{V+U} = \text{specificity} = 1 - \text{false-positive rate,}$$

$$\frac{S}{T+S} = \text{sensitivity} = 1 - \text{false-negative rate,}$$

$$\frac{S}{V+S} = \text{positive predictive value} = 1 - \text{false discovery rate,}$$

$$\frac{U}{T+U} = \text{negative predictive value} = 1 - \text{false omission rate.}$$

2.10 Summary

The null hypothesis (H_0) and alternative hypothesis (H_1) are distinguished in the context of statistical significance testing. The outcomes of a significance test are classified in terms of the true hypothesis (H_0 or H_1) and the conclusion from the evidence (H_0 or H_1), and the 2×2 confusion matrix is introduced as a tool to present the four possible combinations of true hypothesis and conclusion.

The meanings of the p-value and the false discovery rate (FDR) are explained in terms of the confusion matrix, and the distinction between the two is shown.

The Benjamini–Hochberg (BH) FDR criterion (the BH-FDR criterion) is introduced as a criterion for controlling the FDR while maximising the statistical power of the tests, P(H_0 rejected|H_1 is true), and, equivalently, minimising the false-negative rate, P(H_0 accepted|H_1 is true) $= 1 - $ P(H_0 rejected|H_1 is true).

The BH step-down procedure is introduced as a tool for implementing the BH-FDR criterion.

These concepts are illustrated in a simulated set of p-values from tests of $m = 50$ hypotheses.

In the context of significance testing, the distribution of the ordered p-values is compared with the Uniform(0, 1) distribution expected on H_0. Two graphical presentations, the histogram and the quantile–quantile (Q–Q) plot, are used for this purpose.

The Q–Q plot is used to show that the BH step-down FDR criterion is consistent with intuition.

The more general context for the use of Q–Q plots is briefly described, in particular their use for diagnostic plots of residuals, following the fitting of a statistical model to data. The use of the Q–Q plot to compare the distribution of the ordered observations with the quantiles of a formal distribution expected on the model is explained.

Besides the BH-FDR criterion, other criteria that control the FDR are introduced. If discoveries are announced on the basis of a significance threshold α, or a quantile k/m, the FDR achieved can be determined, but the discovery criterion is then not *specified* in terms of control of the FDR.

The BH-FDR identifies the largest subset of tests consistent with control of the FDR at level q^*, and hence maximises the statistical power consistent with this criterion.

The consequences of positive correlations among the p-values for the m hypotheses tested are explored. The variance of the p-values over the hypotheses is then less than the variance of the Uniform(0, 1) distribution, even if H_0 is true for every test.

This means that the *nominal* number of tests for which H_0 is true, m_0, is equivalent to a smaller *effective* number of tests.

In certain special cases, this effective number of tests can be precisely specified. If the m_0 tests comprise several groups, and the tests within each group are completely equivalent, effectively testing the same hypothesis, then the effective number of tests is the number of groups.

The distinction between the false-positive rate and the FDR is relevant not only to statistical significance tests, but to any type of test that can give either a false-positive or a false-negative result, such as a medical diagnostic test. This is illustrated in the context of a test used in routine screening for colorectal cancer.

The distinction between the false-positive rate and the FDR has important implications for the interpretation of the test results obtained: the false-positive rate is low, yet the FDR is high. The advice given to patients takes account of this.

The potentially great difference between the false-positive rate and the FDR in this case shows the care that must be taken in interpreting the values in a confusion matrix – for advising patients, for interpreting evidence of guilt in legal cases, and for other purposes. The many ways of interpreting the four values in the matrix are briefly reviewed.

References

American Cancer Society (2020). *Colorectal Cancer Facts & Figures 2020–2022*. Atlanta: American Cancer Society, 42 pp.

Benjamini, Y. and Hochberg, Y. (1995). Controlling the false discovery rate: a practical and powerful approach to multiple testing. *Journal of the Royal Statistical Society B* 57: 289–300.

D'Souza, N. (2019). Editorial. Faecal immunochemical testing in general practice. *British Journal of General Practice* 69: 60–61.

Fenton, N., Neil, M., and Berger, D. (2016). Bayes and the law. *Annual Review of Statistics and Its Application* 3: 51–77. https://doi.org/10.1146/annurev-statistics-041715-033428.

Hacking, I. (2001). *An Introduction to Probability and Logic*. Cambridge: Cambridge University Press, 302 pp.

Moore, D.S. and McCabe, G.P. (1999). *Introduction to the Practice of Statistics*, 3e. New York: W.H. Freeman and Company, 825 pp.

3

Graphical Presentation of the FDR

3.1   Presentation of the Q–Q Plot on the −log$_{10}$(p) Scale

When using a Q–Q plot to inspect the distribution of p-values, it is conventional to plot, not $p_{(i)}$ and i/m themselves as in Figure 2.5 (Chapter 2, Section 2.5), but $-\log_{10}(p_{(i)})$ against $-\log_{10}(i/m)$. The p-values of greatest interest are the smallest ones, and in the plot of $p_{(i)}$ against i/m, these are bunched together close to the origin. However, in the corresponding plot of $-\log_{10}(p_{(i)})$ against $-\log_{10}(i/m)$ (Figure 3.1), the points representing these p-values are spread out in the upper-right-hand region, much more convenient for inspection and interpretation. The H_0 line still has unit slope and passes through the origin, but if H_0 is true for all tests, the points are no longer approximately equally spaced along this line: points representing $p = 0.1$ and 0.01 are much further apart than points representing $p = 0.9$ and 0.99. In Figure 2.5 (Chapter 2), q^* is represented by the line

$$p_{(i)} = q^*(i/m),\qquad(3.1)$$

and the corresponding line on the new plot is

$$-\log_{10}\left(p_{(i)}\right) = -\log_{10}(q^*) - \log_{10}(i/m),\qquad(3.2)$$

that is, a line of unit slope with intercept $-\log_{10}(q^*)$. Whereas $p_{(k)}$ is the *largest* value of $p_{(i)}$ that lies *below* the line defined by Equation (3.1), $-\log_{10}(p_{(k)})$ is the *smallest* value of $-\log_{10}(p_{(i)})$ that lies *above* the line defined by Equation (3.2), so the point $(-\log_{10}(p_{(k)}), -\log_{10}(k/m))$ and those above and to the right of it represent the test results declared significant. The boundary of these significant results is marked by the line CD, and the line AB now lies to the right of this significance threshold. The area to the right of AB holds the number of false-positive significant test results expected by chance, and the area between AB and CD holds the additional number of significant results obtained. The horizontal distance between these lines,

$$AD = -\log_{10}\left(p_{(k)}\right) - (-\log_{10}(k/m)) = -\log_{10}\left(\frac{p_{(k)}}{k/m}\right) \geq -\log_{10}(q^*),$$

The False Discovery Rate: Its Meaning, Interpretation and Application in Data Science, First Edition.
N.W. Galwey.
© 2025 John Wiley & Sons Ltd. Published 2025 by John Wiley & Sons Ltd.
Companion website: www.wiley.com/go/falsediscoveryrate

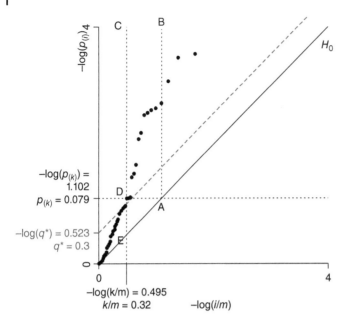

Figure 3.1 Q–Q plot, transformed to the $-\log_{10}$ scale, of the p-values presented on the original scale in Figure 2.5 (Chapter 2).

corresponds to the value at which the FDR is controlled, and, because the line specified in Equation (3.2) and the H_0 line both have unit slope, it is the same as the vertical distance between the point representing the largest significant test result and the H_0 line, *DE*.

When the Q–Q plot is presented on the original, untransformed scale, the FDR is represented by the ratio of the slope of the line given by Equation (3.1) to that of the H_0 line. After transformation to the logarithmic scale, it is represented by the difference between the intercepts of these lines, and, hence, as the intercept of the H_0 line is 0, by that of the line given by Equation (3.2), that is, $-\log_{10}(q^*)$ (Figure 3.1).

3.2 Association of the BH-FDR with Individual *p*-Values

The BH-FDR can not only be used to focus on the set of significant test results identified by a particular value of q^*, but also to consider the whole range of possible values of q^*, from 0 to 1, and to identify the set of test results identified by each value. Each p-value can then be associated with the smallest value of q^* that places it within the significant set. It is this approach that is used when a set of p-values is presented in parallel with an associated set of FDR values by standard statistical software, such as the function p.adjust() with the option setting 'method = "fdr"' in R (R Core Team 2021). This approach is central to the practical application of FDRs, so we will examine it in some detail. For each ordered p-value $p_{(i)}$, we identify $q_{(i)}$, the smallest value of q^*

that will cause $p_{(i)}$ to be included among those considered significant. The corresponding $p_{(i)}$ and $q_{(i)}$ values for the present set of hypotheses are presented in Table 3.1. Note that while $q_{(i)}$ is often the value that will cause $p_{(i)}$ to be set as the threshold for significance $p_{(k)}$, this is not always the case. For example, when we apply the BH step-down procedure and reach $p_{(8)}$, we note that $\dfrac{p_{(8)}}{8/50} = 0.01931$, and as no larger value of i has given a smaller value of $\dfrac{p_{(i)}}{i/50}$, this value becomes $q_{(8)}$. However, moving on to $p_{(7)}$, we find that $\dfrac{p_{(7)}}{7/50} = 0.02029$, and this is larger than $q_{(8)}$, and hence $q_{(7)} = q_{(8)} = 0.01931$. The same

Table 3.1 BF-FDR $(q_{(i)})$ associated with each ordered p-value presented in Table 2.4 (Chapter 2).

i	$p_{(i)}$	i/m	$\dfrac{p_{(i)}}{i/m}$	$q_{(i)}$	i	$p_{(i)}$	i/m	$\dfrac{p_{(i)}}{i/m}$	$q_{(i)}$
1	0.00029	0.02	0.01450	0.00825	26	0.23433	0.52	0.45063	0.45063
2	0.00033	0.04	0.00825	0.00825	27	0.26797	0.54	0.49624	0.49624
3	0.00083	0.06	0.01383	0.01383	28	0.27948	0.56	0.49907	0.49907
4	0.00197	0.08	0.02463	0.01931	29	0.31911	0.58	0.55019	0.53703
5	0.00233	0.10	0.02330	0.01931	30	0.32222	0.60	0.53703	0.53703
6	0.00258	0.12	0.02150	0.01931	31	0.34050	0.62	0.54919	0.54919
7	0.00284	0.14	0.02029	0.01931	32	0.44156	0.64	0.68994	0.68994
8	0.00309	0.16	0.01931	0.01931	33	0.46724	0.66	0.70794	0.70794
9	0.00616	0.18	0.03422	0.03422	34	0.49395	0.68	0.72640	0.72640
10	0.00790	0.20	0.03950	0.03950	35	0.51841	0.70	0.74059	0.74059
11	0.02138	0.22	0.09718	0.09718	36	0.54795	0.72	0.76104	0.76104
12	0.02990	0.24	0.12458	0.12458	37	0.66271	0.74	0.89555	0.88933
13	0.03513	0.26	0.13512	0.13512	38	0.69420	0.76	0.91342	0.88933
14	0.07595	0.28	0.27125	0.24688	39	0.71578	0.78	0.91767	0.88933
15	0.07895	0.30	0.26317	0.24688	40	0.71867	0.80	0.89834	0.88933
16	0.07900	0.32	0.24688	0.24688	41	0.72925	0.82	0.88933	0.88933
17	0.10690	0.34	0.31441	0.31100	42	0.79081	0.84	0.94144	0.94144
18	0.11475	0.36	0.31875	0.31100	43	0.86287	0.86	1.00334	0.98361
19	0.11818	0.38	0.31100	0.31100	44	0.86558	0.88	0.98361	0.98361
20	0.12869	0.40	0.32173	0.31145	45	0.93158	0.90	1.03509	0.99766
21	0.13081	0.42	0.31145	0.31145	46	0.95185	0.92	1.03462	0.99766
22	0.14529	0.44	0.33020	0.33020	47	0.95563	0.94	1.01663	0.99766
23	0.17801	0.46	0.38698	0.38698	48	0.96820	0.96	1.00854	0.99766
24	0.19151	0.48	0.39898	0.39898	49	0.98225	0.98	1.00230	0.99766
25	0.22049	0.50	0.44098	0.44098	50	0.99766	1.00	0.99766	0.99766

argument applies to $q_{(6)}$, $q_{(5)}$ and $q_{(4)}$. Only when we reach $p_{(3)}$ do we find that $\dfrac{P_{(3)}}{3/50} = 0.01383$, and this is smaller than $q_{(8)}$, and hence becomes $q_{(3)}$.

3.3 Distinctive Plotting Symbols for Plotting of BH-FDR Values

So far, all the *p*-values presented on a Q–Q plot have been represented by the same symbol. However, this need not be the case, and when the points in Figure 3.1 are re-plotted, colour-coded according to their associated FDR, namely, $q_{(i)}$, the Q–Q plot acquires further power as a tool for the interpretation of significance tests (Figure 3.2). In this dataset, the values of $-\log_{10}(p)$, ranked in ascending order (corresponding to *p*-values ranked in descending order), diverge rapidly and consistently upwards from the H_0 line, so that smaller *p*-values are associated with a smaller FDR, with a few exceptions like those noted in Section 3.2. This can be indicated clearly by plotting them in different colours, for example, using a palette from blue for large FDR values, through white, to red for small FDR values. Provided that strong colours are used at the two ends of the palette, and pale colours at the middle, this palette will remain informative even if the plot must be presented in monochrome (as in the printed version of this book), because intermediate FDR values represented by pale colours will always occupy intermediate positions on the plot.

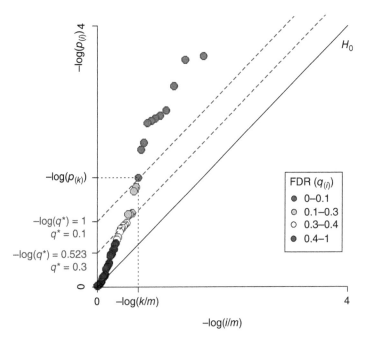

Figure 3.2 Q–Q plot on the $-\log_{10}$ scale, with different plotting symbols used to distinguish between low and high BH-FDR values for the hypotheses tested.

The meaning of the colour coding is further illustrated by marking alternative q^* boundaries on the plot. If the relatively stringent value $q^* = 0.1$ is specified (a BH-FDR boundary commonly used in practice), 11 of the 50 p-values will be declared significant, and these are readily identified by their deep-red (or dark grey) plotting symbol. On this basis, $k/m = 11/50 = 0.22$ and $p_{(k)} = p_{(11)} = 0.02138$. The coordinates of this significance-threshold point are marked on the plot. The p-values for points coloured light red (or light grey) will be declared significant only if the BH-FDR boundary is relaxed to $q^* = 0.3$. The p-values declared significant when $q^* = 0.1$ are also within the larger subset identified when $q^* = 0.3$, and are again declared significant.

3.4 Non-Monotonicity of the BH-FDR: Detection of Correlation Among p-Values from the $-\log_{10}$-Transformed Q–Q Plot

It may seem intuitive that smaller p-values should be associated with smaller FDRs, but we have already seen that this is not necessarily the case: in the present dataset $p_{(4)}...p_{(8)}$ are in increasing order by definition (assuming that the p-values are sampled from a continuum and there are no true ties), whereas $q_{(4)}...q_{(8)}$ all have the same value. Such not-strictly-monotonic relationships can have much more striking effects than the short runs of identical $q_{(i)}$ values in the present dataset. Such effects typically occur when the assumption of independence between the tests, in the cases in which H_0 is true, is not satisfied, and there are positive correlations between the p-values for different tests. The consequence is a deficiency of extreme p-values close to 0 or 1, relative to the Uniform(0, 1) distribution, as was shown in Chapter 2, Section 2.8. Therefore, a simple way to simulate p-values from such a scenario is to produce m test statistics from the non-standard normal distribution

$$Z \sim N(\mu, \sigma), \tag{3.3}$$

where $\mu = 0$ when H_0 is true, $\mu = \mu_1 > 0$ when H_1 is true, and, importantly, $\sigma < 1$ in all cases. The p-value from a one-sided Z-test is then obtained for each test statistic. The next set of results to be explored graphically here has been obtained in this way.

The results comprise $m = 100$ p-values, only $m_0 = 10$ of which come from tests in which H_0 is true. The test statistics are sampled from Distribution (3.3), with $\mu_1 = 1.1$ and $\sigma = 0.7$. The Q–Q plot of the $-\log_{10}$-transformed p-values is presented in Figure 3.3. If $q^* = 0.3$ is specified for this dataset, then $p_{(k)} = p_{(34)} = 0.10011$ and a proportion $k/m = 34/100 = 0.34$ of the tests are declared significant. All p-values to the right of $p_{(34)}$ are declared significant *conditional on the specified value of* q^*, *whether or not they are above the BH-FDR line*. This is due to the 'step-down' nature of the BH procedure. The sequence of p-values smaller than the significance threshold $p_{(34)} = 0.10011$ curves back towards the H_0 line, so none of them achieves a lower FDR – and this is indicated by their light-red (or light-grey) plotting symbol. A slightly lower choice for the BH-FDR, $q^* = 0.295$, is the minimum attainable in this dataset: if a lower value of q^* is specified, none of the p-values is declared significant. Contrary to the pattern seen in the previous dataset (Figure 3.2), specification of

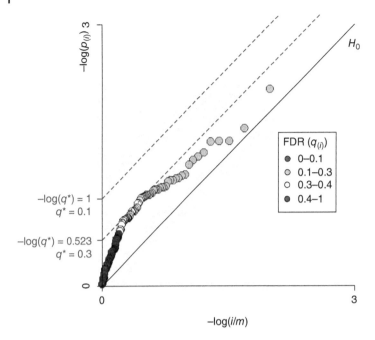

Figure 3.3 Q–Q plot on the $-\log_{10}$ scale, for a set of tests with positive correlations between the p-values, and H_1 true for most tests ($m_0 = 0.1m$).

a more stringent significance threshold will not result in greater confidence that the 'discoveries' announced are true-positives. This representation of the p-values on the negative-logarithmic scale, color-coded by the corresponding values of $q_{(i)}$, makes clear the relationship between the p-values declared significant and the full set – and one important message that this representation conveys is that the BH-FDR criterion, q^*, identifies a *set* of p-values, and is not a property of any individual value.

Another important message is that the BH-FDR criterion (and any other discovery criterion based on p-values) may seriously overestimate the false discovery rate. In the present case, based on simulated data, we know that even if we set the significance threshold at $\alpha = 1$ and announced *all* the significance-test results as discoveries, the expected FDR would only be $m_0/m = 0.1$. Many real-world situations are like this: it is quite likely that H_0 is false, and real effects are present, for a large majority of the m hypotheses tested, but in most cases these effects are too small to be reliably detected by any conventional level of the significance threshold α (Figure 3.3).

In the next example, $m = 100$ and $m_0 = 100$: that is, H_0 is true in every case. Once again, there are positive correlations between the p-values: in this case, $\sigma = 0.9$. The Q–Q plot on the $-\log_{10}$ scale (Figure 3.4) shows that all the points lie *below* the H_0 line: all the p-values are even larger than one would expect on H_0, conditional on their rank. Therefore, there is no significance threshold that will result in an FDR less than one (100%): indeed, such data suggest that the FDR would be *more* than 100%, if such a thing were possible. The positive correlation between the p-values reduces the number of extreme p-values close to zero, and there are no cases in which H_1 is true, to compensate for this effect.

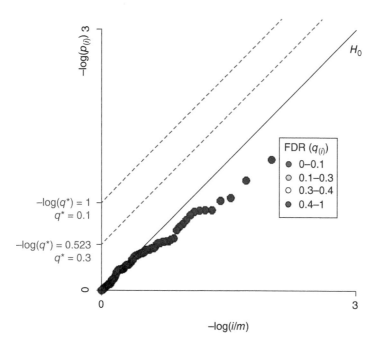

Figure 3.4 Q–Q plot on the $-\log_{10}$ scale, for a set of tests with positive correlations between the p-values, and H_0 true for all tests.

3.5 Summary

The Q–Q plot of a set of p-values, introduced in Chapter 2, is transformed to the $-\log_{10}(p)$ scale. The relationship between features of this plot and the corresponding features of the untransformed plot is explored.

In particular, the p-values of greatest interest, the smallest ones, which were bunched together near the origin in the untransformed plot, are now spread out in the upper-right-hand region, more convenient for inspection and interpretation.

The H_0 line still has unit slope and passes through the origin, and the level q^* at which the FDR is controlled is still represented by the relationship between this line and another line. In the untransformed plot, it is represented by the slope of the line given by Equation (3.1), which is q^*. In the $-\log_{10}$-transformed plot, it is represented by the intercept of the line given by Equation (3.2), which is $-\log_{10}(q^*)$.

Each p-value from a set of hypothesis tests can be associated with a BH-FDR value. To achieve this, for each ordered p-value $p_{(i)}$, we identify $q_{(i)}$, the smallest value of q^* that will cause $p_{(i)}$ to be included among those considered significant.

$q_{(i)}$ is often the value that will cause $p_{(i)}$ to be set as the threshold for significance $p_{(k)}$, but this is not always the case. When the BH step-down procedure is applied, it may be found that the next value of $p_{(i)}$ is not associated with a smaller value of $\dfrac{p_{(i)}}{i/m}$. The value $q_{(i+1)}$ is then also $q_{(i)}$. This argument may apply recursively.

Different plotting symbols (e.g., different colours) can be used for different ranges of values of $q_{(i)}$ on a $-\log_{10}$-transformed Q–Q plot, and the plot then acquires further power as a tool for the interpretation of significance tests.

This can be combined with lines marking alternative q^* boundaries on the plot. For example, the set of p-values that achieves a specified FDR (e.g., $q^* = 0.1$) can be represented by a particular plotting symbol (e.g., a deep-red symbol), and the boundary of this set can be marked on the plot. The set that meets a less stringent criterion (e.g., $q^* = 0.3$) can be represented by a different plotting symbol (e.g., light-red), but this set will also include those meeting the more stringent criterion.

Smaller p-values are not necessarily associated with smaller FDRs: a sequence of ordered p-values may all be associated with the same value of $q_{(i)}$. Such sequences typically occur when the assumption of independence between the tests, in the cases in which H_0 is true, is not satisfied, and there are positive correlations between the p-values for different tests. This situation can be simulated by sampling test statistics Z from Distribution (3.3), specifying that $\sigma < 1$ in all cases. The p-value from a one-sided Z-test is then obtained for each test statistic.

In the resulting $-\log_{10}$-transformed Q–Q plot, it is specified that the FDR is to be controlled at $q^* = 0.3$. The points representing the sequence of p-values smaller than the corresponding significance threshold $p_{(k)}$ then curve back towards the H_0 line, so that none of them achieves a lower FDR – and this is indicated by their all having the same (light-red or light-grey) plotting symbol.

If a value $q^* < 0.295$ is specified, none of the p-values from this dataset are declared significant. Specification of a more stringent significance threshold will not result in greater confidence that the 'discoveries' announced are true-positives.

This representation of p-values and $q_{(i)}$-values makes it clear that the BH-FDR criterion, q^*, identifies a *set* of p-values, and is not a property of any individual value.

The BH-FDR criterion (and any other discovery criterion based on p-values) may seriously overestimate the false discovery rate. In many real-world situations, real effects may be present for a large majority of the m hypotheses tested, but these effects may mostly be too small to be reliably detected by any conventional level of the significance threshold α.

An example is presented in which H_0 is true in every case, and again, there are positive correlations between the p-values. All points on the resulting $-\log_{10}$-transformed Q–Q plot lie *below* the H_0 line: all the p-values are even larger than one would expect on H_0, conditional on their rank. Therefore, there is no significance threshold that will result in an FDR less than one (100%): indeed, these results suggest that the FDR would be *more* than 100%, if such a thing were possible.

Reference

R Core Team (2021). *R: A Language and Environment for Statistical Computing*. Vienna, Austria: R Foundation for Statistical Computing. https://www.R-project.org/.

4

Application of the FDR to Multiple Hypothesis Testing in Real-World Data

4.1 Collation of Gene-Expression Data from the Plant-Genetics Model Organism *Arabidopsis thaliana*

The concepts introduced so far will now be illustrated in the context of a dataset reported by Chan et al. (2011) and made publicly available *via* the Gene Expression Omnibus (GEO) database (Edgar et al. 2002; Barrett et al. 2013; https://www.ncbi.nlm.nih.gov/geo/, accessed 16 April 2024). At the time of writing, this illustrative dataset can be retrieved from GEO by the following steps:

- Choose the tool 'Search for Gene Expression at GEO Profiles'.
- Within the 'GEO Profiles' page, choose the tool 'DataSet Browser'.
- Within the 'DataSet Browser' page, search for the unique identifier 'GDS3927'.
- Follow the link to Reference Series 'GSE16765'.
- Follow the links to 12 individual samples within this series.
- Follow the link to 'View full table...' for each sample.
- Cut and paste the values from each table into a text file.

DataSet Record GDS3927, displayed in the 'DataSet Browser' page, provides the following background information on these data tables:

Title: Salt stress effect on multiple genotypes: leaf
Summary: Analysis of leaf from salt-stressed plants with genotypes Wassilewskija (Ws), Columbia (Col) and single gene mutation (glabrous, gl1-1) in the Col background. Ws plants had the least salt injury. Results provide insight into molecular mechanisms underlying variation in salt stress responses.

The tables comprise data from three genotypes of *Arabidopsis thaliana* grown in two environmental conditions, each combination in two replications, giving $3 \times 2 \times 2 = 12$ gene expression profiles. *A. thaliana* is a small herbaceous plant with a short life cycle, amenable to self-fertilisation, controlled hybridisation and other forms of genetic manipulation, and has therefore become a favourite model organism for research in plant genetics and genomics. Treatment details of the 12 samples are presented in Table 4.1. The genotypes Ws and

The False Discovery Rate: Its Meaning, Interpretation and Application in Data Science, First Edition.
N.W. Galwey.

Table 4.1 Details of 12 samples of *Arabidopsis thaliana* used in a gene expression study.

Sample	Genotype/variation	Stress	Title
	Factors		
GSM420232	Ws	Untreated	Ws_leaf_0mM NaCl_rep1
GSM420233	Ws	Untreated	Ws_leaf_0mM NaCl_rep2
GSM420234	Ws	NaCl	Ws_leaf_100mM NaCl_rep1
GSM420235	Ws	NaCl	Ws_leaf_100mM NaCl_rep2
GSM420236	Col	Untreated	Col_leaf_0mM NaCl_rep1
GSM420237	Col	Untreated	Col_leaf_0mM NaCl_rep2
GSM420238	Col	NaCl	Col_leaf_100mM NaCl_rep1
GSM420239	Col	NaCl	Col_leaf_100mM NaCl_rep2
GSM420240	Col(gl)	Untreated	Col(gl)_leaf_0mM NaCl_rep1
GSM420241	Col(gl)	Untreated	Col(gl)_leaf_0mM NaCl_rep2
GSM420242	Col(gl)	NaCl	Col(gl)_leaf_100mM NaCl_rep1
GSM420243	Col(gl)	NaCl	Col(gl)_leaf_100mM NaCl_rep2

Col are wild-type (WT) lines, and the third genotype, Col(gl), is a mutant obtained from Col as described in the above-mentioned summary. The genotype Col will later be referred to as Col(WT) to distinguish it from this mutant genotype. The two environmental conditions were salt-stressed (NaCl) and unstressed (untreated). The factor 'genotype/variation' will later be referred to simply as 'genotype', for conciseness and because the special character '/' causes problems when used in object names in the R programming language.

The gene expression pattern in each sample was determined by hybridising cRNA extracted from the *A. thaliana* tissue sample with the 'Affymetrix Arabidopsis ATH1 Genome Array' [ATH1-121501]. This microarray includes 22,810 oligonucleotide 'probe-sets', each probeset being a set of short DNA sequences (probes) chosen to record expression of the same specific gene. Information on the gene with which each probeset is associated was obtained *via* the web server DAVID, which provides functional annotation tools for genomics research (Huang et al. 2009; Sherman et al. 2022; https://david.ncifcrf.gov/tools.jsp, accessed 16 April 2024). The first few rows of the probeset 'Name' table returned by DAVID are as shown in Table 4.2.

The first few rows of the normalised gene expression data obtained from GEO for sample GSM420232 (the sample described in the first row of Table 4.1) are shown in Table 4.3. The column headed 'Value' lists the expression level of the corresponding gene in the sample. Note that the probeset IDs are not in the same order in Tables 4.2 and 4.3, so the two tables must be collated: that is, each row of the gene-annotation table must be paired with the appropriate row of the expression-data table using the unique probeset identifiers.

When the expression data from the 12 samples are combined in one dataset, the first few rows of the resulting gene-expression dataset are as shown in Table 4.4. Each of the 12 samples corresponds to one column in this table. Hence, each row of expression values in this dataset can be subjected to a statistical analysis, testing one or more null hypotheses relating

Table 4.2   First rows of information on gene 'names' associated with probesets on Affymetrix array ATH1-121501.

AFFYMETRIX_3PRIME_IVT_ID (Probeset ID)	Name	Species
266603_at	ARID/BRIGHT AND ELM2 DNA-binding domain-containing protein(AT2G46040)	*Arabidopsis thaliana*
266602_at	Pentatricopeptide repeat (PPR-like) superfamily protein (AT2G46050)	*Arabidopsis thaliana*
266601_at	transmembrane protein-like protein (AT2G46060)	*Arabidopsis thaliana*
266600_at	mitogen-activated protein kinase 12 (MPK12)	*Arabidopsis thaliana*
266926_at	LDL receptor wingless signaling/trafficking chaperone (AT2G46000)	*Arabidopsis thaliana*
⋮		⋮

Table 4.3   First rows of gene expression data for sample GSM420232.

ID_REF (Probeset ID)	Value
244901_at	5.163424
244902_at	5.250736
244903_at	6.455655
244904_at	5.51682
244905_at	4.163055
⋮	⋮

to differences in the expression of the gene associated with the corresponding probeset in the different genotypes and environmental conditions.

Quality control and normalisation of gene expression data are generally completed using all available data, to take account of the observed variation across the whole of the micro-array, and the gene expression values presented here have already been normalised on this basis, so comparisons between samples for a given probeset will compare like with like. Null hypotheses concerning differential gene expression are also generally tested for all probesets on an array. However, to produce a manageable example, and a coherent set of hypotheses to which to apply the BH-FDR criterion, we can confine attention to a limited set of probesets, for which the 'Name' text indicates that the corresponding gene may affect the plant's response to NaCl (sodium chloride, common salt).

Table 4.4 First rows of the combined gene-expression data from the 12 samples of *A. thaliana*.

ID_REF	GSM420232	GSM420233	GSM420234	GSM420235	GSM420236	GSM420237	GSM420238	...
244901_at	5.163424	4.973995	4.587746	5.364583	4.772528	4.770687	4.047456	
244902_at	5.250736	4.9395	4.897091	5.68938	4.963313	4.632684	4.365484	
244903_at	6.455655	6.691439	5.629086	6.903891	6.322043	5.985387	5.693574	...
...								...

	...	GSM420239	GSM420240	GSM420241	GSM420242	GSM420243
		5.37732	4.804126	4.89806	5.017702	5.331564
		5.653987	4.839977	4.428501	5.254513	5.190689
	...	6.674524	6.233372	6.125815	6.505519	6.997801
						...

Table 4.5 First rows of information on probesets on Affymetrix array ATH1-121501 with names that contain character strings potentially related to response to salt.

AFFYMETRIX_3PRIME_IVT_ID	Name	Species
259081_at	sodium hydrogen exchanger 2(NHX2)	*Arabidopsis thaliana*
258735_at	Low-temperature and salt-responsive protein family (RCI2A)	*Arabidopsis thaliana*
258751_at	Low-temperature and salt-responsive protein family (RCI2B)	*Arabidopsis thaliana*
258907_at	sodium hydrogen exchanger 4 (NHX4)	*Arabidopsis thaliana*
258959_at	cationic amino acid transporter 7 (CAT7)	*Arabidopsis thaliana*
257662_at	cation exchanger 2 (CAX2)	*Arabidopsis thaliana*
⋮		⋮

To identify such probesets, we use the R function `grep()` to find 'Name' texts that contain any of the following character strings: 'salt', 'sodium', 'chloride', '^cation', ' cation' and/or 'anion'. The character '^' in a `grep()` string indicates that the string must come at the beginning of the line. Thus, specifying the strings '^cation' and ' cation', rather than 'cation', ensures that words like 'translocation' and 'detoxification' will not be returned as correct matches. There are 83 probeset names that contain one or more of these character strings, and the first few rows of the matching subset of the probeset 'Name' table are presented in Table 4.5. The corresponding rows of the gene-expression dataset are presented in Table 4.6.

4.2 Hypotheses Concerning Multiple Response Variables in the Analysis of a Balanced Experimental Design

For an introduction to the statistical analysis of balanced experimental designs such as that specified in the 'sample details' dataset, see, for example, Mead (1988, Chapters 3 and 4). A typical process, applied to the row of expression values for probeset 259081_at, is as follows. A table of means for the six genotype.stress combinations, with margins holding the overall means for each genotype and each stress level, and the grand mean, is obtained, and is presented in Table 4.7. An analysis of variance (anova) is performed to determine whether there are significant differences between the means for the six genotype.stress combinations, and gives the results shown in Table 4.8. That is, the null hypothesis that the true mean is the same for all genotype.stress combinations can be rejected at the significance level $p = 0.01049$.

When the corresponding p-value is obtained for all 83 probesets in the specified subset (which will here be loosely referred to as identifying 'salt-related genes'), they give the histogram presented in Figure 4.1. There is a large excess of p-values close to zero, relative to

Table 4.6 First rows of gene expression data from the 12 samples of *A. thaliana*, for probesets potentially related to response to salt.

ID_REF	GSM420232	GSM420233	GSM420234	GSM420235	GSM420236	GSM420237	GSM420238	...
259081_at	9.322727	9.35052	7.785384	9.030625	9.133842	9.189921	7.104237	
258735_at	8.846864	8.84854	11.146963	11.156304	10.36918	10.432625	12.095383	
258751_at	4.533911	4.008014	6.027713	6.017422	4.682446	4.940537	6.841039	
258907_at	5.77133	5.501366	4.968255	5.496353	5.417722	5.682063	5.080149	
258959_at	5.292391	5.255642	4.54796	4.525304	4.814288	4.780494	4.337468	
257662_at	7.941314	7.855778	7.784695	7.894857	7.265053	7.798374	7.938075	...
...								...

...	GSM420239	GSM420240	GSM420241	GSM420242	GSM420243
	7.984277	7.282263	7.335651	7.418055	7.051764
	12.100559	12.289012	12.376067	12.47245	12.361743
	6.3785	4.572177	4.723533	4.747185	4.25245
	5.121928	5.071933	5.403335	5.293722	5.304764
	4.289223	5.127065	5.119845	4.956516	4.605176
...	7.74843	7.839388	7.933743	7.784643	7.499084
...					...

Table 4.7 Mean expression levels for probeset 259081_at in genotype. stress combinations.

Genotype	Stress		Mean
	Untreated	NaCl	
Ws	9.34	8.41	8.87
Col(WT)	9.16	7.54	8.35
Col(gl)	7.31	7.23	7.27
Mean	8.60	7.73	8.17

Table 4.8 Anova of expression level for probeset 259081_at in the 12 samples of *A. thaliana*, without partitioning of the 'genotype.stress combination' term.

Source of variation	Degrees of freedom (DF)	Sum of squares (SS)	Mean square (MS)	F	p
Genotype.stress combination	5	8.8174	1.76348	8.5814	0.01049
Residual	6	1.233	0.2055		

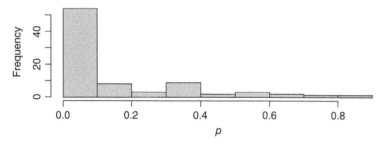

Figure 4.1 Histogram of *p*-values for differences between genotype.stress combinations in salt-related genes.

the uniform distribution expected on H_0, indicating that real differences in gene expression between the genotype.stress combinations are almost certainly present for some of the genes in the subset. The corresponding Q–Q plot, on the $-\log_{10}$ scale, is presented in Figure 4.2. Nearly all the points lie well above the H_0 line, confirming that the *p*-values are generally much smaller than is expected on the basis of their rank order on H_0. If it is specified that the FDR is to be controlled at $q^* = 0.1$, the corresponding significance threshold is $\alpha = 0.06136$, and gene expression is announced to be significantly associated with genotype.stress combinations for 52 of the 83 probesets, that is, $100 \times 52/83 = 63\%$ of the probesets.

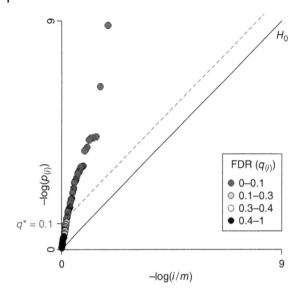

Figure 4.2 Q–Q plot, on the $-\log_{10}$ scale, of p-values for differences between genotype.stress combinations in salt-related genes.

4.3 Partitioning of Model Terms in a Balanced Experimental Design: Hypotheses Concerning Individual Terms

Having established that not all genotype.stress combinations have the same effect on gene expression, we can go on to explore where the differences between them lie. This is done by partitioning the 'global' model term 'genotype.stress combination' in the anova table into terms for the main effect of genotype, the main effect of stress and the genotype.stress interaction, as shown in Table 4.9. Note that the degrees of freedom (DF) and sum of squares (SS) values for these three terms sum to the corresponding values for the 'genotype.stress combination' term in Table 4.8:

- $2 + 1 + 2 = 5.$
- $5.3329 + 2.2886 + 1.1959 = 8.8174.$

Table 4.9 Anova of expression level for probeset 259081_at in the 12 samples of *A. thaliana*, with partitioning of the 'genotype.stress combination' term into main effects and interaction.

Source of variation	Degrees of freedom (DF)	Sum of squares (SS)	Mean square (MS)	F	p
Genotype	2	5.3329	2.66646	12.9753	0.006622
Stress	1	2.2886	2.28864	11.1368	0.015666
Genotype.stress interaction	2	1.1959	0.59794	2.9097	0.130821
Residual	6	1.233	0.2055		

That is, the variation has been partitioned between these terms. Each model term has an associated *p*-value, indicating whether the corresponding part of the variation in expression among genotype.stress combinations is larger than would be expected by chance.

When this partitioning of the model into three terms is performed for each of the 83 probesets, three sets of 83 *p*-values are obtained. In the histogram of the *p*-values for the main effect of stress (Figure 4.3), there is once again a strong concentration of values close to zero, and the points in the corresponding Q–Q plot (Figure 4.4) lie well above the H_0 line. Clearly, the expression level of salt-related genes is not the same between the 'NaCl' and 'untreated' samples. However, similar patterns are obtained from the set of 83 *p*-values for the main effect of genotype, and also from the set for the genotype.stress interaction (results not shown). This indicates that the differences in the tables of genotype.stress combination means are not fully accounted for by differences confined to either the 'genotype' or the 'stress' margin of the table.

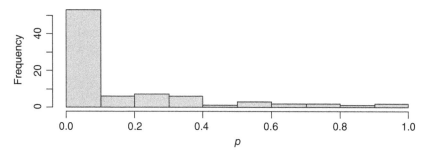

Figure 4.3 Histogram of *p*-values for the main effect of stress in salt-related genes.

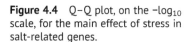

Figure 4.4 Q–Q plot, on the $-\log_{10}$ scale, for the main effect of stress in salt-related genes.

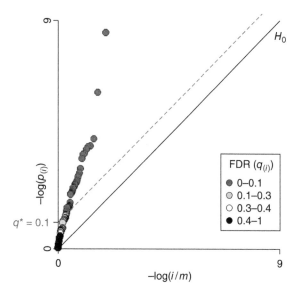

The pattern of differences among the genotype.stress means can be explored further, by further partitioning of the variation accounted for by the model into 'contrasts' that specify more detailed comparisons between particular means. This is done by applying an appropriate set of coefficients to the combinations. Two contrasts that are worth examining to see if they give distinctive patterns of p-values are:

- NaCl versus untreated in the Col(WT) genotype.
- NaCl versus untreated in the Col(gl) genotype.

Together, these contrasts effectively ask the question, 'Does the presence of the (gl) mutation affect the pattern of gene expression produced in response to salt stress?' The appropriate contrast coefficients for specifying each of these comparisons are as shown in Table 4.10.

A two-sided significance test for each of these contrasts is performed using a t statistic: that is, a large value of t, positive or negative, is considered significant. However, these contrasts are not quite the same thing as simple t-tests to compare the two genotype.stress combinations in question. Each contrast is based not just on the variation between replicate samples for those two combinations, but on the 'Residual' MS from the anova table, which is a pooled estimate based on all six combinations, and hence gives a more powerful significance test.

Two more sets of 83 p-values for the salt-related genes are now obtained, one set for each contrast. The histogram and Q–Q plot for the 'NaCl versus untreated in Col (WT)' comparison are presented in Figures 4.5 and 4.6, respectively, and those for the 'NaCl versus untreated in Col(gl)' comparison in Figures 4.7 and 4.8. The histogram and Q–Q plot for 'NaCl versus untreated in Col(WT)' are similar to those obtained for the other sets of p-values considered, but those for 'NaCl versus untreated in Col(gl)' are clearly different. Though there is still a bias in the histogram towards small values of p, these are not concentrated close to zero as in the previous histograms, and the pattern of points in the Q–Q plot does not depart strongly and consistently upwards from the H_0 line. None of the p-values is associated with an FDR below $q^* = 0.1$, and only a few with $q^* < 0.3$. Comparison of the two histograms and the two Q–Q plots indicates that the effect of NaCl stress on the expression of genes in this subset is consistently reduced by the presence of the 'gl' mutation.

Table 4.10 Contrast coefficients to specify comparison of NaCl versus untreated stress levels in the Col(WT) and Col(gl) genotypes.

	Genotype.stress combination					
Comparison	Ws untreated	Ws NaCl	Col(WT) untreated	Col(WT) NaCl	Col(gl) untreated	Col(gl) NaCl
NaCl versus untreated in Col(WT)	0	0	−1	+1	0	0
NaCl versus untreated in Col(gl)	0	0	0	0	−1	+1

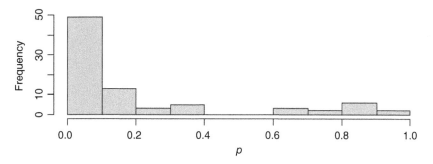

Figure 4.5 Histogram of *p*-values for the NaCl versus untreated contrast in genotype Col(WT), in salt-related genes.

Figure 4.6 Q–Q plot, on the $-\log_{10}$ scale, for the NaCl versus untreated contrast in genotype Col(WT), in salt-related genes.

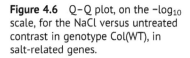

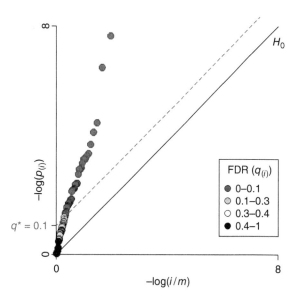

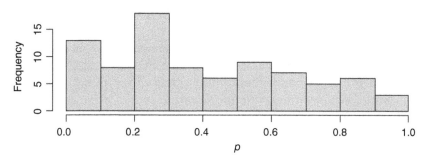

Figure 4.7 Histogram of *p*-values for the NaCl versus untreated contrast in genotype Col(gl), in salt-related genes.

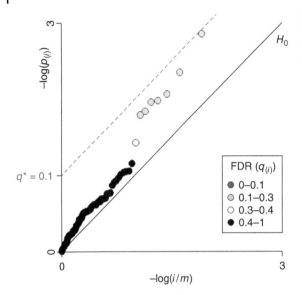

Figure 4.8 Q–Q plot, on the $-\log_{10}$ scale, for the NaCl versus untreated contrast in genotype Col(gl), in salt-related genes.

4.4 Comparison of the Results of Multiple Testing for Contrasting Subsets of Response Variables

It must not be assumed that this pattern of effects of genotype, stress, genotype.stress inter-action and the two contrasts on gene expression is seen because we have chosen a subset of genes with functions potentially related to salt stress: the same pattern might be seen in any or all of the probesets on the array. To explore this possibility, we can turn our attention to another subset of genes, those related to ubiquitin, which is:

> ...an evolutionarily conserved protein found in nearly all eukaryotic organisms. It is highly conserved and virtually identical across all life forms, whether human, yeast, or plant... Ubiquitination (also known as ubiquitylation) is a form of post-translation modification (PTM) in which ubiquitin is attached to a target protein. (according to Hui Jun Guo, Nader Rahimi and Prasanna Tadi in the US National Library of Medicine: https://www.ncbi.nlm.nih.gov/books/NBK556052/, accessed 16 April 2024)

To find the expression values of genes related to the synthesis or function of ubiquitin, we search for probesets for which the 'Name' text contains the character string 'ubiquitin'. There are 196 probeset names that contain this string, and the first few rows of the matching subset of the probeset 'Name' table are shown in Table 4.11.

The histograms of the p-values and the corresponding Q–Q plots for the unpartitioned model, the main effects of genotype and stress and the genotype.stress interaction are fairly similar to those for the 'salt-related' subset, but with one distinctive feature, which is most clearly evident in the main effect of stress (corresponding results for genotype and genotype. stress not shown). As in the case of the 'salt-related' genes, the histogram (Figure 4.9) shows a large excess of p-values close to zero, and the Q–Q plot (Figure 4.10) shows numerous

Table 4.11 First rows of information on probesets on Affymetrix array ATH1-121501 with names that contain the character string 'ubiquitin'.

AFFYMETRIX_3PRIME_IVT_ID	Name	Species
266604_at	ubiquitin-conjugating enzyme 6 (UBC6)	*Arabidopsis thaliana*
266768_s_at	ubiquitin 6 (UBQ6)	*Arabidopsis thaliana*
258574_at	F-box associated ubiquitination effector family protein (AT3G04250)	*Arabidopsis thaliana*
256393_at	F-box associated ubiquitination effector family protein (AT3G06280)	*Arabidopsis thaliana*
258520_at	E3 ubiquitin ligase (AT3G06710)	*Arabidopsis thaliana*
259243_at	histone H2A deubiquitinase (DUF3755) (AT3G07565)	*Arabidopsis thaliana*
⋮		⋮

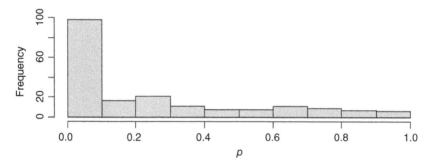

Figure 4.9 Histogram of *p*-values for the main effect of stress in ubiquitin-related genes.

Figure 4.10 Q–Q plot, on the $-\log_{10}$ scale, of *p*-values for main effect of stress in ubiquitin-related genes.

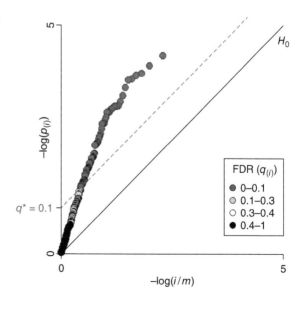

probesets with the FDR controlled at $q^* = 0.1$. But the pattern of points also shows a clear curvature back towards the H_0 line at large values of $-\log_{10}(p)$. That is, the smallest p-values, though smaller than would be expected by chance alone if H_0 were true for all probesets, are not as small as might be expected on the basis of the distribution of the larger p-values (i.e., smaller values of $-\log_{10}(p)$). This suggests that there are positive correlations among the expression values of the probesets, which would be present even if all the samples were of the same genotype at the same stress level, and hence that the effective number of tests is less than the nominal value of $m = 196$.

The histogram and Q–Q plot for the 'NaCl versus untreated in Col(WT)' comparison in the 'ubiquitin-related' genes are presented in Figures 4.11 and 4.12, respectively, and those for the 'NaCl versus untreated in Col (gl)' comparison in Figures 4.13 and 4.14. There is a difference in the patterns of the two Q–Q plots rather similar to that seen in the corresponding plots for the 'salt-related' genes, but not as strong, with a clear concentration of p-values close to zero, corresponding to an FDR controlled at $q^* = 0.3$ or better, for *both* contrasts, not

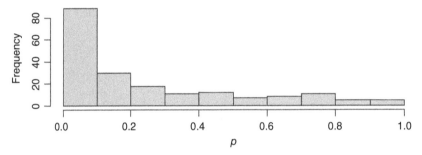

Figure 4.11 Histogram of p-values for the NaCl versus untreated contrast in genotype Col(WT), in ubiquitin-related genes.

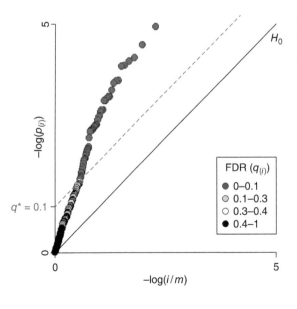

Figure 4.12 Q–Q plot, on the $-\log_{10}$ scale, for the NaCl versus untreated contrast in genotype Col(WT), in ubiquitin-related genes.

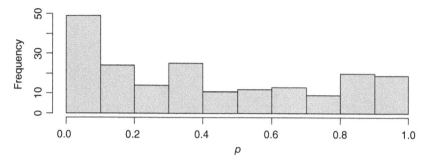

Figure 4.13 Histogram of p-values for the NaCl versus untreated contrast in genotype Col(gl), in ubiquitin-related genes.

Figure 4.14 Q–Q plot, on the $-\log_{10}$ scale, for the NaCl versus untreated contrast in genotype Col(gl), in ubiquitin-related genes.

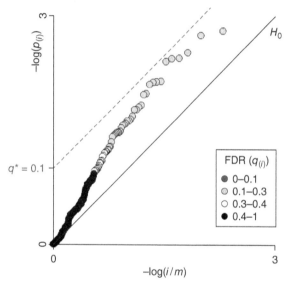

just the contrast in the WT genotype. This suggests that the difference in gene expression pattern caused by the 'gl' mutation may indeed be rather specific to the 'salt-related' genes.

The $-\log_{10}$-transformed p-values for the NaCl versus untreated contrast in genotype Col(gl) are plotted against those in genotype Col(WT), in Figure 4.15a for the salt-related genes and in Figure 4.15b for the ubiquitin-related genes. The plotted points are colour-coded according to the FDR ($q_{(i)}$ value) associated with the Col(WT) p-value (the $q_{(i)}$ values for this genotype are indicated because they cover a wider range and are hence of more interest than those associated with Col(gl)). These plots show that there is very little relationship between the p-values for Col(gl) and those for Col(WT), either among the salt-related genes (correlation between $-\log_{10}(p)$ values: $r = 0.152$) or among the ubiquitin-related genes ($r = 0.142$). Evidently, the 'gl' mutation causes radical changes in the effect of NaCl on gene expression, and these changes are not confined to genes directly related

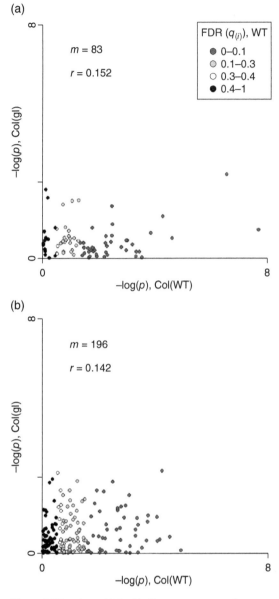

Figure 4.15 $-\log_{10}(p)$ for NaCl versus untreated contrast, in genotype Col(gl) versus genotype Col(WT). (a) Salt-related genes. (b) Ubiquitin-related genes.

to the metabolism of salts. However, the most highly significant effects of NaCl are seen in some of the salt-related genes in the Col(WT) genotype. There are highly significant effects among the ubiquitin-related genes in the Col(WT) genotype also, but inspection of Figures 4.6 and 4.12 shows that the points representing the most extreme salt-related genes not only represent smaller p-values, but also smaller $q_{(i)}$ values (i.e., they lie further from the H_0 line) than the corresponding points for ubiquitin-related genes. One may speculate that there are certain genes with an adaptive response to NaCl stress, and that the expression of this response (which might be either up-regulation or down-regulation of the gene's transcript) is disrupted by the 'gl' mutation.

It is important to note that such disruption is not confined to the gene whose genetic sequence is actually altered by the 'gl' mutation: the weak correlations between $-\log_{10}(p)$ values for Col(gl) and Col(WT) show that this mutation changes the effect of NaCl stress on the expression level of many or most genes, including those involved in basic metabolism. In a more detailed study of these effects of NaCl stress and the 'gl' mutation on gene expression, the next step might be to identify, among both the salt-related and the ubiquitin-related genes, one or more genes of each of the following types:

- Genes that show a large and/or highly significant effect of NaCl stress in Col(WT) only.
- Genes that show a large and/or highly significant effect of NaCl stress in Col(gl) only.
- Genes that show a large and/or highly significant effect of NaCl stress in both Col(WT) and Col(gl).
- Genes that show little effect of NaCl stress in either Col(WT) or Col(gl).

4.5 Representation of the FDR on a Volcano Plot: Selection of Hypotheses for Further Investigation

The use of the phrase 'large and/or highly significant' draws attention to the point that small p-values are not always associated with large effects. Large effects generally give rise to small p-values, but small p-values can also occur simply because the amount of random variation in the data is small. The 'volcano plot' (so called because it resembles an upside-down volcano) is a graphical tool that addresses this issue, and is widely used for presenting results from multiple hypothesis testing (Cui and Churchill 2003). It presents the estimated effect size for each hypothesis tested plotted in the horizontal direction, and the p-value in the vertical direction, transformed to the $-\log_{10}$ scale so that small p-values are not clustered near the origin. This allows the researcher to take both factors into account when selecting hypotheses for further investigation, setting cut-off values for both estimated effect size and p-value, and hence allowing a hypothesis associated with a large effect to be selected even if its p-value is not exceptionally small, and conversely a hypothesis with an exceptionally small p-value to be selected even if the associated effect is not very large.

The FDR values associated with the p-values can also be indicated on a volcano plot, by using different plotting symbols for the points and by indicating the p-values corresponding to selected FDR boundaries ($q_{(i)}$ values), and this is done for the contrasts and gene subsets considered here in Figure 4.16. The FDR boundaries represented by dashed horizontal lines are the $p_{(k)}$ values – the largest p-values considered significant – when the FDR is controlled at the values specified in the legend, namely, 0.4, 0.3 and 0.1. For example, in Figure 4.16b, hypotheses with a $q_{(i)}$ value in the range $0.1 \leq q_{(i)} \leq 0.3$ are represented by a specific symbol (light-red-filled in the colour version of the plot), but the largest p-value lying in this range, $p_{(6)} = 0.01444$, is associated with $q_{(6)} = 0.193$, so the corresponding boundary line is marked with this value. Such a representation will allow a researcher, when selecting a hypothesis for further investigation on the basis of a large effect size, to consider the associated FDR as well as the *p*-value.

A volcano plot can also be produced plotting the −log-transformed FDR (the $q_{(i)}$ value), rather than the unadjusted $p_{(i)}$ value, on the vertical axis (Goedhart and Luijsterburg 2020, Figure 3). Such a plot is presented for the NaCl versus untreated contrast, for salt-related

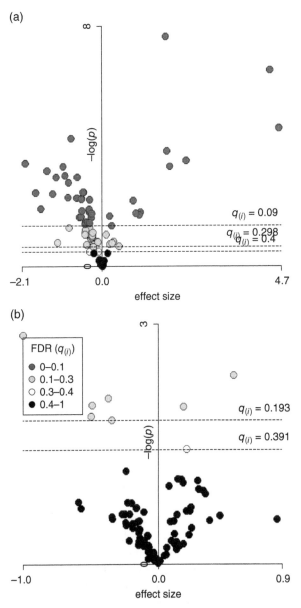

Figure 4.16 Volcano plots for the NaCl versus untreated contrast, for different gene subsets and genotypes, with FDR annotations. (a) Salt-related genes, Col(WT), (b) salt-related genes, Col(gl), (c) ubiquitin-related genes, Col(WT), (d) ubiquitin-related genes, Col(gl).

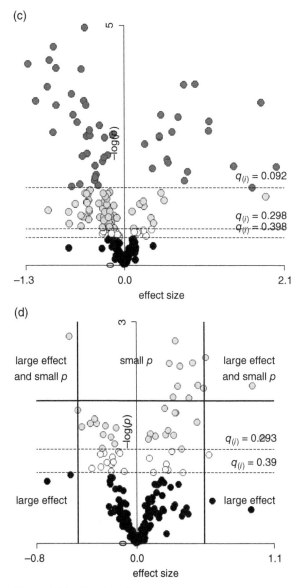

Figure 4.16 (Continued)

genes in genotype Col(gl), in Figure 4.17. Such a plot has some value for the identification of hypotheses of further interest, but it loses information relative to the standard volcano plot, because, as we have seen, sequences of $p_{(i)}$ values may be associated with the same $q_{(i)}$ value: hence, the horizontal arrays of points in the present plot. However, if the positions of points on the volcano plot correspond to unadjusted p-values in the standard manner, and the $q_{(i)}$ values are indicated by plotting symbols and boundary lines as in Figure 4.16, there is no loss of information about the unadjusted p-values, and the FDR information is also clearly displayed.

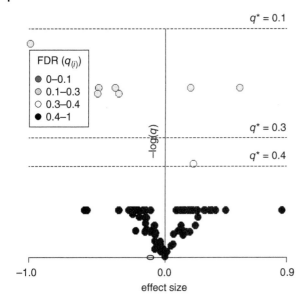

Figure 4.17 Volcano plot for the NaCl versus untreated contrast, for salt-related genes in genotype Col(gl), with $-\log_{10}$-transformed $q_{(i)}$ values, not p-values, on the vertical axis.

The use of the volcano plot to identify hypotheses corresponding to large effects and/or small p-values is illustrated in Figure 4.16d. However, Ebrahimpoor and Goeman (2021) pointed out that if hypotheses are selected simply on this basis, the FDR is not controlled, and they presented methods to take both criteria into account while retaining control of the FDR.

In the present case, when genes for further study have been selected on some combination of effect size, p-value and FDR, further information on their functions could be sought, and they could be submitted to a biochemical pathway analysis such as that offered by MetaCore (MetaCore Login | Clarivate (genego.com), accessed 16 April 2024), to identify the pathways and networks in which their products participate. Probesets on the ATH1-121501 array relating to other genes in these pathways could then be identified, and the corresponding effect sizes and p-values for these probesets examined. In these ways, understanding of the molecular mechanisms in the *Arabidopsis* plant's response to NaCl stress (and by extension that of other plant species) would be advanced.

4.6 Summary

The concepts introduced in previous chapters are illustrated by multiple hypothesis testing in a real-world dataset. The data were obtained from leaf samples of *A. thaliana*, a small herbaceous plant that is a favourite model organism for research in plant genetics and genomics. Three genotypes of *A. thaliana* were grown in two environmental conditions, each combination in two replications, giving $3 \times 2 \times 2 = 12$ samples.

The genotypes were Wassilewskija (Ws), Columbia (Col(WT)) and single gene mutation (glabrous, gl1-1) in the Col genetic background (Col(gl)). The environmental conditions were salt-stressed (NaCl) and unstressed (untreated). In each sample, the expression levels of 22,811 genes were assayed, using a microarray of oligonucleotide 'probesets'.

For each probeset, there was a 'Name' text giving information about the corresponding gene. A subset of probesets was identified for which the 'Name' text included character strings that indicated that the corresponding gene might affect the plant's response to NaCl (sodium chloride, common salt). The specified strings were 'salt', 'sodium', 'chloride', '^cation', ' cation' and 'anion'. There were 83 probesets in this salt-related subset.

An anova was performed on the 12 expression-level values for each probeset in the salt-related subset, to determine whether there were significant differences between the means for the six genotype.stress combinations. H_0: true mean is the same for all combinations. The p-value from this anova was obtained.

The 83 p-values from the salt-related subset are presented in a histogram and in a $-\log_{10}$-transformed Q–Q plot. These plots indicated that there is a large excess of p-values close to zero, associated with low FDR values, relative to the expectation on H_0.

Partitioning of the variation among the genotype.stress combination means, to explore where the differences between them lay, was therefore justified. The variation was partitioned into the following terms:

- Main effect of genotype.
- Main effect of stress.
- Genotype.stress interaction.
- NaCl versus untreated two-sided contrast in Col(WT).
- NaCl versus untreated two-sided contrast in Col(gl).

H_0: true mean is the same for the combinations compared by the term.

The 83 p-values from the salt-related subset were obtained for each partitioned term. A histogram and a $-\log_{10}$-transformed Q–Q plot of the p-values were obtained for each term.

These plots showed a strong concentration of p-values close to zero for the main effect of genotype, the main effect of stress and the genotype.stress interaction. This indicates that the differences in the tables of genotype.stress combination means are not fully accounted for by differences on the 'genotype' or the 'stress' margin.

The histograms and Q–Q plots also showed a strong concentration of p-values close to zero for the NaCl versus untreated contrast in genotype Col(WT), but not in Col(gl).

In order to explore whether the patterns seen here were specific to the salt-related subset of probesets, another subset was identified, related to the protein ubiquitin, which is highly evolutionarily conserved and virtually identical across all life forms. This subset was identified by searching for probesets for which the 'Name' text included the character string 'ubiquitin', and comprised 196 probesets.

The histograms and Q–Q plots obtained for the ubiquitin-related subset were generally similar to those for the salt-related probeset, except that the plots for the NaCl versus untreated contrast in Col(gl) *do* show a clear concentration of p-values close to zero and associated with an FDR below $q^* = 0.3$. This suggests that the difference in gene expression pattern caused by the 'gl' mutation may indeed be rather specific to the 'salt-related' genes.

This possibility was explored further by plotting the $-\log_{10}$-transformed p-values for the NaCl versus untreated contrast in genotype Col(gl) against those in genotype Col(WT), in separate plots for the salt-related genes and the ubiquitin-related genes. The plotted points are colour-coded according to the FDR ($q_{(i)}$ value) associated with the Col(WT) p-value. These plots show that there is very little relationship between the p-values for Col(gl) and those for Col(WT). This indicates that the 'gl' mutation causes radical changes in the effect of NaCl on gene expression, not confined to genes directly related to the metabolism of salts. However, the most highly significant effects of NaCl are seen in some of the salt-related genes in the Col(WT) genotype.

It is speculated that there are certain genes with an adaptive response to NaCl stress, and that the expression of this response is disrupted by the 'gl' mutation. This disruption is not confined to the gene whose genetic sequence is actually altered by the 'gl' mutation: the weak relationship between p-values for Col(gl) and Col(WT) shows that this mutation changes the effect of NaCl stress on the expression level of many or most genes, including those involved in basic metabolism.

Suggestions are made for further exploration of the effects of NaCl stress and the 'gl' mutation on gene expression. Salt-related and ubiquitin-related genes with distinctive patterns of these effects might be identified from the analyses presented here.

A 'volcano plot' can help to identify such genes (i.e., hypotheses for further investigation), allowing small p-values due to large effect sizes to be distinguished from those due to low levels of random variation. A volcano plot can be annotated with information about FDR values, and this is preferable to plotting the $q_{(i)}$ values themselves.

Further information on the functions of genes chosen for further investigation could be sought, and these genes could be submitted to a biochemical pathway analysis. Probesets relating to other genes in the same pathways could then be identified, and their p-values from the present analyses examined. In these ways, understanding of the molecular mechanisms in response to NaCl stress, in *A. thaliana* and other plant species, would be advanced.

References

Barrett, T., Wilhite, S.E., Ledoux, P. et al. (2013). NCBI GEO: archive for functional genomics data sets—update. *Nucleic Acids Research* 41 (Database issue): D991–D995.

Chan, Z., Grumet, R., and Loescher, W. (2011). Global gene expression analysis of transgenic, mannitol-producing, and salt-tolerant *Arabidopsis thaliana* indicates widespread changes in abiotic and biotic stress-related genes. *Journal of Experimental Botany* 62: 4787–4803. PMID: 21821598.

Cui, X. and Churchill, G.A. (2003). Statistical tests for differential expression in cDNA microarray experiments. *Genome Biology* 4: 210. https://doi.org/10.1186/gb-2003-4-4-210. PMCID: 154570. PMID: 12702200.

Ebrahimpoor, M. and Goeman, J.J. (2021). Inflated false discovery rate due to volcano plots: problem and solutions. *Briefings in Bioinformatics* 22 (5): https://doi.org/10.1093/bib/bbab053.

Edgar, R., Domrachev, M., and Lash, A.E. (2002). Gene expression Omnibus: NCBI gene expression and hybridization array data repository. *Nucleic Acids Research* 30 (1): 207–210.

Goedhart, J. and Luijsterburg, M.S. (2020). VolcaNoseR is a web app for creating, exploring, labeling and sharing volcano plots. *Scientific Reports* 10: 20560. https://doi.org/10.1038/s41598-020-76603-3.

Huang, D.W., Sherman, B.T., and Lempicki, R.A. (2009). Systematic and integrative analysis of large gene lists using DAVID bioinformatics resources. *Nature Protocols* 4: 44–57.

Sherman, B.T., Hao, M., Qiu, J. et al. (2022). DAVID: a web server for functional enrichment analysis and functional annotation of gene lists. *Nucleic Acids Research* 50 (W1): W216–W221. https://doi.org/10.1093/nar/gkac194.

5

Alternative Approaches to the Multiple-Testing Problem

5.1 An FDR Is Not a *p*-Value: The Formal Distinction

The FDR is sometimes referred to as a *p*-value adjusted or corrected for multiplicity, but this is misleading. The illustration of the relationship of these two statistics to the confusion matrix (Figure 2.1, Chapter 2) shows that they have a different conceptual basis. A *p*-value is the probability of a false-positive result conditional on *the null hypothesis* (H_0) being *true*, whereas an FDR is the probability of a false-positive result conditional on *the alternative hypothesis* (H_1) being *accepted*. The same distinction can be expressed more informally: a *p*-value is the probability that when there is nothing really going on, you announce a discovery and make a fool of yourself; whereas an FDR is the probability that when you announce a discovery, there is nothing really going on and you make a fool of yourself. (If you ever intend to announce a discovery, you must accept that both risks will exist with finite probability.)

Besides the BH-FDR ($q_{(i)}$), several other functions of a set of *p*-values are widely used to take account of multiplicity. These alternatives, which *can* be viewed as adjusted or corrected *p*-values, will be briefly reviewed here.

5.2 Retaining the *p*-Value Conceptual Basis: The Šidák and Bonferroni 'Corrections'

The basic problem concerning significance-testing of multiple hypotheses is that the more hypotheses are tested, the greater the probability that some of them will give 'significant' *p*-values by chance, even when H_0 is true for all tests. The best-known method for seeking to take account of this is the 'Bonferroni correction' (Bonferroni 1936), which is applied to each *p*-value in turn, and relates to the probability that, by chance alone, at least one of the *p*-values would be less than the *p*-value in question. (The term 'Bonferroni correction' is given in quotation marks in this paragraph because it is potentially misleading. It suggests that there is something 'incorrect' about the original *p*-values, whereas in fact both the 'uncorrected' and the 'corrected' p-value are valid on their own terms. The alternative terminology 'Bonferroni adjustment' and 'Bonferroni-adjusted p-value' is sometimes used.) The Bonferroni correction is often considered as a possible alternative to the FDR in multiple-testing situations, so it is worth considering its conceptual basis in some detail. It is performed as follows. If H_0 is true for all the m tests, the probability that any one test will give a p-value less than or equal to p is, by definition, p. Therefore, the probability that it will give a p-value greater than p is $(1 - p)$. If all the tests are mutually independent, the probability that all of them will give p-values greater than p is $(1 - p)^m$. Therefore, the probability that at least one of them will give a p-value less than p is

$$P_{\text{corrected}} = 1 - (1-p)^m. \tag{5.1}$$

This is the Šidák-corrected p-value (Šidák 1967), a recognised correction in its own right, but also a stepping stone on the way to the Bonferroni correction,

$$P_{\text{corrected}} = mp. \tag{5.2}$$

The final step is to note that for all values of p and m,

$$1 - (1-p)^m \leq mp, \tag{5.3}$$

and that when p is small and m is large,

$$1 - (1-p)^m \approx mp. \tag{5.4}$$

That is:

- the Bonferroni-corrected p-value is always larger than the Šidák-corrected value: thus, the Bonferroni correction is conservative, underestimating the significance of each result, and
- when p is small and m is large, the Bonferroni- and Šidák-corrected p-values are approximately equal.

If the significance tests are not mutually independent and there are positive correlations between the p-values, then the probability of obtaining a smaller p-value by chance is less than that given by Equation (5.1), and both the Šidák and the Bonferroni correction are conservative.

As an alternative to 'correcting' the p-value, one can keep the original p-value but 'correct' the significance threshold from α to α/m. Formal definitions of the Bonferroni correction are usually presented in terms of this change to the significance threshold rather than a change to the p-value, but statistical software (e.g., the function p.adjust() in R (R Core Team 2021)) offers the user Bonferroni-adjusted p-values.

When a 'family' of m significance tests is considered jointly in this way, the probability that at least one of them will give a significant result, even when H_0 is true for every hypothesis tested, is called the *family-wise error rate* (FWER). A procedure such as the Bonferroni or Šidák correction that ensures that the FWER will be below a specified significance threshold α is said to *control the FWER* at level α.

5.3 Multiple Testing of Pairwise Comparisons Among Groups of Samples

When the Šidák or Bonferroni correction is applied, the p-values entered into this procedure have typically been obtained from separate statistical analyses – for example, each of a set of Y-variates considered in turn in a univariate regression analysis with the same X-variate, as discussed in Chapter 2, Section 2.8. However, a single, more elaborate analysis can give rise to more than one null hypothesis, and there is then a case for making corrections for multiplicity within such an analysis. The methods that have been devised for doing so will be reviewed here in the context of a one-way analysis of variance (anova), which compares the means of several groups of observations, typically obtained from different experimental treatments, $\text{Trt}_1...\text{Trt}_k$, where k is the number of groups, or from different levels of some other type of categorical variable, such as crop varieties (Fisher 1925, republished 1990, Section 48, Technique of plot experimentation). The one-way anova produces an F statistic that tests the global null hypothesis ($H_{0,\text{global}}$) that the true mean value of the response variable is the same for all groups (i.e., $\mu_1 = \mu_2 = ... = \mu_k = \mu$, where μ_j is the true mean response to Trt_j): that is, the differences between the observed group means arise only from random variation among the observations within each group. However, it is often also of interest to make pairwise comparisons between the group means, with the null hypothesis that there is no difference between the true means for the two groups under consideration. A single comparison of this kind closely resembles an independent-samples t test, and indeed is performed using the t statistic, but it differs from the standard t test in that, although only two of the means are being compared, the estimate of residual variance and the degrees of freedom of the t statistic are obtained using information from all the groups. For a fuller account of these methods, see, for example, Moore and McCabe (1999, Chapter 12, One-way analysis of variance, pp. 743–797).

For example, suppose that a study to compare six experimental treatments, Trt_1 to Trt_6, each applied to $n = 5$ experimental units in a fully randomised design, has given the results shown in Table 5.1, and hence the treatment-mean values presented in Table 5.2.

The population variance between observations on the same treatment is assumed to be the same for all treatments, and the estimate of this residual variance from Trt_j is

$$s_j^2 = \frac{\sum\limits_{i=1}^{n}\left(y_{ij} - \overline{T_j}\right)^2}{n-1}, \tag{5.5}$$

where

y_{ij} = the response value of the ith unit receiving treatment Trt_j,
$\overline{T_j}$ = the mean of the response values in treatment Trt_j,

and

n = the number of units receiving each treatment = 5.

For example, the estimate of the residual variance from Trt_1 is

$$s_1^2 = \frac{(10.53 - 15.504)^2 + \cdots + (14.96 - 15.504)^2}{5-1} = 10.33.$$

Table 5.1 Individual-unit data from an experiment with six treatment groups.

Trt$_1$		Trt$_2$		Trt$_3$	
Unit ID	y	Unit ID	y	Unit ID	y
5	10.53	24	23.99	7	21.39
30	15.58	22	33.09	28	14.88
19	19.08	25	28.78	13	23.26
3	17.37	26	25.10	27	22.77
21	14.96	11	24.34	1	20.29

Trt$_4$		Trt$_5$		Trt$_6$	
Unit ID	y	Unit ID	y	Unit ID	y
15	13.47	9	26.45	6	23.09
2	18.67	17	26.82	20	11.44
14	13.65	12	25.72	8	14.28
29	10.36	10	26.22	23	17.61
16	9.43	4	22.40	18	24.67

Table 5.2 Group means from the experiment with six treatment groups.

	Treatment					
	Trt$_1$	Trt$_2$	Trt$_3$	Trt$_4$	Trt$_5$	Trt$_6$
Mean response	15.504	27.060	20.518	13.116	25.522	18.218

Provided that n is the same for every treatment, the pooled estimate of the residual variance is then

$$s^2 = MS_{\text{Resid}} = \frac{\sum_{j=1}^{k} s_j^2}{k} = \frac{10.33 + 15.00 + 11.30 + 13.11 + 3.20 + 31.80}{6} = 14.122,$$

(5.6)

where

$k = $ number of treatments $= 6$.

The degrees of freedom of this estimate, obtained from the experimental design, are

$$DF_{\text{Resid}} = k(n-1) = 6 \times (5-1) = 24.$$

(5.7)

The mean square for variation between treatments is obtained as

$$MS_{Treat} = \frac{n \sum_{j=1}^{k} (\overline{T}_j - \overline{T}.)^2}{k-1} = \frac{5 \times \left[(15.504 - 19.9897)^2 + ... + (18.218 - 19.9897)^2\right]}{6-1} = 151.383,$$

(5.8)

where

$\overline{T}_j$ = the mean of the response values in treatment Trt_j,

and

$\overline{T}.$ = the grand mean of all the response values.

The degrees of freedom of MS_{Treat} are

$$DF_{Treat} = k - 1 = 6 - 1 = 5.$$

(5.9)

(There are more computationally efficient ways to perform these calculations, but they are presented using the formulae provided in this paragraph for clarity.) H_0 is tested using the F statistic,

$$F = MS_{Treat}/MS_{Resid} = 151.383/14.122 = 10.72,$$

with DF_{Treat}, DF_{Resid} degrees of freedom. The corresponding p-value is obtained from standard statistical software, for example, the R function `pf (q = 10.72, df1 = 5, df2 = 24, lower.tail = FALSE, ...)`.

In the present case,

$$F_{5, 24} = 10.72, p = 0.0000168.$$

These numerical results can be conveniently summarised in a one-way analysis of variance (one-way anova) table, as in Table 5.3.

The null hypothesis that the true treatment means are all the same can be confidently rejected, but this does not mean that each treatment mean is different from all the others: it is usually of interest to explore the differences between group means in more detail. The difference between every pair of group means in this experiment is presented in Table 5.4.

The significance of the difference between any pair of treatment means, $\overline{T}_j$ and $\overline{T}_{j'}$, without reference to any other comparison, can be tested by calculating the appropriate t statistic,

$$t_\nu = \frac{\overline{T}_j - \overline{T}_{j'}}{\sqrt{\left(\frac{1}{n} + \frac{1}{n}\right)s}},$$

(5.10)

Table 5.3 One-way anova of the experiment with six treatment groups.

Source of variation	Degrees of freedom (DF)	Mean square (MS)	F	p
Treatment	5	151.383	10.72	0.0000168
Residual	24	14.122		

Table 5.4 Differences between every pair of group means in the experiment to compare six treatment groups.

	Trt$_1$	Trt$_2$	Trt$_3$	Trt$_4$	Trt$_5$
Trt$_2$	11.556				
Trt$_3$	5.014	−6.542			
Trt$_4$	−2.388	−13.944	−7.402		
Trt$_5$	10.018	−1.538	5.004	12.406	
Trt$_6$	2.714	−8.842	−2.300	5.102	−7.304

where

$$\nu = \mathrm{DF_{Resid}} = \text{the degrees of freedom of } s.$$

The interpretation of this statistic depends on whether a 'two-sided' or a 'one-sided' significance test is to be conducted, as follows:

- If a two-sided test is specified, then a large difference between $\overline{T}_j$ and $\overline{T}_{j'}$, *whether positive or negative*, will be considered significant: that is, the alternative hypothesis is H_1: $\mu_{j'} - \mu_j \neq 0$. The p-value is then given by $P(|T_\nu| > |t_\nu|)$, where T_ν is the random variable having a t distribution with ν degrees of freedom (not to be confused with the symbols $\overline{T}_j$ and $\overline{T}_{j'}$ representing treatment means).
- if a one-sided test is specified, then only a large difference between $\overline{T}_j$ and $\overline{T}_{j'}$ in a specified direction will be considered significant: that is, if positive differences are expected, the alternative hypothesis is H_1: $\mu_{j'} - \mu_j > 0$, and any negative difference will be considered non-significant. The p-value is then given by $P(T_\nu > t_\nu)$. (If negative differences are expected, the alternative hypothesis is H_1: $\mu_{j'} - \mu_j < 0$, any positive difference will be considered non-significant, and the p-value is given by $P(T_\nu < t_\nu)$.)

For example, to compare the means for treatments Trt$_6$ and Trt$_4$, we calculate

$$t_{24} = \frac{\overline{T}_6 - \overline{T}_4}{\sqrt{\left(\frac{1}{n} + \frac{1}{n}\right)s}} = \frac{18.218 - 13.116}{\sqrt{\left(\frac{1}{5} + \frac{1}{5}\right)} \times 14.122} = \frac{5.102}{\sqrt{\left(\frac{1}{5} + \frac{1}{5}\right)} \times 14.122} = 2.146.$$

whence, with a two-sided test,

$$p = P(|T_{24}| > 2.146) = P(T_{24} > 2.146) + P(T_{24} < -2.146) = 2 \times 0.0211 = 0.0421.$$

With a one-sided test, and the alternative hypothesis H_1: $\mu_4 - \mu_6 > 0$,

$$p = P(T_{24} > 2.146) = 0.0211.$$

The one-sided test with the other alternative hypothesis, H_1: $\mu_4 - \mu_6 < 0$, is irrelevant, because the observed difference, $\overline{T}_4 - \overline{T}_6 = 5.102$, is in the 'wrong' direction for that hypothesis. A similar comparison can be made for every pair of means in the study, and the p-values can be displayed in a table of the same form as Table 5.4, with highlighting to indicate those that meet the chosen significance criterion, so that the pattern of differences between the means is revealed, as shown in Table 5.5.

Table 5.5 *p*-Values for two-sided pairwise comparisons, based on the *t* distribution, between the experimental group means presented in Table 5.2.

	Trt$_1$	Trt$_2$	Trt$_3$	Trt$_4$	Trt$_5$
Trt$_2$	0.000059				
Trt$_3$	0.04551	0.01108			
Trt$_4$	0.32504	0.0000047	0.00472		
Trt$_5$	0.00031	0.5237	0.0459	0.000024	
Trt$_6$	0.26476	0.00106	0.34284	0.04214	0.00521

p-values for differences that are significant at the $\alpha = 0.05$ level are highlighted.

The smallest difference between the two means that will give a *p*-value smaller than α when this test is performed is referred to as Fisher's least significant difference (LSD) – with the important qualification that it should not be attributed to R.A. Fisher unless it conforms to his stipulation that the global test to compare the complete set of means has been performed first, and has given a significant result. In the present case, rearranging Equation (5.10) and taking into account that large values of $\left|\overline{T}_{j'} - \overline{T}_j\right|$ *whether positive or negative* are significant, we find that the least significant difference between the means for treatments j and j' is

$$\left|\overline{T}_{j'} - \overline{T}_j\right| = t_{\frac{\alpha}{2},\nu}\sqrt{\left(\frac{1}{n} + \frac{1}{n}\right)}s, \tag{5.11}$$

where

$t_{\frac{\alpha}{2},\nu} =$ the $\left(1 - \frac{\alpha}{2}\right)$ quantile of the *t* distribution with ν degrees of freedom.

Specifying the usual significance threshold $\alpha = 0.05$, we note that

$t_{\frac{0.05}{2},24} = t_{0.025,24} = 2.0639,$

and substituting numerical values into Equation (5.11), we obtain

$$\left|\overline{T}_j - \overline{T}_{j'}\right| = 2.0639 \times \sqrt{\left(\frac{1}{5} + \frac{1}{5}\right)} \times 14.122 = 4.905. \tag{5.12}$$

Comparison of Tables 5.4 and 5.5 confirms that all the differences between means larger than the LSD correspond to *p*-values smaller than 0.05, and all those smaller than the LSD to *p*-values larger than 0.05. Having first obtained a highly significant *F* statistic for the global test, we conclude that this difference is significant.

However, if this procedure is followed with no correction for multiplicity, as here, the probability that at least one of these $m = k(k-1)/2$ tests will produce a significant result by chance alone is of course larger than the significance threshold α specified for each individual test. If $k = 3$, Fisher's stipulation that the result of the global test must be significant is a sufficient defence against this, but for $k > 3$, additional measures are required.

Before proceeding to the general case, it is instructive to explore in more detail why $k = 3$ is a special case. The argument can be expressed using set-theory notation, in which $A \cap B$ indicates the intersection of sets A and B, that is, the elements that are present in both sets. In the present context, a set comprises one or more hypotheses such as '$\mu_1 = \mu_2$' or '$\mu_1 = \mu_3$'. The intersection of these sets, '$\mu_1 = \mu_2 \cap \mu_1 = \mu_3$', then means '$\mu_1 = \mu_2$ and $\mu_1 = \mu_3$'. Conversely, $A \cup B$ indicates the union of sets A and B, that is, the elements that are present in one set, or the other, or both. Thus, '$\mu_1 = \mu_2 \cup \mu_1 = \mu_3$' means '$\mu_1 = \mu_2$ and/or $\mu_1 = \mu_3$', that is, 'either $\mu_1 = \mu_2$ is true, or $\mu_1 = \mu_3$ is true, or both are true'.

The global null hypothesis in this case is $\mu_1 = \mu_2 = \mu_3$, and this can be rewritten as the intersection of three *minimal hypotheses*,

$$\mu_1 = \mu_2 \cap \mu_1 = \mu_3 \cap \mu_2 = \mu_3.$$

But this intersection hypothesis implies three simpler intersection hypotheses, $\mu_1 = \mu_2 \cap \mu_1 = \mu_3$ etc., and these in turn imply the three minimal null hypotheses, $\mu_1 = \mu_2$, etc. The simpler intersection hypotheses can be presented as the middle level of a hierarchy, with the global null hypothesis at the top and the minimal null hypotheses at the bottom, as shown in Figure 5.1. Hypotheses at successive levels that have component hypotheses in common are connected by lines: that is, the hypothesis at the upper end of the line implies the hypothesis at the lower end. An arrowhead at the lower end of a line indicates that rejection of the hypothesis at the tail of the arrow implies rejection of the hypothesis at its point. We undertake not to consider any null hypothesis for rejection unless we have rejected all the null hypotheses that imply it. Thus, we will not test the null hypothesis '$\mu_1 = \mu_2$' – that is, consider it for rejection – unless we have already rejected both $\mu_1 = \mu_2 \cap \mu_1 = \mu_3$ and $\mu_1 = \mu_2 \cap \mu_2 = \mu_3$. But we see that rejection of the global null hypothesis implies rejection of these simpler hypotheses: we do not need to test them explicitly. The same argument applies to the other two minimal intersection hypotheses.

Another way of looking at this argument is to note that in the special case of $k = 3$, the global null hypothesis not only implies the simpler intersection hypotheses, it is also *implied by* them. If $\mu_1 = \mu_2 \cap \mu_1 = \mu_3$ is true, then $\mu_2 = \mu_3$ must also be true, and the global null hypothesis is true.

But we have stipulated that we will never reject $\mu_1 = \mu_2$ (or either of the other two minimal hypotheses) unless we have already rejected the global hypothesis. So the probability that we incorrectly reject *even one* minimal hypothesis is no greater than the probability that we incorrectly reject both this minimal hypothesis *and* the global hypothesis. This argument can be expressed more formally, as follows. Regarding each value p as a realisation of a

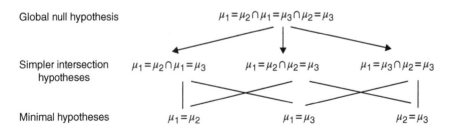

Figure 5.1 Hierarchy of hypotheses for comparisons between three group means.

random variable P (see Chapter 2, Section 2.4), and specifying the significance threshold as α, define the event

'B' = at least one minimal test gives $P \leq \alpha$, although the corresponding null hypothesis is true

$$= (P_{12} \leq \alpha | H_{0,12}) \cup (P_{13} \leq \alpha | H_{0,13}) \cup (P_{23} \leq \alpha | H_{0,23}).$$

Then, keeping our resolution to consider tests of the minimal hypotheses only if we have rejected the global hypothesis,

$$\text{P(incorrectly reject at least one minimal hypothesis)} = \text{P}\left(\left(P_{\text{global}} \leq \alpha \,|\, H_{0,\text{global}}\right) \cap \text{'B'}\right),$$
(5.13)

and from the laws of probability (see, for example, Hacking 2001, Chapter 6, The basic rules of probability, pp 58–68),

$$\text{P}\left(\left(P_{\text{global}} \leq \alpha \,|\, H_{0,\text{global}}\right) \cap \text{'B'}\right) = \text{P}\left(\text{'B'} \,|\, P_{\text{global}} \leq \alpha, H_{0,\text{global}}\right) \cdot \text{P}\left(P_{\text{global}} \leq \alpha \,|\, H_{0,\text{global}}\right).$$
(5.14)

But

$$\text{P}\left(\text{'B'} \,|\, P_{\text{global}} \leq \alpha, H_{0,\text{global}}\right) \leq 1,$$
(5.15)

and substituting Inequality (5.15) into Equations (5.14) and (5.13),

P(incorrectly reject at least one minimal hypothesis) $\leq$

$$\text{P}\left(P_{\text{global}} \leq \alpha \,|\, H_{0,\text{global}}\right).$$
(5.16)

Thus, if $p_{12} < p_{\text{global}}$, we can reject the hypothesis $\mu_1 = \mu_2$, not at the significance level $\alpha = p_{12}$, the p-value that we obtain for our direct test of it, which is still subject to the constraint of multiplicity, but at $\alpha = p_{\text{global}}$, the p-value that we obtained from the test of the global null hypothesis.

If $p_{12} > p_{\text{global}}$, we can reject the hypothesis at any significance level down to p_{12}, and still satisfy Inequality (5.16), but not at any more stringent level, because at any level below $\alpha = p_{12}$ our test will of course fail the simple significance criterion

$$\text{P}(P_{12} \leq \alpha \,|\, H_{0,12}) = \alpha.$$
(5.17)

Combining Inequality (5.16) and Equation (5.17), we conclude that we can reject the hypothesis $\mu_1 = \mu_2$ at the level

$$\alpha = \max\left(p_{\text{global}}, p_{12}\right),$$
(5.18)

that is, whichever is the larger of these two p-values. The same argument applies to the other two minimal hypotheses.

To see that this argument does not extend to more than three groups, consider the case $k = 4$. The hierarchy of hypotheses is then too complicated to present completely and conveniently, but part of it is shown in Figure 5.2. The simplest intersection hypotheses no longer imply the global null hypothesis, because each of them admits the possibility of inequality between some pairs of means. For example, $\mu_1 = \mu_2 \cap \mu_1 = \mu_3$ allows $\mu_4 \neq \mu_1 = \mu_2 = \mu_3$, and $\mu_1 = \mu_2 \cap \mu_3 = \mu_4$ allows $\mu_1 = \mu_2 \neq \mu_3 = \mu_4$. Hence, rejection of the global null hypothesis

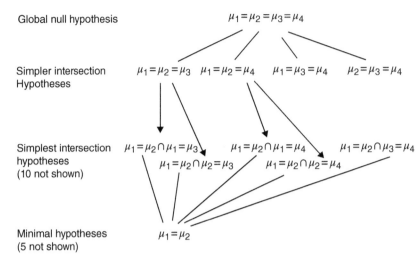

Global null hypothesis $\mu_1=\mu_2=\mu_3=\mu_4$

Simpler intersection Hypotheses $\mu_1=\mu_2=\mu_3$ $\mu_1=\mu_2=\mu_4$ $\mu_1=\mu_3=\mu_4$ $\mu_2=\mu_3=\mu_4$

Simplest intersection hypotheses (10 not shown)
$\mu_1=\mu_2\cap\mu_1=\mu_3$
$\mu_1=\mu_2\cap\mu_2=\mu_3$
$\mu_1=\mu_2\cap\mu_1=\mu_4$
$\mu_1=\mu_2\cap\mu_2=\mu_4$
$\mu_1=\mu_2\cap\mu_3=\mu_4$

Minimal hypotheses (5 not shown) $\mu_1=\mu_2$

Figure 5.2 Part of the hierarchy of hypotheses for comparisons between four group means.

does not imply rejection of the simplest intersection hypotheses, and we cannot proceed directly to test the minimal hypotheses.

For an example of how the argument is applied when the number of groups *does* equal 3, suppose that attention is confined to observations from Treatments 2, 3 and 5 in the dataset introduced in Table 5.1, the means of which are presented again in Table 5.6 for convenience, and that a one-way anova is performed on this subset, giving the results shown in Table 5.7. The results of the two-sided significance tests, performed using the *t* statistic without any adjustment for multiplicity, are then as shown in Table 5.8.

Table 5.6 Means of treatment groups 2, 3 and 5 from the experiment presented in Tables 5.1 and 5.2.

	Treatment		
	Trt_2	Trt_3	Trt_5
Mean response	27.060	20.518	25.522

Table 5.7 One-way anova of an experiment with three treatment groups.

Source of variation	Degrees of freedom (DF)	Mean square (MS)	F	p
Treatment	2	58.503	5.9498	0.0160
Residual	12	9.833		

Table 5.8 Two-sided significance tests for the pairwise comparisons from the analysis of the subset of treatment groups presented in Table 5.6.

Comparison	Difference	t (DF = 12)	p
Trt_3 versus Trt_2	−6.542	−3.299	0.0064
Trt_5 versus Trt_2	−1.538	−0.776	0.4530
Trt_5 versus Trt_3	5.004	2.523	0.0268

Because the global null hypothesis can be rejected at the significance level $p = 0.0160$, the minimal hypothesis $\mu_2 = \mu_3$ may also be rejected at this significance level: if the global H_0 $\mu_2 = \mu_3 = \mu_5$ is true, the probability of obtaining $p \leq 0.0160$ from the global test *and even one* case of $p \leq 0.0160$ from the pairwise tests is less than 0.0160. However, this minimal hypothesis may not be rejected at the level of its own, smaller p-value, $p = 0.0064$.

The minimal hypothesis $\mu_3 = \mu_5$ can also be rejected at any significance threshold down to $\alpha > 0.0268$: below this, its own p-value will not allow it to be rejected. Some care must be taken concerning what is meant if we say that '$\mu_3 = \mu_2$ can be rejected at $p < 0.0160$ and $\mu_3 = \mu_5$ can be rejected at $p = 0.0268$'. A more rigorous statement is that we can reject both $\mu_3 = \mu_2$ and $\mu_3 = \mu_5$ while conserving the FWER at $\alpha = 0.0268$, but that if we reject only $\mu_3 = \mu_2$ we can conserve it at the more stringent level of $\alpha < 0.0160$.

The minimal hypothesis $\mu_3 = \mu_5$ cannot be rejected by setting any threshold below $\alpha > 0.4530$, a value much too generous to be used in practice. It cannot be rejected solely on the grounds that the global null hypothesis has been rejected at a stringent level: that rejection may be driven by the value of μ_2, which does not contribute to this minimal hypothesis.

For the general situation in which $k > 3$, several methods have been proposed to take account of the increased probability that at least one pairwise comparison will be significant by chance. There is no arithmetic obstacle to the application of the Bonferroni correction to the p-values for comparisons between means. We could simply note that $m = 6 \times (6 - 1)/2 = 15$ hypotheses have been tested, and adjust the p-values accordingly, to

$$p_{adjusted} = \min(mp, 1).$$

For example, for Trt_2 versus Trt_1,

$$p_{adjusted} = 15 \times 0.000059 = 0.00088.$$

The results of doing so are shown in Table 5.9. Note that in the case of, for example, Trt_6 versus Trt_1, $mp = 15 \times 0.32504 = 4.8756 > 1$, and therefore $p_{adjusted} = 1$. We could make the corresponding change to the calculation of the LSD, using the $\left(1 - \frac{\alpha}{2m}\right)$ quantile of the t statistic. In the present case,

$$t_{\frac{0.05}{2 \times 15}, 24} = t_{0.001667, 24} = 3.2584,$$

and substituting this value into Equation (5.11), we obtain $\left|\overline{T}_j - \overline{T}_{j'}\right| = 7.7443$. Comparison of Tables 5.4 and 5.9 confirms that the significant differences that survive this 'correction' are those that exceed this value.

Table 5.9 Bonferroni-corrected p-values for pairwise comparisons, based on the differences between experimental group means presented in Table 5.4.

	Trt$_1$	Trt$_2$	Trt$_3$	Trt$_4$	Trt$_5$
Trt$_2$	0.00088				
Trt$_3$	0.68260	0.16624			
Trt$_4$	1.00000	0.00007	0.07083		
Trt$_5$	0.00458	1.00000	0.68856	0.00036	
Trt$_6$	1.00000	0.01597	1.00000	0.63206	0.07819

Bonferroni-corrected p-values for differences that are significant at the $m\alpha = 0.05$ level are highlighted.

However, this approach takes no account of the non-independence of the comparisons between the treatment means. $m = k(k-1)/2$ tests have been made for comparisons among only k entities, and this induces positive correlations among the p-values. This makes the Bonferroni correction conservative, and its use is not recommended in this context. A criterion that does take account of this non-independence is Tukey's honestly significant difference (HSD), and this is perhaps the simplest widely used adjustment for multiplicity in comparisons between means, and the most neutral in its approach to all the comparisons. The test statistic for this approach is

$$q_s = \frac{|\overline{T}_j - \overline{T}_{j'}|}{\sqrt{\frac{2}{n}s}}.$$ (5.19)

This is closely related to the formula for the t statistic for an individual pairwise comparison (Equation 5.10), with the differences that:

- it is a function of the absolute difference between $\overline{T}_j$ and $\overline{T}_{j'}$, stripped of its plus or minus sign: that is, it corresponds to the two-sided t test, in which the direction of the difference does not matter; and
- the statistic is referred to not as t but as q_s, to indicate that it is not to be compared to the t distribution but to the related Studentised range distribution.

(N.B. The symbol q_s is not to be confused with the symbol q representing an FDR – see Chapter 2, Section 2.4.) The precise shape of the Studentised range distribution, like that of the t distribution, depends on the value of ν, but it also depends on the value of k. Whereas the t distribution is related to the distribution of the difference between two sample means, $\overline{T}_1$ and $\overline{T}_2$, taken from the same population, so that by definition $H_0{:}\mu_2 = \mu_1$ is true, the Studentised range is related to the difference between the maximum and minimum of k sample means, $\overline{T}_{min}$ and $\overline{T}_{max}$, again taken from the same population, so that by definition $H_0{:}\mu_{max} = \mu_{min}$ is true. Since the difference between $\overline{T}_{min}$ and $\overline{T}_{max}$ is expected to be larger by chance than that between $\overline{T}_1$ and $\overline{T}_2$ (unless of course $k = 2$), the Studentised range distribution is wider than the corresponding t distribution for $k \geq 3$.

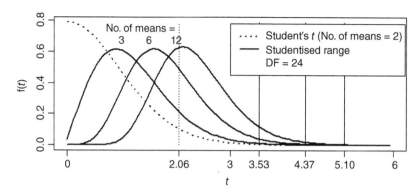

Figure 5.3 Probability distribution of the Studentised range distribution.

Note that the distribution of q_s also requires that n should be a constant – that is, the number of replications is the same for every value of j. The same constraint applies to other methods for the comparison of k means discussed later in this section.

The distribution of q_s is available from published tables or from software, for example, the R function `ptukey()`: the effect of the value of k on its width and shape is shown in Figure 5.3. In the special case of $k = 2$, it is the same as the distribution of abs(t) – that is, the positive half of the t distribution – and in this case only the probability density has a maximum at $q_s = 0$. Larger values of k shift the distribution to the right: that is, the larger the number of means compared, the more probable it is that the difference between the largest and smallest means will be wide. The Studentised range values corresponding to the significance threshold $\alpha = 0.05$ are marked by vertical lines, and are larger for larger values of k. That for $k = 2$ is the same as the threshold for the two-sided t test, namely, 2.06 when $\nu = 24$.

In the present example, with $\nu = 24$ and $k = 6$, the Studentised range distribution gives the p-values shown in Table 5.10. In every case, the p-value from the test using the Studentised range distribution is substantially larger than that obtained from the two-sided test using the standard t distribution, presented in Table 5.5. Tukey's HSD is obtained by likewise replacing the quantile of the t distribution with that of the Studentised range distribution in the formula for the LSD. In the present case,

$$q_{s,\frac{0.05}{2},k=6,\nu=24} = 3.091931,$$

Table 5.10 p-values for pairwise comparisons, using the Studentised range distribution, based on differences between experimental group means presented in Table 5.4.

	Trt$_1$	Trt$_2$	Trt$_3$	Trt$_4$	Trt$_5$
Trt$_2$	0.000749				
Trt$_3$	0.315815	0.101058			
Trt$_4$	0.911819	0.000063	0.047637		
Trt$_5$	0.003681	0.98598	0.317845	0.00031	
Trt$_6$	0.858935	0.012061	0.923690	0.29830	0.05206

and substituting this value into Equation (5.11), we obtain

$$|\overline{T}_j - \overline{T}_{j'}| = 3.091931 \times \sqrt{\left(\frac{1}{5} + \frac{1}{5}\right) \times 14.122} = 7.348656.$$

As expected, this is substantially larger than the unadjusted LSD, 4.905, but somewhat smaller than the value obtained from the Bonferroni correction, 7.7443. Comparison of Tables 5.4 and 5.10 confirms that the significant differences that survive this adjustment from LSD to Tukey's HSD are those that exceed this value.

Neither the simple LSD nor Tukey's HSD takes any account of the rank order of the means contributing to the set of pairwise comparisons. For example, the difference $\overline{T}_6 - \overline{T}_4 = 18.218 - 13.116 = 5.102$ and the difference $\overline{T}_5 - \overline{T}_3 = 25.522 - 20.518 = 5.004$ are very similar, and they give similar p-values: on the simple LSD basis, 0.04214 and 0.04590 respectively, and on the Tukey's HSD basis, 0.29830 and 0.31785, respectively. But $\overline{T}_3$ and $\overline{T}_5$ are adjacent in the ranking of treatment means, whereas $\overline{T}_4$ and $\overline{T}_6$ are separated by the mean of $\overline{T}_1$, 15.504. Intuition suggests that conditional on two means being adjacent in the ranking, it is less probable that they will be widely separated than if they are at widely separated ranks. This consideration is taken into account by Duncan's multiple range test (Duncan, 1955). The procedure for this test is to arrange the group means in rank order, then obtain the p-value for every possible pair of means, determined in relation to the Studentised range distribution (each pair of means being the minimum and maximum observed value in relation to the means that lie between them). All subsets of the means that do not differ significantly are then identified. It can happen that two means differ significantly when they are considered as the minimum and maximum values of the set lying between them, but nevertheless both lie within a larger set of means that do not differ significantly. In this case, the difference between the two means is not declared significant (https://en.wikipedia.org/wiki/Duncan%27s_new_multiple_range_test, accessed 11 May 2024). Subsets of means that do not differ significantly are often identified by placing a common letter next to each mean within the subset. Means that are not joined by a common letter are then recognised as significantly different from each other. When this test is applied to the example presented in Tables 5.1 to 5.3, with the significance threshold set at $\alpha = 0.05$, the results shown in the column headed 'Duncan' in Table 5.11 are obtained. Note that of the two pairs of means noted earlier as having similar differences:

- Trt$_5$ and Trt$_3$, adjacent in the ranking, have no subset indicated to which both belong – that is, they differ significantly, whereas
- Trt$_4$ and Trt$_6$, separated in the ranking by Trt$_1$, are both in subset 'c', indicating that they do not differ significantly according to this test.

The system of using a common letter to identify sets of means that do not differ significantly is not confined to Duncan's multiple range test: it can also be applied to the simple LSD or Tukey's HSD, although these methods are not *based on* the identification of subsets of means. The results of doing so are also presented in Table 5.11. The groups of not-significantly-different means identified by the simple LSD are smaller than those identified by Tukey's HSD or Duncan's multiple range test, that is, more differences between means are identified as significant, because no additional caution is introduced to take account of multiplicity.

Table 5.11 Ranked treatment means from Table 5.2, with the identification of not-significantly-different subsets on different criteria.

Rank	Treatment	Mean	Subset definition criterion		
			Duncan	Tukey's HSD	LSD (Student's *t*)
1	Trt_2	27.060	a	a	a
2	Trt_5	25.522	a	ab	a
3	Trt_3	20.518	b	abc	b
4	Trt_6	18.218	bc	bcd	bc
5	Trt_1	15.504	bc	cd	cd
6	Trt_4	13.116	c	d	d

These systems of subsets of not-significantly-different means may be helpful, but they do present difficulties of interpretation. The practitioner who is told that (according to Duncan's multiple range test or Tukey's HSD) there is no significant evidence that Trt_3 differs from Trt_1, nor Trt_1 from Trt_4, but that there is nevertheless significant evidence that Trt_3 differs from Trt_4, may reasonably complain that they are receiving mixed messages. In addition, Duncan's multiple range test has been criticised on the grounds that it does not control the FWER. The Wikipedia article on this test states:

> Duncan's test has been criticised as being too liberal by many statisticians including Henry Scheffé, and John W. Tukey. Duncan argued that a more liberal procedure was appropriate because in real world practice the global null hypothesis H_0 = "All means are equal" is often false and thus traditional statisticians overprotect a probably false null hypothesis against type I errors. According to Duncan, one should adjust the protection levels for different p-mean comparisons according to the problem discussed. The example discussed by Duncan in his 1955 paper is of a comparison of many means (i.e. 100), when one is interested only in two-mean and three-mean comparisons, and general p-mean comparisons (deciding whether there is some difference between p-means) are of no special interest (if p is 15 or more for example). Duncan's multiple range test is very "liberal" in terms of Type I errors. (https://en.wikipedia.org/wiki/Duncan%27s_new_multiple_range_test, accessed 11 May 2024).

That is, when Duncan's multiple range test is applied, even if $(\mu_1 = \mu_2 = ... = \mu_k = \mu)$, so that H_0: $\left(\mu_j - \mu_{j'} \right) = 0$ is true for all the $m = k(k-1)/2$ pairwise comparisons between the means, the probability that at least one comparison will give significant evidence of a difference may remain greater than α. The Wikipedia article then gives a detailed numerical illustration of this 'liberality', even on Duncan's own terms.

It is sometimes the case that one of the groups in a one-way anova is identified *a priori* as a control treatment, with which each of the other groups is to be compared, but that there is no *a priori* structure among the other groups: all the $(k-1)$ comparisons with the control are of equal interest, and there are no special expectations in relation to any particular comparison. Multiplicity is still present, but the number of tests in the family under consideration is reduced from the $m = k(k-1)/2$ pairwise comparisons taken into account by the Studentised range test and Duncan's multiple range test, to $m = (k-1)$. A method for controlling the FWER in this situation is provided by Dunnett's test (Dunnett 1955, 1964).

The test statistic is obtained using the same formula as for the t statistic (Equation (5.10)), and Dunnett's test, like the simple pairwise comparison using the t distribution (but unlike the Studentised range test or Duncan's multiple range test), requires a choice between specification of a two-sided or a one-sided test.

Software to obtain the distribution of Dunnett's test statistic does not appear to be generally available, but the two-sided version of the test has been implemented in the software R, in the function `DunnettTest()` within the `"DescTools"` package (https://cran.r-project.org/web/packages/DescTools/DescTools.pdf, accessed 12 May 2024). In this implementation, the null distribution against which the observed statistic value is to be tested is obtained by simulation using values produced by a random number generator, and the precise p-value obtained depends on the results of this simulation process. In order to obtain identical results from successive runs of the same `DunnettTest()` function, it is necessary to specify a particular arbitrary 'seed' value to start the simulation process. The R commands used to analyse the dataset presented in Table 5.1 are therefore as follows:

```
set.seed(79480)
DunnettTest(x = t.data$y, g = t.data$t, control = 1)
```

The data object `t.data$y` holds the values of the response variable y, `t.data$t` holds the specification of the treatment groups, and the option setting 'control = 1' indicates that Trt_1 is the control against which the other treatments are to be compared.

These commands give the results presented in Table 5.12. The interpretation of these two-sided p-values is similar to that of a Bonferroni-corrected p-value: if $H_0: (\mu_j - \mu_1) = 0$ is true for all $j = 2...6$, then the probability that a difference as large as or larger than $(\overline{T}_2 - \overline{T}_1) = 11.556$ will be observed for at least one of the five tests is $p = 0.00024$, and so on. That is, the FWER is controlled. However, like the Studentised range test, Dunnett's test avoids the conservatism of the Bonferroni correction, because it takes account of the non-independence of the

Table 5.12 Results from Dunnett's tests on the means presented in Table 5.2.

Comparison	$\overline{T}_j - \overline{T}_1$	t	Two-sided test: p-value	One-sided test: significance level[*]
$\mu_2 - \mu_1$	11.556	4.862	0.00029	$p < 0.01$
$\mu_3 - \mu_1$	5.014	2.110	0.16227	NS
$\mu_4 - \mu_1$	−2.388	−1.005	0.77122	Not applicable (effect in 'wrong' direction)
$\mu_5 - \mu_1$	10.018	4.215	0.00143	$p < 0.01$
$\mu_6 - \mu_1$	2.714	1.142	0.67975	NS

[*] NS = Not significant, that is, $p > 0.05$.

tests. Moreover, the p-values are smaller than the corresponding p-values from the Studentised range test ($p = 0.00075$, etc.) because fewer comparisons are made.

There does not appear to be a readily available implementation of the one-sided version of Dunnett's test. However, Dunnett (1955) published tables for the critical values of the test statistic for particular values of α, k and ν. In the present case, that is, for $k = 6$ and $\nu = 24$, the one-sided critical values of the test statistic with the alternative hypothesis $(\mu_j - \mu_1) > 0$ are $t = 2.36$ for $\alpha = 0.05$, and $t = 3.17$ for $\alpha = 0.01$. Hence, the significance levels for the comparisons between means are as shown in Table 5.12.

5.4 Repeated Testing in Interim Analyses Before Study Completion: Alpha Spending

Our willingness to tolerate false-positive results, measured by the significance threshold α, can be regarded as a 'resource', and the methods for taking account of multiplicity that control the FWER at level α can be regarded as 'spending' this resource on the m tests within the family in question. The Bonferroni correction divides α equally between the tests, 'spending' a false-positive rate of α/m on each one, but other divisions are possible. For example, one might, in principle, decide that in a family of four null hypotheses tested in different experiments, Null Hypothesis 1 was more likely to be false than the others, or if it were false, would indicate a more interesting effect. One might then wish to test it with more statistical power, to give it a greater probability of being selected for further investigation. To achieve this, one could set a significance threshold of $\frac{2}{5}\alpha$ for Null Hypothesis 1, but $\frac{1}{5}\alpha$ for the other three null hypotheses, and still control the FWER at

$$\frac{2}{5}\alpha + 3 \times \left(\frac{1}{5}\alpha\right) = \alpha.$$

Such explicit 'alpha spending' is rarely performed in practice for tests on separate datasets, but the concept is regularly applied in the context of clinical trials, when one or more pre-planned interim analyses may be conducted on the results from patients for whom data collection is complete, while other patients are still being recruited and/or contributing data, to determine whether the trial has already effectively met its objectives, and should be 'terminated for efficacy'. (An alternative, precautionary strategy is to determine whether the trial is unlikely ever to reach its objectives, and should be 'terminated for futility'.) For example, suppose that a single interim analysis was to be conducted when half the planned number of patients had been recruited, and the overall Type-I error rate was to be controlled at $\alpha = 0.05$. Naïvely, one might set the significance threshold at $\alpha/2 = 0.025$, both at the interim analysis, and at the final analysis if the result of the interim analysis is non-significant and the trial therefore continues. But this would be conservative, not only because of the conservatism of the Bonferroni correction relative to the Šidák correction (Section 5.2), but also because the two tests are not independent: the trials that continue on this basis will be those with large interim p-values, and since the patients who contributed to the interim analysis will also contribute to the final analysis, this will bias the final p-value upwards. The extent of this bias, and the measures needed to correct it, can be explored as follows.

The trial sample comprises two non-overlapping, independently recruited subsets of patients:

- those that contribute to both the interim and final analyses, and
- those that contribute only to the final analysis.

Consider a somewhat idealised scenario in which separate analyses could be performed on each of these subsets, each analysis producing a Z statistic which, on H_0, would be distributed

$$Z \sim N(0, 1).$$

Now suppose, for the moment, that the trial is continued and data from the second subset of patients is collected regardless of the outcome of the interim analysis of the first subset. Because the two subsets are independently sampled, the probability density of obtaining the result Z_1 from the analysis of the first subset and Z_2 from the analysis of the second is then given by

$$f(Z_1, Z_2) = f(Z_1) \cdot f(Z_2),$$

and the bivariate distribution of Z_1 and Z_2 is as shown in the contour plot in Figure 5.4. The value of the Z statistic from the final analysis of the two subsets combined will be

$$Z_{1,2} = \frac{1}{\sqrt{2}}(Z_1 + Z_2).$$

(In this idealised scenario this relationship is exact, not an approximation, as the variance among patients receiving the same treatment is assumed to be known, not estimated from the data.) We note that on H_0,

$$\text{mean}(Z_{1,2}) = \frac{1}{\sqrt{2}}(\text{mean}(Z_1) + \text{mean}(Z_2)) = \frac{1}{\sqrt{2}}(0 + 0) = 0,$$

$$\text{var}(Z_{1,2}) = \frac{1}{2}(\text{var}(Z_1) + \text{var}(Z_2)) = \frac{1}{2}(1 + 1) = 1,$$

and hence

$$Z_{1,2} \sim N(0, 1),$$

as expected. This result can be obtained from the contour plot as follows:
Define two new variables, $Z_{1,2}$ and $W = \frac{1}{\sqrt{2}}(Z_1 - Z_2)$.

- At each value of $Z_{1,2}$, integrate $f(Z_1, Z_2)$ over the range of W, $[-\infty, +\infty]$, to obtain the marginal distribution of $Z_{1,2}$.
- This integration can be envisaged as 'sweeping up' the probability density in the contour plot, from bottom right to top left, and the marginal distribution can therefore appropriately be plotted at the top left-hand corner of the contour plot, with the axes rotated by 45° relative to those of the contour plot.
- The symmetry of the contour plot indicates that the marginal distribution of $Z_{1,2}$ is normal, and calculation confirms that mean $(Z_{1,2}) = 0$, var $(Z_{1,2}) = 1$.

Now consider the effect on the contour plot when the trial is terminated for efficacy if Z_1 is significant, according to a two-sided test with threshold $\alpha/2 = 0.025$ (Figure 5.5).

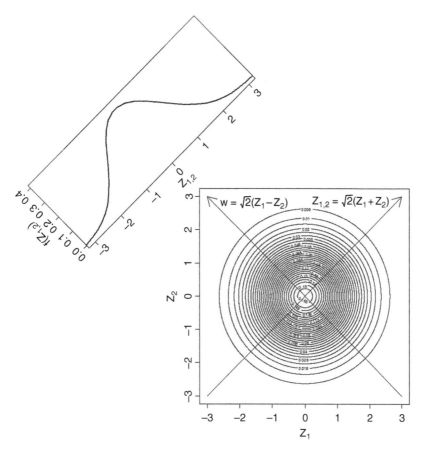

Figure 5.4 Bivariate and marginal distributions of test statistics on H_0, from independent analyses of pre- and post-interim subsets of patients in a clinical trial.

A proportion 0.025 of the probability (i.e., of the volume under the contour function) is cut off from the extremes of Z_1, 0.0125 at each end. If a trial falls in this category, its contribution to the probability density of the contour plot is zero. This has an effect on the marginal distribution of $Z_{1,2}$. The effect is too small to be readily detected from the plot of this marginal distribution at the top left-hand corner of the contour plot, but is just visible when the unconditional distribution of $Z_{1,2}$ and the distribution conditional on the interim analysis are presented in the same plot (Figure 5.6).

The total area under the conditional-distribution curve is slightly smaller, since it represents only a proportion $(1 - 0.025) = 0.975$ of the total probability distribution of the trial outcome: there is a probability 0.025 that the trial is terminated following the interim analysis, and never produces a value of $Z_{1,2}$. Because it is extreme values of Z_1 that are missing, the reduction in probability density is greatest at extreme values of $Z_{1,2}$. The quantile that cuts off a proportion 0.025 of the unconditional distribution of $Z_{1,2}$, namely, $Z_{1,2} = \pm2.241$, cuts off only a proportion 0.0178 of the conditional distribution. Hence, if H_0 is true, a significant result will be obtained at either the interim or the final analysis with probability $0.025 + 0.0178 = 0.0428$, a more stringent significance criterion than the intended threshold $\alpha = 0.05$.

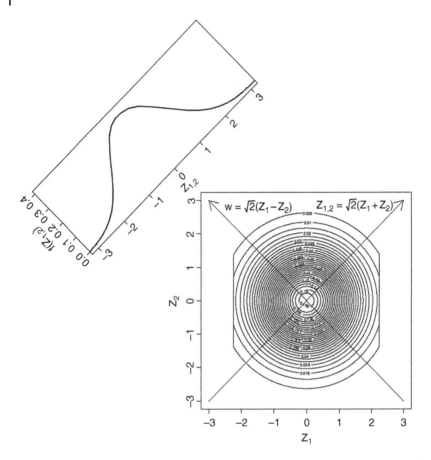

Figure 5.5 Bivariate and marginal distributions of test statistics on H_0, from analyses of pre- and post-interim subsets of patients in a clinical trial, the second analysis conditional on the outcome of the first.

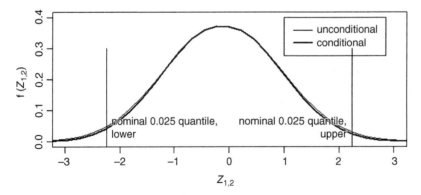

Figure 5.6 Comparison of the marginal distributions of test statistics on H_0, from unconditional and conditional analyses of pre- and post-interim subsets of patients in a clinical trial.

Numerical exploration over a range of values of α is required to determine the amount of relaxation of the nominal significance threshold that is required to compensate for this phenomenon. Such exploration shows that the required change is a relaxation of the nominal threshold at each analysis, designated by α', from $\alpha' = \alpha/2 = 0.025$ to $\alpha' = 0.0294$. The absolute value of the significance threshold for each test statistic (Z_1 and $Z_{1,2}$) is thereby reduced from $|Z| = 2.241$ to $|Z| = 2.178$. On H_0, the probability that the trial will continue to the final analysis *and* give a significant result in that analysis is then 0.0206, and the total probability of a significant result is therefore $\alpha = 0.0294 + 0.0206 = 0.05$, as intended.

The corresponding values for the significance threshold $\alpha = 0.01$ are relaxation of the nominal threshold from $\alpha' = \alpha/2 = 0.005$ to $\alpha' = 0.0056$, giving a reduction of the test-statistic significance threshold from $|Z| = 2.807$ to $|Z| = 2.770$, and a probability of a significant final-analysis result of 0.0044, whence $\alpha = 0.0056 + 0.0044 = 0.01$, as required.

On the basis outlined here, but using advanced numerical methods for accurate determination of tail areas of probability-density distributions, Pocock (1977), building on work by Armitage et al. (1969), presented the appropriate values of α' for trials with total numbers of equally spaced statistical analyses (interim and final) ranging from 2 to 20, in order to achieve an overall significance threshold $\alpha = 0.05$ or 0.01. He also showed how, when H_1 is true, a larger number of interim analyses reduce the average total number of patients that will be sampled before the trial is terminated (either for efficacy at an interim analysis or because the final analysis has been reached), which will reduce the cost of the trial and the demands on patients and researchers. Besides presenting results on the basis of the Z statistic, he considered the more usual case in which the between-patient variance of a normally distributed continuous variable must be estimated from the data (i.e., in which the Z statistic is replaced by the t statistic), and also other types of response variable – exponential, binary and rank (non-parametric). In the subsequent decades, further generalisations of the alpha-spending approach to interim analyses have been developed, including non-equally spaced analyses (DeMets and Gordon Lan 1994). Alpha spending and other strategies for control of the FWER can be presented and explored graphically: conventions for doing so were presented and applied by Bretz et al. (2009).

5.5 Is Control of the Family-Wise Error Rate (FWER) a Desirable Goal?

With the exception of the FDR, all the adjustments and corrections for multiplicity considered here – the Bonferroni and Šídák corrections, Tukey's honestly significant difference, Duncan's multiple range test, Dunnett's test and alpha spending – have the same conceptual basis as a simple p-value: the probability that H_0 will be rejected when it is true. Those methods that are based on the control of the FWER seek to maintain this probability below a specified level in relation to a specified 'family' of tests. All such methods are vulnerable to two problems. Firstly, if the number of tests in the family is large, control of the FWER results in excessively stringent significance thresholds for the individual tests, reducing the power of each test and causing non-significant results in many cases in which H_1 is true. Secondly, it is often difficult to decide what 'family' of tests would be appropriate. Suppose that I plan to perform a study today that will result in m significance tests. I may decide to protect myself against making a fool of myself by setting the significance threshold for the individual tests at a level such that the FWER for the whole set is controlled at $\alpha = 0.05$. But what if I perform a similar, independent study tomorrow? If H_0 is true for all hypotheses in both studies, the probability that I mistakenly announce a discovery on one day or the other is now $1 - (1 - 0.05)^2 = 0.0975$. To control the FWER at the same level in the enlarged two-day 'family', I must set my threshold for each day to something like $\alpha = 0.05/2 = 0.025$, giving $1 - (1 - 0.025)^2 = 0.049375$ for the whole family. To achieve a low probability of *ever* mistakenly announcing a discovery over my whole research career, I would have to set my significance threshold to an immensely stringent level, probably causing me to miss many opportunities for a true discovery. In the case of corrections for multiplicity applied to a set of pairwise comparisons or a series of interim analyses within a single study, there is a natural specification for the family of tests, but this does not in itself indicate why we should be interested in controlling the FWER within this particular family.

The important consequences of the choice of specification for the 'family' of tests to be considered when controlling the FWER can be illustrated in the context of the *Arabidopsis thaliana* data introduced in Chapter 4. Suppose it is decided that the distinction between the salt-related and ubiquitin-related subsets of genes is unimportant, and that these should be combined in a single family for testing purposes. The p-values obtained from the anova to test the global null hypothesis that the mean expression level is the same in all six genotype.stress combinations, illustrated in Table 4.8 (Chapter 4), can be considered. The p-values from the 83 probesets in the salt-related subset of genes can be specified as a 'family', as can the 196 p-values from the ubiquitin-related subset, or alternatively the $83 + 196 = 279$ p-values from the two subsets combined.

The unadjusted p-values, Bonferroni-corrected p-values and BH-FDR values ($q_{(i)}$ values) for the salt-related subset of genes, the ubiquitin-related subset and the combined subsets are summarised numerically in Table 5.13, and the log-transformed Q–Q plots for the three subsets are presented in Figure 5.7 (the plot for the salt-related subset being repeated from

Table 5.13 Numerical summary of unadjusted and adjusted p-values, and $q_{(i)}$ values, for differences between genotype.stress combinations in expression levels of different subsets of genes in *Arabidopsis thaliana*.

Subset of genes	m	Unadjusted p-values		Bonferroni-corrected p-values		BH-FDR ($q_{(i)}$ values)	
		Number significant	Proportion significant	Number significant	Proportion significant	Number significant	Proportion significant
Salt-related	83	47	0.566	13	0.157	52	0.627
Ubiquitin-related	196	91	0.464	9	0.046	90	0.459
Salt + ubiquitin combined	279	138	0.495	15	0.054	138	0.495

Significance is specified at the threshold $\alpha = 0.05$ for unadjusted or Bonferroni-corrected p-values, and $q^* = 0.1$ for $q_{(i)}$ values.

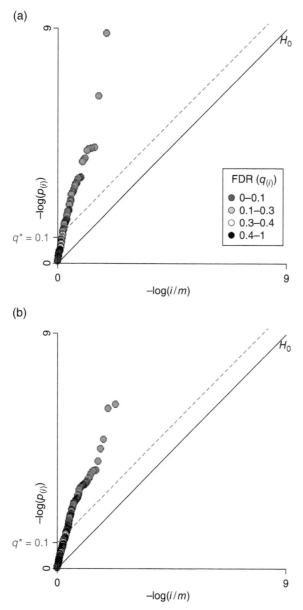

Figure 5.7 Q–Q plot, on the $-\log_{10}$ scale, of p-values for differences between genotype.stress combinations in different subsets of genes. (a) Salt-related genes, (b) ubiquitin-related genes, (c) salt- and ubiquitin-related genes combined.

(c)

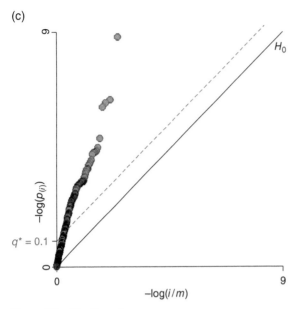

Figure 5.7 (Continued)

Figure 4.2 (Chapter 4) for ease of reference). The proportion of unadjusted p-values significant at the threshold $\alpha = 0.05$ in the salt-related and ubiquitin-related subsets is fairly similar, and the proportion in the combined subsets is the average of the two, weighted by the
size (m) of each subset. However, after application of the Bonferroni correction, the proportion significant in the larger (ubiquitin-related) subset is considerably the smaller of the two,
and the number significant in the combined subsets, 15, is smaller than the sum of the numbers in the two component subsets, $13 + 9 = 22$. Is there a good reason for losing interest in
some hypotheses simply because the two families of tests have been considered jointly, as a
single family? In contrast, the proportion that are significant on the BH-FDR criterion at the
threshold $q^* = 0.1$ (strictly, at whatever p-value corresponds to $q^* = 0.1$) is fairly similar
between the two subsets, and the proportion for the combined subsets is intermediate
between the two. All these proportions are much higher than any of the proportions for
the Bonferroni-corrected p-values, and they are therefore expected to give a much larger
harvest of true-positive results. The Q–Q plots confirm the conclusions from the numerical
summary of the BH-FDR values, showing a similar pattern for the salt-related and ubiquitin-related subsets, and a pattern for the combined subsets that is similar to both. Altogether, the BH-FDR seems like a better basis than either the unadjusted or the adjusted
p-values on which to proceed to selection of hypotheses for further investigation.

   Such considerations, in a research environment where large numbers of significance tests
can be conducted every day, have driven the increasing interest in the FDR as an alternative to
an adjusted p-value that controls the FWER. Moreover, 'How often will there be no real effect
present when I announce a discovery?' is surely often a more important question than 'How
often will I announce a discovery when there is no real effect present?' The researcher's integ-
rity and reputation, and the value for money obtained from follow-up investigations, depend

more directly on the answer to the former question, which can be re-formulated as 'What proportion of the discoveries I announced will, if pursued, turn out to be false-positives?' However, in order to predict the answer to this question, there is a price to be paid: information must be available, or assumptions must be made, about the proportion of tests undertaken for which H_0 is true, and the magnitude of the effects present in the cases in which it is false. The BH-FDR is effectively a source of guidance on this issue, but not the only one: other possible methods for specifying appropriate values are explored in Chapter 6, Sections 6.1 and 6.3.

In view of the problem of specifying an appropriate family of tests, what merit is there in methods of hypothesis testing that control the FWER? One context in which they are of value is in establishing a 'level playing field' between families of tests. A straightforward example of this occurs in genetics research, in which it is desired to identify which of many genes are associated with a particular phenotype, typically a disease. A number of genetic loci at which variant forms are present (*polymorphic loci*) are identified in each gene, the variant forms at a particular locus (typically two per locus) being referred to as the *alleles* at that locus. Significance tests are performed at each locus, to determine whether either of the alleles is positively associated with the occurrence of the phenotype. A common way of summarising the evidence of association for a particular gene is by the lowest p-value obtained for any locus in the gene. However, genes vary in length, and longer genes typically have more polymorphic loci. A correction for varying degrees of multiplicity in different genes is therefore needed, and an adjustment is applied to the lowest single-locus p-value in each gene so as to control the FWER for the gene.

One further refinement required in the genetics context must be mentioned. The adjustment for multiplicity cannot be performed simply by replacing p by mp, where m is the number of polymorphic loci in the gene, because some of the polymorphic loci are in close proximity along the gene. Different individuals tend to carry the same combination of alleles at such *linked* loci, which results in positive correlation between the p-values for these loci. The effective number of tests is then less than m, as discussed in Chapter 2, Section 2.8. Moreover, the average closeness of linkage varies between genes, so it cannot be assumed that the proportional reduction in the effective number of tests will be the same for every gene. Various methods have been proposed to determine the effective number of tests on the basis of the observed correlations between the alleles at different loci within a gene (Wen and Lu 2011), and one or other of these methods is used to adjust the value of m before the correction for multiplicity is applied.

In practice, great importance is attached to control of the FWER in confirmatory research studies, as part of a more general policy of rigorous control of the Type-I error rate (the false-positive rate) in such studies. In the exploratory phase of a research programme, hypotheses are often chosen for further study on the basis of small p-values, and this results in downward bias of the p-values: even among the chosen cases in which H_0 is true, the p-values will be small. But the hypotheses to be pursued are chosen on the basis of comparisons among the p-values, not their absolute value, so this bias does not greatly matter. In confirmatory research, however, such bias is carefully avoided, so that each p-value can be taken literally. There is already evidence that the hypothesis under consideration is worth further investigation, and the focus is on ensuring that few 'losers' are announced to be 'winners' at this second stage. In clinical trials, this is done by strict prior specification of the criteria required to establish the efficacy of an intervention, including appropriate allowance for multiplicity.

For example, if it was agreed in advance that a clinical intervention was to be considered efficacious if any one of three outcomes was achieved (e.g., lowering of blood pressure *or* reduction of the frequency of cardiovascular events *or* reduction in mortality), then it would be appropriate to apply a Bonferroni correction to the three *p*-values reported. (If, as is often the case, there were positive correlations between the three outcomes, this would be a conservative precaution.) Similar arguments can be deployed when a trial fails to demonstrate efficacy overall, but gives nominally significant efficacy in a particular subgroup of patients, for example, older males. The use of an alpha-spending criterion, to correct for multiplicity when efficacy may be considered to be demonstrated at any one of several interim analyses, rests on the same logical basis.

In the analysis of a confirmatory study, if any correction for multiplicity is required, there is a natural basis for specification of the appropriate family for control of the FWER, namely, all tests to be conducted in the study in question, and only those tests. Does this mean that the resulting *p*-value can be interpreted without further qualification? For guidance on this question, we can reason as follows:

- If only the smallest of a family of m *p*-values, $p_{(1)}$, is considered significant (i.e., if α is specified such that $\alpha/m = p_{(1)}$), then the Bonferroni-corrected value $mp_{(1)}$ is the level at which the FWER is controlled (see Section 5.2).
- The conventional calculation of an FDR requires a fairly large set of *p*-values to provide context for each other, whereas a single confirmatory study, after control of the FWER, produces only a single *p*-value.
- Hence, for a single confirmatory study, considered in isolation, after taking account of any within-study multiplicity, $m = 1$.
- The proportion of *p*-values expected to be less than or equal to p by chance is p. If a single confirmatory trial gives a significant result, the observed proportion is $k/m = 1/1 = 1$. Hence, from Inequality (2.19, Chapter 2), the FDR is controlled at

$$E\left(\frac{V}{V+S}\right) \leq \frac{p_{(k)}}{k/m} = p/(1/1) = p.$$

In this context, the *p*-value *is* the level at which the FDR is controlled.

The title of Section 5.1 should therefore perhaps be unpackaged as a more nuanced statement: An FDR is not (conceptually speaking) a *p*-value (though in some circumstances it is numerically equal to one).

On the basis of this argument, control of the Type-I error rate seems to be a fairly sound basis for the interpretation of a confirmatory study. The study will not then have an unfair advantage in relation to another study that has reported a single outcome: a 'level playing field', as specified earlier in this section, will be achieved. Moreover, this approach allows the researchers to indicate the importance of their findings in terms of *p*-values, which are familiar to their audience, while maintaining a defence against 'cherry-picking' of significant results. Corrections for multiplicity are often used in this way in the reporting of clinical trials, when the criteria for success are required to be specified in advance, as in the three-outcomes scenario described earlier in this section.

The relationship between exploratory and confirmatory statistical analyses is a major aspect of the problem of multiplicity. It is the subject of an extensive literature, and there are contexts in which the relationship is treated formally. One of these is multivariable regression analysis, in which explanatory variables are selected for inclusion in a final model. The model-building process inevitably introduces bias away from the null hypothesis in the coefficients of the final model, as variables that have large estimated effects by chance are more likely to be included. Therefore, large datasets are routinely divided into 'training' and 'validation' subsets: the model-building process is carried out on the training set, and the final model, with some explanatory variables retained and others discarded, is then re-fitted to the validation set, to obtain unbiased estimates of regression coefficients and p-values. Ideally, it is then further evaluated in a test set, to assess the 'generalization error' of the final chosen model. For a good introduction to these methods, see Hastie, Tibshirani, and Friedman (2009, Chapter 7, Model Assessment and Selection). In a Bayesian context, the appropriate criterion for concluding that a discovery has been validated has been explored by Held (2020).

The relationship between the FDR and the Bonferroni-corrected p-value when the threshold for significance is set at $\alpha = p_{(1)}$ can be illustrated further by reference to the confusion matrix of the counts of the possible test outcomes, presented in Table 2.2, Chapter 2, and repeated here (Table 5.14), now with symbols for the marginal-total values.

In the notation of this table,

$$\text{FDR} = \frac{V}{R}. \tag{5.20}$$

Suppose that the m hypotheses tested are a random sample from an effectively infinite population of hypotheses available for testing, as suggested in Chapter 2, Section 2.3, and that H_0 is true in a proportion π_0 of this population, and H_1 is true in the proportion $\pi_1 = 1 - \pi_0$. We can then regard this FDR as a realisation of a random variable, and enquire about its expected value. Next, suppose that we specify $p_{(1)}$ as the significance threshold, so that the corresponding null hypothesis is the only one rejected. Then $R = 1$, and the expected counts in the cells of the table are as shown in Table 5.15. Note also that

$$\pi_0 \leq 1, \tag{5.21}$$

and that from the definition of a p-value,

$$P\left(P < p_{(1)} \mid H_0\right) = p_{(1)}. \tag{5.22}$$

Table 5.14 Symbols for the values in the confusion matrix, including marginal values.

True hypothesis	Conclusion from evidence		Total
	H_0	H_1	
H_0	U	V	m_0
H_1	T	S	m_1
Total	$m - R$	R	m

Table 5.15 Expected values in the cells of the confusion matrix when only one null hypothesis is rejected.

	Conclusion from evidence		
True hypothesis	H_0	H_1	Total
H_0	$m\pi_0 \cdot (1 - P(P < p_{(1)}\mid H_0))$	$m\pi_0 \cdot P(P < p_{(1)}\mid H_0)$	$m\pi_0$
H_1	$m\pi_1 \cdot (1 - P(P < p_{(1)}\mid H_1))$	$m\pi_1 \cdot P(P < p_{(1)}\mid H_1)$	$m\pi_1$
Total	$m - 1$	1	m

Hence, substituting values from Table 5.15, Inequality (5.21) and Equation (5.22) into Equation (5.20),

$$E(FDR) = E\left(\frac{V}{R}\right) = \frac{m\pi_0 p_{(1)}}{1} \leq m p_{(1)}, \tag{5.23}$$

that is, the FDR is controlled at the Bonferroni-corrected p-value.

If such a Bonferroni-corrected p-value is to be interpreted as a rate at which the FDR is controlled, it is important to bear in mind that if $\pi_0 = 1$, then $E(m p_{(1)}) = 1$ and $FDR = 1$. Only if $\pi_0 < 1$ and

$$P\left(P < p_{(1)} \mid H_1\right) > P\left(P < p_{(1)} \mid H_0\right), \tag{5.24}$$

does the expected value of $m p_{(1)}$ fall below 1. That is:

- H_1 must be true in some cases, and
- the probability of a significant test result must be larger when H_1 is true,

in order for the expected FDR to fall below 100%.

5.6 Holm's Method: A Generalisation of the Bonferroni Correction

The equivalence between the Bonferroni correction and the FDR when only the smallest p-value is considered significant is a special case of a more general relationship between the FDR and adjustments for multiplicity that control the FWER. It can be controlled at level α not only by the Bonferroni criterion, namely,

- any p-value in the family is significant if, and only if, $p < \alpha/m$,

but also by a related but less stringent criterion, proposed by Holm (1979), namely,

- all p-values among the smallest k values in the family, $p_{(h)}$, $h = 1...k$, are significant if, and only if,

$$p_{(h)} < \frac{\alpha}{m - (h - 1)} \text{ for all } h.$$

When $k = 1$, this reduces to application of the Bonferroni criterion. Holm's criterion not only controls the FWER, but also controls the FDR, at level

$$q_{(k)} = \frac{P_{(k)}}{k/m}.$$

(5.25)

The reasoning is as follows.

Consider, as in Chapter 2, Section 2.4, a family of m p-values, p_i, $i = 1...m$, sorted in ascending order, $p_{(1)}...p_{(m)}$, obtained from tests of null hypotheses $H_{(1)}...H_{(m)}$, of which $m_0 \leq m$ are true and m_1 are false, that is, $m = m_0 + m_1$. The null hypotheses giving small values of $p_{(i)}$ are rejected, and for the smallest values these are true-positive results, but the hth null hypothesis in the ranking is true, and its rejection is a false-positive. This scenario is illustrated in Table 5.16. Note that the null hypotheses $H_{(h+1)}... H_{(m)}$ may be either true or false: it does not affect the argument.

To control the FWER, we need to ensure that

P(one or more of the $m - (h - 1)$ null hypotheses $H_{(h)}... H_{(m)}$ is rejected, even when all these hypotheses are true) $= \alpha$.

We require to find the value of α', the adjusted individual-test significance threshold, that meets this criterion. The argument from here on is the same as for the Šidák correction (Section 5.2). For an individual true null hypothesis,

$$P(p \leq \alpha') = \alpha',$$

and if we assume the p-values to be independent, we therefore specify that

$$1 - (1 - \alpha')^{(m - (h - 1))} = \alpha.$$

(5.26)

Rearranging Equation (5.26), we obtain

$$\alpha' = 1 - (1 - \alpha)^{1/(m - (h - 1))}.$$

(5.27)

Table 5.16 Scenario in which hypotheses $H_{(1)}$ ... $H_{(h-1)}$ of m null hypotheses, ordered according to their p-values, are rejected.

Hypothesis	Conclusion from evidence	p-value of ith hypothesis ($p_{(i)}$)
$H_{(1)}$	FALSE	$p_{(1)}$
$H_{(2)}$	FALSE	$p_{(2)}$
$\vdots$		$\vdots$
$H_{(h-1)}$	FALSE	$p_{(h-1)}$
$H_{(h)}$	TRUE	$p_{(h)}$
$H_{(h+1)}$	?	$p_{(h+1)}$
$H_{(h+2)}$	?	$p_{(h+2)}$
$\vdots$		$\vdots$
$H_{(m)}$	?	$p_{(m)}$

For any specified value α', we then test each ranked p-value in turn, starting from $p_{(1)}$, to determine whether it meets the significance criterion

$$p_{(h)} < \alpha'.$$

When we have identified the largest p-value that does so, $p_{(k)}$, we declare $p_{(1)}...p_{(k)}$ to be significant. Using the relationship between the Šidák correction and the Bonferroni correction, we can replace Equation (5.27) with a simpler approximation:

$$\alpha' = \frac{\alpha}{m - (h-1)}. \tag{5.28}$$

This value is slightly smaller than that obtained from Equation (5.27), making the significance test slightly conservative, and slightly less powerful, if the p-values are in fact independent. It is also conservative if the p-values are positively correlated, because the effective number of tests is then less than the nominal number (see Chapter 2, Section 2.8). Only if there are negative correlations among the p-values is the test anti-conservative.

To obtain adjusted p-values for direct comparison with α, we first substitute the observed p-value $p_{(h)}$ for α', and $p^*_{(h)}$, a provisional adjusted value, for α, in Equation (5.28), and rearrange this equation to obtain

$$p^*_{(h)} = p_{(h)}(m - (h-1)). \tag{5.29}$$

This equation can give a value greater than 1, in which case a further adjustment is made, to $p^*_{(h)} = 1$. However, the values of $p^*_{(h)}$ do not necessarily increase monotonically with h, and yet a further adjustment is therefore needed, which can be illustrated with a numerical example.

Consider a family of 12 p-values, $p = 0.0062, 0.0058, 0.0095, 0.0006, 0.0081, 0.0038, 0.0542, 0.0431, 0.0077, 0.0049, 0.0117, 0.0469$. These are sorted into ascending order in the second column of Table 5.17.

Table 5.17 Numerical illustration of Holm's method.

h	$p_{(h)}$	$\alpha'_{(h)}$	$p_{(h)} < \alpha'_{(h)}$	Decision	$p^*_{(h)}$	$p_{adj(h)}$
1	0.0006	0.00417	TRUE	Reject $H_{(1)}$	0.0072	0.0072
2	0.0038	0.00455	TRUE	Reject $H_{(2)}$	0.0418	0.0418
3	0.0049	0.00500	TRUE	Reject $H_{(3)}$	0.0490	0.0490
4	0.0058	0.00556	FALSE	Accept $H_{(4)}$	0.0522	0.0522
5	0.0062	0.00625	TRUE	Accept $H_{(5)}$	0.0496	0.0522
6	0.0077	0.00714	FALSE	Accept $H_{(6)}$	0.0539	0.0539
7	0.0081	0.00833	TRUE	Accept $H_{(7)}$	0.0486	0.0539
8	0.0095	0.01000	TRUE	Accept $H_{(8)}$	0.0475	0.0539
9	0.0117	0.01250	TRUE	Accept $H_{(9)}$	0.0468	0.0539
10	0.0431	0.01667	FALSE	Accept $H_{(10)}$	0.1293	0.1293
11	0.0469	0.02500	FALSE	Accept $H_{(11)}$	0.0938	0.1293
12	0.0542	0.05000	FALSE	Accept $H_{(12)}$	0.0542	0.1293

Cases in which $p_{(h)} < \alpha'$ but $H_{(h)}$ is accepted are highlighted.

The third column of the table gives the appropriate adjusted value $\alpha'_{(h)}$ against which to test each p-value when the threshold $\alpha = 0.05$ is specified, and the next column indicates whether the criterion $p_{(h)} < \alpha'_{(h)}$ is met. The next column, headed 'Decision', indicates whether the null hypothesis $H_{(h)}$ can be rejected, on the basis of the criterion $p_{(h)} < \alpha'$, for values of h up to and including the one under consideration. In the present case, for $h = 1, 2$ and 3, $p_{(h)} < \alpha'$ is true, and $H_{(h)}$ can be rejected. But for $h = 4$, $p_{(h)} < \alpha'$ is false: hence, $k = 3$, and for $h > k$, $H_{(h)}$ must be accepted regardless of whether $p_{(h)} < \alpha'$ is true or false. The cases in which $p_{(h)} < \alpha'$ is true but $H_{(h)}$ is nevertheless accepted are highlighted.

In these and some other cases, a further adjustment of $p^*_{(h)}$ is required: the final adjusted value $p_{\text{adj}(h)}$ is obtained by replacing the value of $p^*_{(h)}$ under consideration by the largest value above it. This step can be expressed more formally as

$$p_{\text{adj}(h)} = \max\left(p^*_{(i)}, i = 1...h\right).$$

The justification of this step is the same as that related to the adjustment for multiplicity of p-values for pairwise comparisons when the number of group means being compared is three (Section 5.3). We consider the value $p^*_{(h)}$ requiring further adjustment, and the largest p-value above it, $p^*_{(k)}$, and regard both of them as realisations of random variables, $P^*_{(h)}$ and $P^*_{(k)}$, respectively. We then note that the event

$$\left(P^*_{(k)} = p^*_{(k)}\right) \cap \left(P^*_{(h)} = p^*_{(h)}\right)$$

has occurred, and that from the laws of probability,

$$P\left(\left(P^*_{(k)} \leq p^*_{(k)}\right) \cap \left(P^*_{(h)} \leq p^*_{(h)}\right)\right) = P\left(P^*_{(k)} \leq p^*_{(k)}\right) \cdot P\left(\left(P^*_{(h)} \leq p^*_{(h)}\right) \mid \left(P^*_{(k)} \leq p^*_{(k)}\right)\right).$$

But

$$P\left(\left(P^*_{(h)} \leq p^*_{(h)}\right) \mid \left(P^*_{(k)} \leq p^*_{(k)}\right)\right) \leq 1.$$

Hence,

$$P\left(\left(P^*_{(k)} \leq p^*_{(k)}\right) \cap \left(P^*_{(h)} \leq p^*_{(h)}\right)\right) \leq P\left(\left(P_{(k)} \leq \alpha'_{(k)}\right)\right).$$

Expressing the same idea in English: the probability of obtaining a value as extreme as $p^*_{(h)}$ and one as extreme as $p^*_{(k)}$ is less than or equal to $p^*_{(k)}$. Hence, though we cannot reject $H_{(h)}$ at significance level $p^*_{(h)}$ while adjusting for multiplicity, we can at least do so at level $p^*_{(k)}$.

The relationship between the Holm and BH-FDR criteria can also be illustrated by an example, with $m = 50$ simulated p-values, presented in Table 5.18. The relationship is presented visually in Figure 5.8.

The H_0 line and the line indicating $q^* = p_{(i)}/(i/m) = 0.1$ and hence $-\log_{10}(q^*) = 1$ are marked. Starting from $i = m = 50$ and working downwards, inspecting the BH-FDR step-down criterion, we note that for $i = 50...41$ (points close to the origin, plotted blue in the colour version of the figure), $p_{(i)}/(i/m) = p_{(i)}m/i = 0.1259$, and the FDR criterion $q^* = 0.1$

Table 5.18 Ordered p-values illustrating the relationship between the Holm and BH-FDR criteria.

i	$p_{(i)}$	m/i	$p_{(i)}*m/i$	BH $q_{(i)}$	$m-(i-1)$	$p_{(i)}*(m-(i-1))$	Holm's $p_{adj(i)}$
1	0.000710	50.00	0.0355	0.0355	50	0.0355	0.0355
2	0.002010	25.00	0.0502	0.0502	49	0.0985	0.0985
3	0.003692	16.67	0.0615	0.0615	48	0.1772	0.1772
4	0.005684	12.50	0.0710	0.0710	47	0.2671	0.2671
5	0.007943	10.00	0.0794	0.0794	46	0.3654	0.3654
6	0.015107	8.33	0.1259	0.0794	45	0.6798	0.6798
7	0.017625	7.14	0.1259	0.0794	44	0.7755	0.7755
8	0.020143	6.25	0.1259	0.0794	43	0.8661	0.8661
9	0.022661	5.56	0.1259	0.0794	42	0.9517	0.9517
10	0.025179	5.00	0.1259	0.0794	41	1.0323	1.0000
11	0.027696	4.55	0.1259	0.0794	40	1.1079	1.0000
12	0.030214	4.17	0.1259	0.0794	39	1.1784	1.0000
13	0.032732	3.85	0.1259	0.0794	38	1.2438	1.0000
14	0.035250	3.57	0.1259	0.0794	37	1.3042	1.0000
15	0.037768	3.33	0.1259	0.0794	36	1.3596	1.0000
16	0.040286	3.13	0.1259	0.0794	35	1.4100	1.0000
17	0.042803	2.94	0.1259	0.0794	34	1.4553	1.0000
18	0.045321	2.78	0.1259	0.0794	33	1.4956	1.0000
19	0.047839	2.63	0.1259	0.0794	32	1.5309	1.0000
20	0.050357	2.50	0.1259	0.0794	31	1.5611	1.0000
21	0.052875	2.38	0.1259	0.0794	30	1.5862	1.0000
22	0.055393	2.27	0.1259	0.0794	29	1.6064	1.0000
23	0.057911	2.17	0.1259	0.0794	28	1.6215	1.0000
24	0.060428	2.08	0.1259	0.0794	27	1.6316	1.0000
25	0.062946	2.00	0.1259	0.0794	26	1.6366	1.0000
26	0.062946	1.92	0.1211	0.0794	25	1.5737	1.0000
27	0.062946	1.85	0.1166	0.0794	24	1.5107	1.0000
28	0.062946	1.79	0.1124	0.0794	23	1.4478	1.0000
29	0.062946	1.72	0.1085	0.0794	22	1.3848	1.0000
30	0.062946	1.67	0.1049	0.0794	21	1.3219	1.0000
31	0.062946	1.61	0.1015	0.0794	20	1.2589	1.0000
32	0.062946	1.56	0.0984	0.0794	19	1.1960	1.0000
33	0.062946	1.52	0.0954	0.0794	18	1.1330	1.0000
34	0.062946	1.47	0.0926	0.0794	17	1.0701	1.0000
35	0.062946	1.43	0.0899	0.0794	16	1.0071	1.0000
36	0.062946	1.39	0.0874	0.0794	15	0.9442	1.0000
37	0.062946	1.35	0.0851	0.0794	14	0.8812	1.0000

Table 5.18 (Continued)

i	$p_{(i)}$	m/i	$p_{(i)}*m/i$	BH $q_{(i)}$	$m-(i-1)$	$p_{(i)}*(m-(i-1))$	Holm's $p_{adj(i)}$
38	0.062946	1.32	0.0828	0.0794	13	0.8183	1.0000
39	0.062946	1.28	0.0807	0.0794	12	0.7554	1.0000
40	0.063546	1.25	0.0794	0.0794	11	0.6990	1.0000
41	0.103232	1.22	0.1259	0.1259	10	1.0323	1.0000
42	0.105750	1.19	0.1259	0.1259	9	0.9517	1.0000
43	0.108268	1.16	0.1259	0.1259	8	0.8661	1.0000
44	0.110785	1.14	0.1259	0.1259	7	0.7755	1.0000
45	0.113303	1.11	0.1259	0.1259	6	0.6798	1.0000
46	0.115821	1.09	0.1259	0.1259	5	0.5791	1.0000
47	0.118339	1.06	0.1259	0.1259	4	0.4734	1.0000
48	0.120857	1.04	0.1259	0.1259	3	0.3626	1.0000
49	0.123375	1.02	0.1259	0.1259	2	0.2467	1.0000
50	0.125893	1.00	0.1259	0.1259	1	0.1259	1.0000

Figure 5.8 −log-transformed Q–Q plot, showing the relationship between the BH and Holm FDR criteria in the p-values presented in Table 5.18.

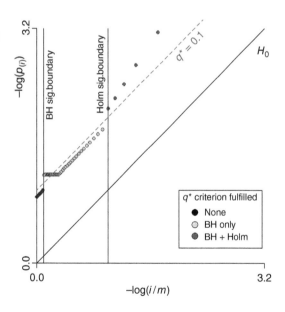

is not met. However, for $i = 40$, $p_{(40)} = 0.063546$, whence $p_{(40)}50/40 = 0.0794$, so for the set of values $i \leq 40$ (light-red and deep-red points), the criterion $q^* = 0.1$ is met. Thus, application of the BH-FDR criterion at this level gives $k = 40$ test results announced as significant at $p_{(40)} = 0.063546$. This BH significance boundary is marked on the figure. (For values in the range $i = 5...1$ (deep-red points), increasingly stringent FDR criteria are also met.)

Alternatively, starting from $i = 1$ and working upwards, we see that for $i = 1...5$, $p_{(i)}m/i <$ 0.1 in every case, so if only p-values in this range are considered significant, the FDR is again controlled at $q^* = 0.1$, though with many fewer null hypotheses rejected, and hence lower statistical power, than when the BH-FDR criterion is used. However, something is gained: the Holm criterion shows that this step-up approach, leading to the specification of a significance threshold at $p_{(5)} = 0.007943$, not only controls the FDR at $q^* = 0.1$, but also controls the FWER, at the (unimpressive) rate of $p_{(5)} \times (50 - (5 - 1)) = 0.3654$, whereas the BH-FDR criterion, which admits points below the $q^* = 0.1$ line among the rejected hypotheses, offers no control of the FWER. This Holm significance boundary is also marked on the figure.

The consequences of other significance thresholds can also be explored. If the threshold is relaxed to $i = 6$, then, noting that $p_{(6)} = 0.015107$, we obtain $p_{(6)} \times 50/6 = 0.1259$: that is, the largest significant p-value lies below the $q^* = 0.1$ line and the FDR is not controlled at this rate. Moreover, setting the threshold at this level gives $p_{(6)} \times (50 - (6 - 1)) = 0.6798$, indicating that very little control of the FWER is achieved: 'significant' results are more likely that not to occur, even if H_0 is true for all hypotheses. If the significance threshold is relaxed to $i = 10$, $p_{(10)} = 0.025179$, then $p_{(10)} \times (50 - (10 - 1)) = 1.0323$, and *no* control of the FWER is achieved. Only if the significance threshold is relaxed as far as $i = 32$, $p_{(32)} = 0.062946$, giving $p_{(32)} \times 50/32 = 0.0984$, is $q^* = 0.1$ again achieved (albeit with no control of the FWER).

Now consider an alternative dataset, with different values of $p_{(i)}$, $i = 1...4$, the values for $i = 5...50$ remaining unchanged. The $p_{(i)}$ values for $i = 1...12$, and associated statistics, are now as shown in Table 5.19, and this alternative dataset is represented visually in Figure 5.9.

As before, the level at which the FWER is controlled, indicated by Holm's $p_{\mathrm{adj}(i)}$, increases (becomes less stringent), over the range $i = 1...5$ (and indeed beyond). However, the points over this range trend upwards in relation to the $q^* = 1$ line, so that the expected FDR when

Table 5.19 Alternative ordered p-values illustrating a contrasting relationship between the Holm and BH-FDR criteria.

i	$p_{(i)}$	m/i	$p_{(i)}*m/i$	BH $q_{(i)}$	$m - (i - 1)$	$p_{(i)}*(m - (i - 1))$	Holm's $p_{\mathrm{adj}(i)}$
1	0.002022	50.00	0.1011	0.0794	50	0.1011	0.1011
2	0.003645	25.00	0.0911	0.0794	49	0.1786	0.1786
3	0.005146	16.67	0.0858	0.0794	48	0.2470	0.2470
4	0.006571	12.50	0.0821	0.0794	47	0.3088	0.3088
5	0.007943	10.00	0.0794	0.0794	46	0.3654	0.3654
6	0.015107	8.33	0.1259	0.0794	45	0.6798	0.6798
7	0.017625	7.14	0.1259	0.0794	44	0.7755	0.7755
8	0.020143	6.25	0.1259	0.0794	43	0.8661	0.8661
9	0.022661	5.56	0.1259	0.0794	42	0.9517	0.9517
10	0.025179	5.00	0.1259	0.0794	41	1.0323	1.0000
11	0.027696	4.55	0.1259	0.0794	40	1.1079	1.0000
12	0.030214	4.17	0.1259	0.0794	39	1.1784	1.0000
$\vdots$							$\vdots$

Figure 5.9 −log-transformed Q−Q plot, showing the relationship between the BH and Holm FDR criteria in the p-values presented in Table 5.19.

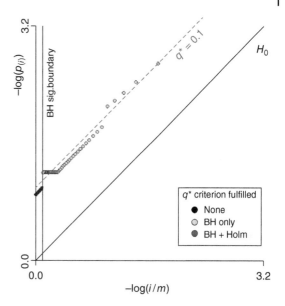

$p_{(i)}$ is specified as the largest significant p-value, $p_{(i)}m/i$, actually decreases as i increases over this range, from 0.1011 to 0.0794. Nevertheless, it does not fall below 0.0794, attained when $i = 5$, $p_{(5)} = 0.007943$, and this value is attained again when $i = 40$ and $p_{(40)} = 0.063546$, giving a much larger harvest of rejected null hypotheses. In conclusion, a demand for stringency in control of the FWER will not consistently achieve a low FDR.

5.7 Summary

The formal distinction between a p-value and an FDR is presented. A p-value is the probability of a false-positive result conditional on the null hypothesis (H_0) being true, whereas an FDR is the probability of a false-positive result conditional on the alternative hypothesis (H_1) being accepted.

Functions of a set of p-values that are widely used to take account of multiplicity – other than the BH-FDR – are reviewed.

The Šidák and Bonferroni 'corrections' (or 'adjustments') control the probability that at least one test result will be found significant when H_0 is true for all tests. Thus, they have the same conceptual basis as the p-value.

The Šidák correction gives the probability on the assumption that the tests are mutually independent, and the mathematically simpler Bonferroni adjustment is the limiting case when p is small and the number of tests (m) is large.

The m tests considered jointly are referred to as a 'family', and the Šidák and Bonferroni adjustments control the family-wise error rate (FWER) at the specified significance threshold α.

In an experiment to compare several treatment groups (k groups, where $k \geq 3$), pairwise comparisons between groups can be made using significance tests. Methods for taking account of this multiple testing are presented.

The mean values of a response variable in each group can first be compared by a one-way analysis of variance, with the global null hypothesis that all the treatment means are equal. If this hypothesis is rejected, every possible pairwise comparison can be tested using the t statistic. The least significant difference (LSD) between treatment means can also be determined on the basis of this distribution.

The p-values for these tests can be adjusted to take account of multiplicity. When $k = 3$, a significant result from the global test, p_{global}, is a sufficient defence. If the p-value for a pairwise comparison is less than p_{global}, it is replaced by p_{global}.

When $k > 3$, there is no arithmetic obstacle to the application of the Bonferroni correction. However, the p-values are not mutually independent: there are positive correlations between them. This will make the Šidák and Bonferroni adjustments conservative, and other methods are more appropriate.

Multiplicity and non-independence can be taken into account by testing the t statistic for each comparison against the Studentised range distribution instead of the standard t distribution. Tukey's honestly significant difference (HSD) between treatment means can also be determined on the basis of this distribution.

The standard t statistic and the Studentised range distribution do not take account of the rank position, among the k means, of the means in each pairwise comparison. An adjustment for multiplicity that does so is provided by Duncan's multiple range test. However, this test does not control the FWER.

The results of the standard t test, the test against the Studentised range distribution and Duncan's multiple range test can be displayed by presenting the group means in rank order and annotating them with letters of the alphabet. Subsets of means that do not differ significantly are connected by the same letter.

In some situations, one of the k groups is identified *a priori* as a control group, to which all the others are to be compared. In this situation, Dunnett's test provides an adjustment for multiplicity that controls the FWER.

The significance threshold α can be regarded as a 'resource', and methods that control the FWER can be regarded as 'spending' this resource on the m tests within the family. For example, the Bonferroni correction divides α equally between the tests, 'spending' a false-positive rate α/m on each one.

The concept of 'alpha spending' is also applicable to situations in which an interim analysis is conducted before a study is complete, to determine whether it has already effectively met its objectives (leading to 'termination for efficacy'), or is unlikely ever to do so (leading to 'termination for futility').

The p-values from interim and final analyses are positively correlated. Therefore, if the significance threshold is set at $\alpha/2$ for each analysis, the overall significance threshold will be more stringent than α. The method for an appropriate adjustment of each threshold is presented.

The question of whether control of the FWER is a desirable goal is considered. Several objections to it are noted, namely:

- If the number of tests in the family is large, control of the FWER results in excessively stringent significance thresholds for the individual tests, reducing their statistical power.
- It is often difficult to decide what 'family' of tests would be appropriate.

- 'How often will there be no real effect present when I announce a discovery?' is often a more important question than 'How often will I announce a discovery when there is no real effect present?'

The important consequences of the choice of specification for the 'family' of tests are illustrated in the context of the *A. thaliana* data introduced in Chapter 4.

However, in order to answer the question 'How often will there be no real effect present when I announce a discovery?', information must be available, or assumptions made, about the proportion of tests undertaken for which H_0 is true, and the magnitude of the effects in the cases in which it is false.

Controlling the FWER can be valuable to create a 'level playing field' when families of tests are to be compared.

Great importance is attached to control of the FWER and the Type-I error rate in confirmatory research studies. It is argued that such control is less important in the exploratory phase of research, in which hypotheses are chosen for further study.

For a single confirmatory study, after any within-study multiplicity has been taken into account, $m = 1$. If the study gives a significant result, then $E(FDR) \leq p/(1/1) = p$, and the p-value *is* the level at which the FDR is controlled. In this context, control of the Type-I error rate seems a sound basis for interpretation.

The relationship between exploratory and confirmatory statistical analyses is a major aspect of the problem of multiplicity. Contexts in which the relationship is treated formally are briefly reviewed.

The relationship between the FDR and the Bonferroni-corrected p-value is illustrated further by reference to the confusion matrix of the counts of the four possible test outcomes, introduced in Chapter 2.

Holm's method, a generalisation of the Bonferroni correction, is introduced. It specifies a criterion on which all of the smallest k p-values, $p_{(h)}$, $h = 1...k$, from a family of m tests, can be judged significantly. Holm's method controls both the FWER and the FDR. However, when the FDR is controlled at level q^*, Holm's method often gives a much smaller set of 'discoveries' than does the BH-FDR. That is, control of the FWER is obtained at a price in statistical power.

References

Armitage, P., McPherson, C.K., and Rowe, B.C. (1969). Repeated significance tests on accumulating data source. *Journal of the Royal Statistical Society, Series A* 132: 235–244.

Bonferroni, C.E. (1936). *Teoria statistica delle classi e calcolo delle probabilità. Pubblicazioni del R Istituto Superiore di Scienze Economiche e Commerciali di Firenze.*

Bretz, F., Maurer, W., Brannath, W., and Posch, M. (2009). A graphical approach to sequentially rejective multiple test procedures. *Statistics in Medicine* 28: 586–604. https://doi.org/10.1002/sim.3495.

DeMets, D.L. and Gordon Lan, K.K. (1994). Interim analysis: the alpha spending function approach. *Statistics in Medicine* 13: 1341–1352.

Duncan, D.B. (1955). Multiple range and multiple *F* tests. *Biometrics* 11: 1–42.

Dunnett, C.W. (1955). A multiple comparison procedure for comparing several treatments with a control. *Journal of the American Statistical Association* 50: 1096–1121. https://doi.org/10.1080/01621459.1955.10501294.

Dunnett, C.W. (1964). New tables for multiple comparisons with a control. *Biometrics* 20: 482–491.

Fisher, R.A. (1925 re-issued in 1990). *Statistical Methods for Research Workers. Re-issued in Statistical Methods, Experimental Design, and Scientific Inference*. Oxford: Oxford University Press 362 pp.

Hacking, I. (2001). *An Introduction to Probability and Inductive Logic*. Cambridge, UK: Cambridge University Press 302 pp.

Hastie, T., Tibshirani, R., and Friedman, J.H. (2009). *The Elements of Statistical Learning: Data Mining, Inference, and Prediction*, 2e 745 pp. New York: Springer.

Held, L. (2020). A new standard for the analysis and design of replication studies. *Journal of the Royal Statistical Society A* 183: 431–448.

Holm, S. (1979). A simple sequentially rejective multiple test procedure. *Scandinavian Journal of Statistics* 6: 65–70. JSTOR 4615733. MR 0538597.

Moore, D.S. and McCabe, G.P. (1999). *Introduction to the Practice of Statistics*, 3e. New York: W.H. Freeman and Company 825 pp.

Pocock, S.J. (1977). Group sequential methods in the design and analysis of clinical trials. *Biometrika* 2: 191–199.

R Core Team (2021). *R: A Language and Environment for Statistical Computing*. Vienna, Austria: R Foundation for Statistical Computing https://www.R-project.org/.

Šidák, Z.K. (1967). Rectangular confidence regions for the means of multivariate normal distributions. *Journal of the American Statistical Association* 62: 626–633. https://doi.org/10.1080/01621459.1967.10482935.

Wen, S.-H. and Lu, Z.-S. (2011). Factors affecting the effective number of tests in genetic association studies: a comparative study of three PCA-based methods. *Journal of Human Genetics* 56: 428–435.

6

The FDR in the Context of Bayesian Statistics

6.1 The Bayesian Interpretation of the BH-FDR

So far we have considered the FDR in terms of *frequentist* statistical concepts, namely the probabilities or probability densities of observed values, or of summary statistics calculated from observed values such as a sample mean or the difference between two sample means, on the basis of assumptions about the values of unknown parameters of the populations from which the observations are drawn, such as the population mean and variance. In particular, we have explored the consequences of the assumption that a null hypothesis H_0 is true – H_0 usually being that some effect, such as the difference between two population means, is zero. The alternative approaches to multiple testing that we have considered, namely the Bonferroni correction and its relations, are also within the frequentist framework, being based on assumptions about population parameters and consequent inferences about the distributions of observations. In the alternative, *Bayesian* framework, the unknown population parameters are not assumed to have specified, fixed values, but instead are regarded as random variables, each with a probability distribution. The core of the Bayesian approach is *Bayes' theorem*, which concerns the relationship between two assertions, one concerning a hypothesis, the other concerning the data, such as:

- Assertion H: H_0 is true.
- Assertion D: $P \leq \alpha$.

(In this context, we once again make the distinction between P, a p-value considered in the abstract as a random variable, and p, an observed realisation of that variable – see Chapter 2, Section 2.4.) Assertion D can be tested by inspecting the data: the assertion is either seen to be true or it is not. However, it can never be known with certainty whether Assertion H is true: one can only obtain a probability that it is true, a statement about one's belief.

Bayes' theorem states that

$$P(H|D) = \frac{P(D|H) \cdot P(H)}{P(D|H) + P(D|H')} = \frac{P(D|H) \cdot P(H)}{P(D)}, \tag{6.1}$$

The False Discovery Rate: Its Meaning, Interpretation and Application in Data Science, First Edition.
N.W. Galwey.
© 2025 John Wiley & Sons Ltd. Published 2025 by John Wiley & Sons Ltd.
Companion website: www.wiley.com/go/falsediscoveryrate

where H' means 'not H', i.e., that Assertion H is false. That is, $P(D)$ is the overall probability of D, not conditional on H. Conversely, $P(H)$ is the probability that Assertion H is true, not conditional on the truth of Assertion D – that is, prior to the inspection of the data to determine the truth or falsehood of D. It is known as the *prior probability* of H. The proof of the theorem is straightforward, and is given, for example, by Hacking (2001, Chapter 7, pp. 69–71).

The major attraction of the Bayesian approach to statistics is that its outcome, $P(H|D)$, is what the researcher primarily wants to know, namely, the probability of the hypothesis in the light of the data, known as the *posterior probability*. But there is a price to pay for this advantage: the Bayesian approach requires the specification of the prior probability of H, and this is a matter of belief. The researcher must specify how credible Assertion H is – the probability that H is true – without reference to the data. This can be done on the basis of previous knowledge, or of expert opinion, or by attempting to specify a neutral value that will 'allow the data to speak for themselves', but all these approaches are open to challenge.

In the context of the FDR, we want to determine the probability that a particular H_0 is true, given that the corresponding test result was announced as significant: that is, given that the hypothesis under consideration is in the set $i = 1...k$, where $p_{(k)}$ is the largest p-value announced as significant. Substituting this specification into Equation (6.1), we obtain

$$P\left(H_0|P \leq p_{(k)}\right) = \frac{P\left(P \leq p_{(k)}|H_0\right) \cdot P(H_0)}{P\left(P \leq p_{(k)}\right)}, \tag{6.2}$$

the left-hand side of this equation being the FDR. Seeking values for the terms on the right-hand side, we note that on H_0,

$$P \sim \text{Uniform}(0, 1),$$

whence

$$P\left(P \leq p_{(k)} |H_0\right) = p_{(k)}. \tag{6.3}$$

We next seek to evaluate $P(P \leq p_{(k)})$, not conditional on H_0, and for this purpose we consider the situation when nothing is known about the distribution of P, and only the ranks of the p-values are available. In this case, the probability that a randomly chosen p-value is among the k lowest-ranked values in the sample of m is

$$P\left(P \leq p_{(k)}\right) = k/m. \tag{6.4}$$

We are effectively using the observed distribution of the ordered p-values, $p_{(i)}, i = 1...m$, as our unconditional distribution of P. Substituting Equation (6.4) into Equation (6.2), we obtain

$$P\left(H_0|P \leq p_{(k)}\right) = \frac{P\left(P \leq p_{(k)}|H_0\right) \cdot P(H_0)}{k/m}. \tag{6.5}$$

We next note that since no probability can be greater than 1,

$$P(H_0) \leq 1 \tag{6.6}$$

by definition. Then substituting Equation (6.3) and Inequality (6.6) into Equation (6.5), we obtain

$$P\left(H_0|P \le P_{(k)}\right) \le \frac{P_{(k)}}{k/m}. \tag{6.7}$$

That is, the FDR is controlled at the same level as the BH-FDR criterion obtained by the frequentist methods used in previous chapters.

6.2 Numerical Equivalence Between a One-Sided *p*-Value and a Posterior Probability

The FDR is not the only statistical concept that can be given either a frequentist or a Bayesian interpretation. Indeed, in certain circumstances, the *p*-value, the frequentist's primary tool for comparing alternative hypotheses, is numerically equivalent to a Bayesian posterior probability. The conditions for such equivalence will be examined here.

Consider a case in which an effect Δ is under investigation, for example, the mean difference in the value of a certain response variable in an experiment to compare two treatments, an active treatment and a control. Δ is estimated by a random variable D, the observed value of which is calculated from the experimental data. In a Bayesian analysis, Δ itself is also regarded as a random variable: its value is unknown, but different values are believed to be more or less probable. Bayes' theorem (Equation (6.1)) tells us that for any given value of Δ, say δ, and for any given value of D, say d,

$$P(\Delta = \delta|D = d) = \frac{P(D = d|\Delta = \delta) \cdot P(\Delta = \delta)}{P(D = d)}. \tag{6.8}$$

Note the use of a Greek letter (Δ, δ) to represent an unobservable parameter, and the corresponding Latin letter (D, d) to represent an observed estimator of that parameter. Note also the use of an upper-case letter (Δ or D) to represent the random variable in the abstract, and the corresponding lower-case letter (δ or d) to represent a realisation of the variable – a particular postulated or observed value. For simplicity, we will specify that D and Δ are both normally distributed:

$$D \sim N(\mu_D, \sigma_D), \tag{6.9}$$

$$\Delta \sim N(\mu_\Delta, \sigma_\Delta). \tag{6.10}$$

The relative weight that we should give to the data and to our prior belief is then inversely proportional to the variance of these two variables, respectively:

$$w_D = \frac{1}{\sigma_D^2}. \tag{6.11}$$

$$w_\Delta = \frac{1}{\sigma_\Delta^2}. \tag{6.12}$$

It can then be shown that the strength of our posterior belief concerning the true value, $P(\Delta = \delta | D = d)$, is expressed by the following distribution:

$$\Delta | (\mu_\Delta, \sigma_\Delta^2, D = d, \sigma_D^2) \sim N\left(\frac{w_\Delta \mu_\Delta + w_D d}{w_\Delta + w_D}, \frac{1}{w_\Delta + w_D}\right). \tag{6.13}$$

That is:

- the mean of the posterior distribution is a weighted mean of the prior mean (μ_Δ) and the estimate from the data (d), and
- the variance of the posterior distribution is inversely related to the weights, and hence directly related to the variances of the component variables (σ_Δ^2 and σ_D^2).

Again for simplicity, we will specify that σ_D is known with sufficient precision that it need not be estimated from the current experiment, and hence that a Z test, rather than a t test, can be used to determine the significance of d. We will make the further simplifying assumption that $\sigma_D = 1$, so that D itself can be used as the test statistic Z without further calculation. That is, for any particular value $\Delta = \delta$,

$$D | (\Delta = \delta, \sigma_D^2 = 1) \sim N(\delta, 1). \tag{6.14}$$

Next, suppose that before inspecting the data we wish to be completely agnostic about the value of Δ, having no information on which to base a prior probability distribution. We can try to express this open-mindedness by specifying that all values in the range $-\infty \leq \Delta \leq +\infty$ are equally probable, that is,

$$\Delta \sim \text{Uniform}(-\infty, +\infty), \tag{6.15}$$

a flat, 'uninformative' prior probability distribution. In terms of the normal distribution, this is equivalent to

$$\Delta \sim N(0, \infty). \tag{6.16}$$

This has the disadvantage that the probability of Δ lying in any finite range is infinitesimal, and the function specifying the distribution cannot be integrated like a conventional probability distribution to give an area of 1. The distribution is therefore known as an 'improper prior'. However, this turns out not to be an insuperable obstacle.

The resulting bivariate distribution of Δ and D is then as shown by the contour plot in Figure 6.1: a ridge of uniform width, the summit of which is an infinite line of uniform height, running from low values of Δ and D to high values of Δ and D. The flat prior probability distribution of Δ is shown immediately to the left of the bivariate distribution, and the distribution of D not conditional on any particular value of Δ – the denominator of the right-hand side of Equation (6.1) – is shown immediately below it. This unconditional distribution of D is obtained by integrating the probability density at each value of D over all values of Δ (that is, 'sweeping up' the probability density in the contour plot from bottom to top), and gives the same (infinitesimal) probability density at each value of D: hence,

$$D \sim \text{Uniform}(-\infty, +\infty). \tag{6.17}$$

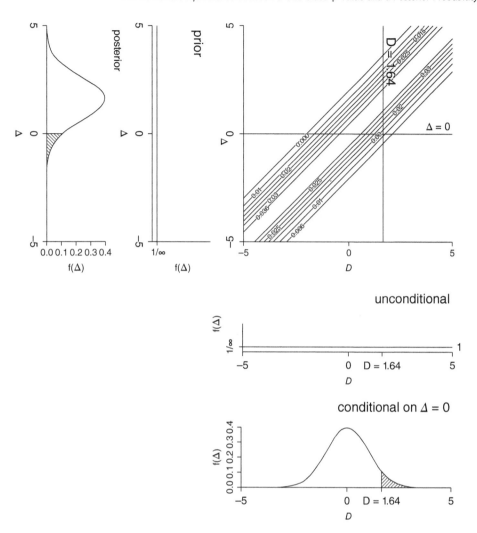

Figure 6.1 Bivariate distribution of an observable variable D conditional on an unobservable parameter Δ: uniform ('uninformative') prior distribution of Δ.

Now suppose that the null hypothesis H_0: $\Delta = 0$ is to be tested, and a mean treatment effect $D = 1.64$ is observed, that is, a value located just at the significance threshold $\alpha = 0.05$ for a one-sided test in which only positive values of D will cause rejection of H_0. The horizontal line representing this null hypothesis and the vertical line representing this observation are marked on the bivariate distribution of Δ and D in Figure 6.1. The distribution of D conditional on H_0 is shown at the bottom of the figure, with shading to indicate the region corresponding to the one-sided p-value, $P(D \geq 1.64|$ $H_0) = 0.05$. Similarly, the distribution of Δ conditional on the observe value $D = 1.64$ is obtained by substituting $\sigma_D^2 \to \infty$ into Distribution (6.9) and hence into Equation (6.11) and Distribution (6.13), giving

$$w_\Delta \to 0,$$

$$\Delta | \left(\mu_\Delta = 0, \sigma_\Delta^2 \to \infty, D = d, \sigma_D^2 = 1 \right) \sim N \left(\frac{0 \times 0 + 1 \times d}{0 + 1}, \frac{1}{0 + 1} \right),$$

$$\Delta | \left(\mu_\Delta = 0, \sigma_\Delta^2 \to \infty, D = d, \sigma_D^2 = 1 \right) \sim N(d, 1). \tag{6.18}$$

This distribution is shown at the extreme left of the figure, with shading to indicate the region corresponding to the posterior probability that Δ is negative, namely,

$$P(\Delta \leq 0 | D = 1.64) = 0.05. \tag{6.19}$$

This is identical to the frequentist p-value from a one-sided Z test: the p-value can thus be reinterpreted as a Bayesian posterior probability. This connection applies also to the one-sided t test, but unfortunately it cannot be extended to the two-sided Z or t test, as it depends on the symmetry of the Z and T distributions. The criterion $\Delta \leq 0$ on which the posterior probability is based may be referred to as a null hypothesis, but note that it is not quite the same as H_0 for the significance test. The distribution of Z (or in the present case D) on which the significance test is based is conditional on $\Delta = 0$, not $\Delta \leq 0$.

6.3 Does the Bayesian Interpretation of a *p*-Value Offer a Solution to the Multiplicity Problem?

Statistical investigation of a parameter of interest, such as the experimental treatment effect Δ in the previous section, concerns the relationship between the parameter value estimated from data and the true, unobservable value. Researchers may explore this relationship using either frequentist or Bayesian statistical methods, and it has sometimes been suggested that a Bayesian approach may overcome the multiplicity problem presented by p-values. For example, Trafimow and Marks (2015) announced in the journal *Basic and Applied Social Psychology* (BASP):

> [A] 2014 Editorial emphasized that the null hypothesis significance testing proce- dure (NHSTP) is invalid, and thus authors would be not required to perform it (Trafimow, 2014). However, to allow authors a grace period, the Editorial stopped short of actually banning the NHSTP. The purpose of the present Editorial is to announce that the grace period is over. From now on, BASP is banning the NHSTP.
>
> ...
>
> Bayesian procedures are more interesting. The usual problem with Bayesian proce- dures is that they depend on some sort of Laplacian assumption to generate numbers where none exist ... However, there have been Bayesian proposals that at least some- what circumvent the Laplacian assumption, and there might even be cases where there are strong grounds for assuming that the numbers really are there ... Conse- quently, with respect to Bayesian procedures, we reserve the right to make case- by-case judgments, and thus Bayesian procedures are neither required nor banned from BASP.

A similar outlook is alluded to, in less prescriptive terms, near the end of the *ASA [American Statistical Association] Statement on Statistical Significance and P-Values* (Wasserstein and Lazar 2016):

> In view of the prevalent misuses of and misconceptions concerning *p*-values, some statisticians prefer to supplement or even replace *p*-values with other approaches. These include methods that emphasize estimation over testing, such as confidence, credibility, or prediction intervals; Bayesian methods; alternative measures of evidence, such as likelihood ratios or Bayes Factors; and other approaches such as decision-theoretic modelling and false discovery rates. All these measures and approaches rely on further assumptions, but they may more directly address the size of an effect (and its associated uncertainty) or whether the hypothesis is correct.

The relationship between Bayesian and frequentist statements about probability in relation to hypotheses and data, and the prospects for a Bayesian route out of the multiplicity problem, will be examined here.

The conclusion of a frequentist analysis is typically given in terms of a *p*-value; that of a Bayesian analysis, in terms of a posterior probability distribution. The meanings of the two conclusions are different: the *p*-value is the probability of an extreme dataset conditional on a null hypothesis concerning the parameter; whereas, conversely, the posterior distribution is that of the unknown parameter, conditional on the data. At first sight, the Bayesian interpretation seems to offer a solution to the multiple testing problem. However, we have seen that in some circumstances a *p*-value and the corresponding posterior probability are numerically identical, and it seems implausible that simply reinterpreting the *p*-value as a posterior probability will be sufficient to overcome the problem. If a *p*-value is vulnerable to multiplicity, surely a numerically identical posterior probability is not immune?

On the frequentist basis, a small *p*-value may be difficult to interpret: it could mean that H_0 is false and can be rejected; or alternatively, it could have occurred, even though H_0 is true, because a large number of similar tests were conducted, and only the few that gave a significant result were reported. If the audience is not informed of the number of tests that have been conducted, such selective reporting of significance tests is sometimes known as 'cherry-picking'. By contrast, the posterior probability is conditional, not on H_0, but on observing a dataset like the one under consideration. The researcher can make a statement about the small probability that the true treatment effect is in the 'wrong' direction – the direction that would not cause the researcher to announce a discovery – and this statement will not be invalidated by the existence of other similar datasets, whether reported or not. If other datasets giving the same posterior probability (Equation (6.19)) have been reported, then the expected percentage in which $\Delta \leq 0$ (i.e., the true effect is in the 'wrong' direction) is 5%, and the more such datasets are observed, the closer to this figure the actual percentage is expected to be. (Though the actual percentage can never be known, as Δ is unobservable.)

But there is a problem. This posterior probability is conditional on the flat, 'uninformative' prior distribution of Δ (Distributions (6.15) and (6.16)), and in many multiple testing situations, this is unrealistic. Studies that lead to multiple testing are often 'fishing expeditions' in which large effects, either positive or negative, are expected to be rare: for most of the hypotheses tested, even if H_0 is not exactly true, the real effects are expected to be close to

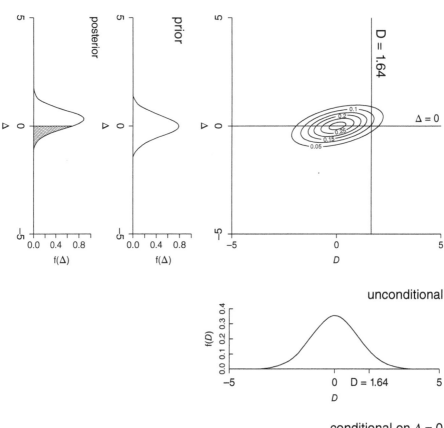

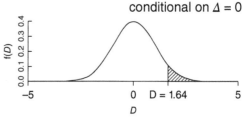

Figure 6.2 Bivariate distribution of an observable variable D conditional on an unobservable parameter Δ: non-uniform ('informative', 'sceptical') prior distribution of Δ.

zero. A prior probability distribution corresponding to such expectations has been termed 'sceptical' by Spiegelhalter et al. (1994). (They specified other priors, characterised as 'enthusiastic', having a positive mean value of Δ; or 'reference', adding as little as possible to the data; or 'clinical', expressing the collective opinion of well-informed individuals.) Figure 6.2 shows the changes to the pattern seen in Figure 6.1 caused by the adoption of a more appropriate prior.

The contour plot of the bivariate distribution now shows an ellipsoidal hill, the long axis of which runs from low values of Δ and D to high values of Δ and D. The prior distribution of Δ, shown immediately to the left of the contour plot, now has the distribution

$$\Delta \sim N(0, 0.5), \tag{6.20}$$

and most values of Δ lie within the range ± 0.5: a 'sceptical' prior as specified by Spiegelhalter, Freedman and Parmar. However, this does not affect the shape of the distribution of D
conditional on $\Delta = 0$, shown at the bottom of the plot – neither its location nor its scale. The
value $D = 1.64$ is still just significant at the threshold $\alpha = 0.05$. The new prior distribution of
Δ does, however, affect the marginal (unconditional) distribution of D, shown immediately
below the contour plot, which now has a maximum at zero. Values of $D \geq 1.64$ are now
rather rare, but when the value $D = 1.64$ does occur, the posterior probability distribution,
at the extreme left of the figure, shows that

$$P(\Delta \leq 0 | D = 1.64) = 0.20. \tag{6.21}$$

The posterior probability that the true effect is in the 'wrong' direction is now much larger
than the p-value. The large observed value of D is not sufficient to overcome the sceptical prior.

Thus, an individual p-value, on its own, is of little use as a guide to the confidence that can
be placed in the announcement of an individual discovery in such a multiple-testing study.
It must be placed in the context of a prior distribution of Δ. If no basis for such a prior distribution external to the study is available, the distribution must effectively be obtained by
considering the individual p-value in the context of the complete set of p-values for the set of
comparable hypotheses tested in the study – and this is what the FDR does.

If an individual significant p-value, or a subset of p-values that achieve statistical
significance, are interpreted as posterior probabilities without due regard for the full
multiple-testing set from which they were taken, the posterior probability of a real effect
in the direction of interest will be overestimated. Steps should be taken to ensure that such
'cherry-picking' does not occur: Bayesian methods provide no intrinsic defence against it.

6.4 Numerical Equivalence of *p*-Value, Posterior Probability and BH-FDR: The Prosecutor's Answer to the Accusation of Fallacy?

It has been noted earlier (Chapter 5, Section 5.5) that when a single significance test is considered in isolation, the p-value obtained is numerically equivalent to the BH-FDR, and the
preceding section (Section 6.3) shows that on the basis of certain assumptions a p-value is
numerically equivalent to a Bayesian posterior probability, and concludes by arguing that
the FDR is conceptually equivalent to a posterior probability.

But in Chapter 2, Section 2.9, the distinction between a p-value and an FDR was illustrated by reference to the Prosecutor's Fallacy, in which the probability of rejecting H_0 when
it is true (the p-value, or some other measure of the Type-I error rate or false-positive rate) is
mistakenly, and perhaps dishonestly, represented as the probability of H_0 being true when it
is rejected (the Bayesian posterior probability or the FDR) (Thompson and Schumann, 1987;
Fenton et al. 2016; RSS Statistics and the Law Section, 2022). Can the prosecutor defend
himself against the accusation of dishonesty by arguing that these different measures of
credibility, though conceptually distinct, have the same numerical value? The circumstances in which this may be the case will be explored here.

We specify the alternative hypotheses:

- H_0: the suspect is innocent, and
- H_1: the suspect is guilty.

We then consider a single significance test, which gives the result

$$P = p,$$

where

P = the p-value considered as a random variable,
p = the observed p-value, a realisation of P.

The significance test is correctly constructed, so that

$$P(P \leq p|H_0) = p \tag{6.22}$$

and

$$P(P \leq p|H_1) > p. \tag{6.23}$$

That is:

- the p-value correctly states the probability of obtaining such an extreme test result if the suspect is innocent, but
- the probability of this outcome is larger if the suspect is guilty.

Further, we stipulate that the ratio $\dfrac{P(P \leq p|H_1)}{P(P \leq p|H_0)}$ increases monotonically as p decreases.

Such a p-value is a *relative* measure of the strength of evidence against the suspect (the smaller the p-value, the stronger the evidence): but it is *only a relative measure*. It is not equal to the Bayesian posterior probability of innocence unless additional criteria are specified, as follows.

Suppose further that α is specified as the significance threshold: a test result $p \leq \alpha$ will be taken as significant evidence of guilt. Substituting these specifications into Bayes' theorem (Equation 6.1), we obtain

$$P(H_0|P \leq \alpha) = \frac{P(P \leq \alpha|H_0) \cdot P(H_0)}{P(P \leq \alpha)} = \alpha \cdot \frac{P(H_0)}{P(P \leq \alpha)}, \tag{6.24}$$

where

$P(H_0)$ = the prior probability that H_0 is true, before we have seen the result of the significance test,

and

$$P(P \leq \alpha) = P(P \leq \alpha|H_0) \cdot P(H_0) + P(P \leq \alpha|H_1) \cdot P(H_1) \tag{6.25}$$

= the overall probability of obtaining the result $P \leq \alpha$, not conditional on either H_0 or H_1.

$P(P \leq \alpha)$ is known as the *base rate* of positive (statistically significant) test results, the overall long-term rate in the sampled population. From Equation (6.24), we see that if

$$P(H_0) = P(P \leq \alpha), \tag{6.26}$$

that is, if our prior belief in H_0 is equal to the overall probability of a significant test result, averaged over H_0 and H_1 weighted according to the prior probabilities of these hypotheses, then

$$P(H_0|P \leq \alpha) = \alpha. \tag{6.27}$$

In this case – and only then – the posterior probability that H_0 is true is the same as the p-value. But there is no *a priori* reason why the two quantities in Equation (6.26) should be the same. Indeed, a perfect test of guilt would be one which always gave a significant result when the suspect was guilty and always gave a negative result when he was innocent, in which case the prior probability of *guilt*, not innocence, would be the same as the overall probability of a significant result:

$$P(H_1) = P(P \leq \alpha). \tag{6.28}$$

If we accept both Equation (6.26) and Equation (6.28), and also keep in mind that

$$P(H_0) + P(H_1) = 1,$$

we arrive at the specification

$$P(H_0) = P(H_1) = P(P \leq \alpha) = \tfrac{1}{2}. \tag{6.29}$$

That is, if:

- the p-value is to be equal to the posterior probability of innocence, and
- the prior probability of guilt is equal to the unconditional probability of a significant result,

then:

- our prior belief must be neutral between H_0 (innocence) and H_1 (guilt), and
- in a hypothetical population of suspects composed of equal proportions of innocent and guilty individuals, the test must give a significant result on half the suspects. It need not be perfect (in the sense specified above), but a low proportion of significant results among the innocent must be matched by a high proportion among the guilty.

This is a highly artificial situation, but it may be instructive to examine the confusion matrix to which it gives rise (Table 6.1).

Table 6.1 A confusion matrix in which the posterior probability of H_0 equals the p-value. Tabulated values are expected proportions.

True hypothesis	Conclusion from evidence		Total
	H_0	H_1	
H_0	$\frac{1}{2}\alpha$	$\frac{1}{2}(1-\alpha)$	$\frac{1}{2}$
H_1	$\frac{1}{2}(1-\alpha)$	$\frac{1}{2}\alpha$	$\frac{1}{2}$
Total	$\frac{1}{2}$	$\frac{1}{2}$	1

This confusion matrix is analogous to the bivariate distribution of D and Δ that made a one-sided p-value numerically equal to the posterior probability of an effect in the 'wrong' direction (Figure 6.1). In both cases, the prior probability distribution of the hypotheses and the unconditional distribution of the observations (values of D or significant versus non-significant test results) are uniform over the range of permitted values. In both cases, the bivariate distribution of probability over combinations of hypothesis and observed value is symmetrical around a diagonal line along which hypothesis and observation agree exactly, from bottom left to top right in the plot of Δ versus D, and from top left to bottom right in the confusion matrix.

As an alternative tactic, the prosecutor might appeal to Inequality (2.19) in Chapter 2, and the arguments presented in Chapter 5, Section 5.5, and argue that when a single significance test is conducted, the p-value is the level at which the FDR is controlled. However, this argument depends on the assumption that in this case, $k/m = 1/1 = 1$ is an unbiased estimate of the unconditional probability $P(P \leq p)$, the overall proportion of test results that are significant at level p. But on the contrary, when a suspect who has produced a significant test result is considered in isolation, k/m equals 1 by definition. As an estimate of $P(P \leq p)$, this is clearly both biased and very imprecise, and to compensate, we must have external information or beliefs concerning the terms $P(H_0)$, $P(H_1)$ and $P(P \leq \alpha|H_1)$ that contribute to $P(P \leq \alpha)$ when $\alpha = p$ is substituted into Equations (6.24) and (6.25). For example, in the context of a confirmatory clinical trial considered in Section 5.5, we are testing the treatment because we have previous evidence that it is likely to work (i.e., $P(H_0)$ is small and $P(H_1)$ is large) and because we believe that if it *does* work, we are likely to get a significant test result (i.e., $P(P \leq \alpha|H_1)$ is large). Likewise, in the forensic context, we must have good reason *other than the significance test* to think that the suspect is likely to be guilty, and we must believe that we are likely to get a significant test result if the suspect is indeed guilty. Only then can a significant test result provide persuasive evidence of guilt.

Having shown that the Prosecutor's Fallacy ceases to be a fallacy in the unusual case in which $P(H_0) = P(P \leq \alpha)$ (Equation 6.26), we will now consider the more usual situation in which $P(H_0)$ and $P(P \leq \alpha)$ are very different. Using the graphical conventions of Figure 2.1 (Chapter 2), Figure 6.3 shows what happens when a test with good performance characteristics is applied in a situation where the prior probability of the suspect's innocence, $P(H_0)$, is large. The test in the scenario illustrated has a low false-positive rate, $P(P \leq \alpha|H_0)$ being fairly small, as indicated by the relative areas of the two rectangles in the upper row in Figure 6.3a. It also has high sensitivity, the probability of obtaining a significant result when H_1 is true, $P(P \leq \alpha|H_1)$, being close to 1, as indicated by the areas of the rectangles in the lower row. However, because the prior probability of H_0, $P(H_0)$, is large (i.e., the combined area of the rectangles in the upper row is much larger than that of the rectangles in the lower row), most of the significant results are false-positives, and the FDR is large, as indicated in Figure 6.3b. This happens when the sampled population is large, but contains only a few cases in which H_1 is true – indeed only one case, if we are considering a crime committed by a single individual. The base rate for positive results, $P(P \leq \alpha)$, is then low, and the majority of positive results are false-positives even though the test has a low false-positive rate. This would be the case if the DNA from a *randomly chosen* individual in a large human population matched DNA found at a crime scene. The genetic variant in question might be rare, but in a large sampled population, most matches would nevertheless be false-positives. *In the absence of other reasons for suspicion*, a match would not be strong evidence of guilt.

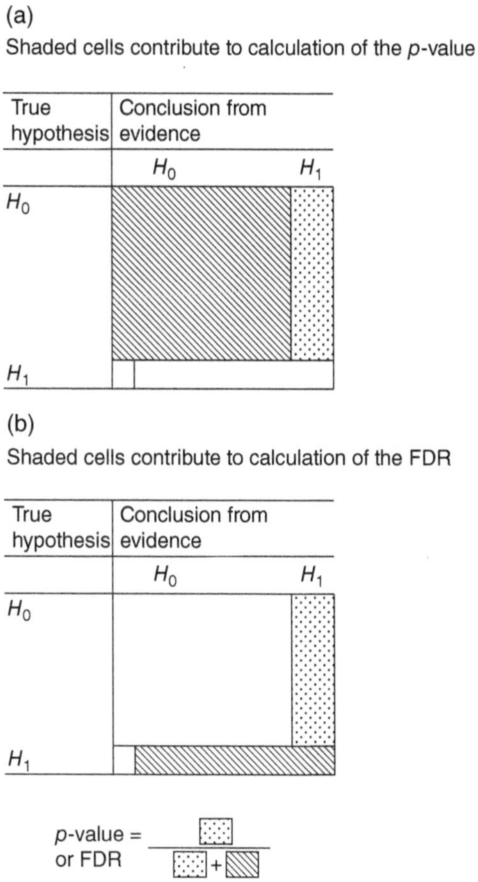

Figure 6.3 (a) and (b) The relationship between the *p*-value and the FDR when the prior probability of H_0 is large but the unconditional probability of a significant result is small.

(a)

Shaded cells contribute to calculation of the *p*-value

(b)

Shaded cells contribute to calculation of the FDR

$$p\text{-value} = \frac{\boxed{}}{\boxed{} + \boxed{}}$$
or FDR

The same reasoning applies to the medical diagnostic test considered in Chapter 2, Section 2.9. The test for colorectal cancer has a fairly low false-positive rate and high sensitivity, but the disease is relatively rare, so in the large sample screened, most positive outcomes are nevertheless false-positives.

It should be noted that although a DNA match between crime scene and suspect is not necessarily strong evidence of guilt, a mismatch is often compelling evidence of innocence. The reasoning, in terms of Bayes' theorem, is then as follows:

$$P(\text{suspect guilty}|\text{DNA mismatch}) = \frac{P(\text{DNA mismatch}|\text{suspect guilty}) \cdot P(\text{suspect guilty})}{P(\text{DNA mismatch})}.$$

(6.30)

If the genetic test has a low false-negative rate, and if the DNA from the crime scene certainly comes from the guilty individual, then P(DNA mismatch|suspect guilty) will be very small. If the population from which the suspect has been sampled is large, yet contains only one guilty individual, then the prior probability P(suspect guilty) will be small, and the unconditional probability P(DNA mismatch) will be close to 1. Substituting these values into the right-hand side of Equation (6.30), the posterior probability P(suspect guilty| DNA mismatch) will be very small.

It is important to note that the Prosecutor's Fallacy is not the only reason why p-values should be treated with caution in a forensic context. Even on the assumption of H_0 (i.e., without reference to the Prosecutor's Fallacy), the p-value or other measure of Type-I error rate quoted should be subjected to careful scrutiny. The quoted probability of a particular observation on the assumption of H_0 may be based on an inappropriate null distribution. For example, a rare genetic variant may be present in DNA found at the crime scene, and the prosecutor may state a probability of this event based on the frequency of the variant in the general population. But what if the individual truly responsible for the crime was a blood-relation of the accused? Or a member of the same small ethnic group? Or, turning to non-genetic evidence, what if the suspect is picked out in an identity parade, in which the other members of the line-up have not been well chosen and the suspect matches the witness's *previous* description of the guilty individual better than any other member? An inappropriately large base-population size, and a correspondingly low base rate, are then used when determining the Type-I error rate: the true probability that an innocent suspect will give a 'significant' test result may be much larger.

There are other mechanisms that can also result in an inappropriate null distribution. Suspicious events of a particular type may be assumed to occur independently, so that

$$P(2 \text{ events occur}) = (P(1 \text{ event occurs}))^2,$$

whereas in fact the events are positively correlated, so that $P(2$ events occur$)$ is larger than this relationship indicates. The p-value will then be an underestimate, and the evidence for H_1 will appear stronger than it really is.

Both of these mechanisms for mis-specification of the null distribution can be expressed in terms of multiplicity. When an inappropriately large base population is specified, the number of possible sampling outcomes is exaggerated, biasing the calculated Type-I error rate downward. When the occurrence of more than one suspicious event is taken as a positive result, if the events are positively correlated, the effective number of events is less than the nominal number, and again the calculated Type-I error rate is biased downward. The importance of an appropriate specification of the distribution of the test statistic on H_0 will be considered further in Chapter 8.

6.5 Summary

Bayes' theorem and the concepts of prior and posterior probability are introduced.

The posterior probability that H_0 is true if the significance threshold is set to $p_{(k)}$ ($P(H_0|P \leq p_{(k)})$) is shown to be closely related to the FDR. It is shown that if the observed distribution of the p-values is taken as the prior distribution of P, then the BH criterion controls $P(H_0|P \leq p_{(k)})$ at the same level as it controls the FDR.

It is shown that in certain circumstances a p-value can be interpreted as a posterior probability that H_0 is true. This is the case when the p-value comes from a one-sided test using the Z- or t-statistic, and the prior distribution of the statistic is specified as the 'uninformative' Uniform$(-\infty, +\infty)$ distribution.

It is sometimes thought that Bayesian statistics can offer a solution to the multiplicity problem. However, simply re-interpreting a p-value as a posterior probability is not a solution.

One reason for this is that the 'uninformative' prior distribution is often unrealistic. Multiple testing studies are often 'fishing expeditions' in which large effects are expected to be rare.

Another reason is that if a subset of significant p-values are interpreted as posterior probabilities without reference to the full multiple-testing set, the posterior probability of a real effect in the direction of interest will be overestimated. Bayesian methods provide no intrinsic defence against such 'cherry-picking'.

Misrepresentation of a p-value as a posterior probability or an FDR is the 'Prosecutor's Fallacy'. It is shown that the p-value and the posterior probability are equal only if our prior belief in H_0 equals the *base rate* of positive (statistically significant) test results. The base rate is the overall (unconditional) probability of a significant test result, averaged over H_0 and H_1, weighted according to the prior probabilities of these hypotheses; that is, the overall long-term rate in the sampled population.

The prosecutor may still argue that a single p-value indicates the rate at which the expected FDR is controlled. However, this argument depends on the assumption that $k/m = 1/1 = 1$ is an unbiased estimate of the unconditional probability $P(P \leq p)$, whereas when a suspect who has produced a significant test result is considered in isolation, $k/m = 1$ by definition. Only if we have good reason other than the significance test to think that the suspect is likely to be guilty, and we believe that we are likely to get a significant test result if the suspect is indeed guilty, can a significant test result provide persuasive evidence of guilt.

If the prior probability of H_0 is large, then even a test with good performance characteristics (low false-positive rate, $P(P \leq \alpha|H_0)$, and high sensitivity, $P(P \leq \alpha|H_1)$) can give a high FDR. This happens when the sampled population is large, but contains only a few cases in which H_1 is true. The base rate for positive results, $P(P \leq \alpha)$, is then low, and the majority of positive results are false-positives. This would be the case if the DNA from a *randomly chosen* individual in a large human population matched DNA found at a crime scene. It is also the case for medical diagnostic tests such as the test for colorectal cancer considered in Chapter 2, Section 2.9.

Although a DNA match between crime scene and suspect is not necessarily strong evidence of guilt, a mismatch is often compelling evidence of innocence. The reasoning leading to this conclusion is presented in terms of Bayes' theorem.

Besides the Prosecutor's Fallacy, there are other reasons why p-values should be treated with caution in a forensic context. The distribution of the test statistic on the assumption of innocence (H_0) should be subject to careful scrutiny. The probability of a 'significant' test result may be much larger for the innocent suspect than for the general population, and suspicious events may not occur independently of each other.

References

Fenton, N., Neil, M., and Berger, D. (2016). Bayes and the Law. *Annual Review of Statistics and Its Application* 3: 51–77. https://doi.org/10.1146/annurev-statistics-041715-033428.

Hacking, I. (2001). *An Introduction to Probability and Logic*. Cambridge: Cambridge University Press, 302 pp.

RSS Statistics and the Law Section (2022). *Healthcare serial killer or coincidence? Statistical issues in investigation of suspected medical misconduct.* London: Royal Statistical Society, 61 pp.

Spiegelhalter, D.J., Freedman, L.S., and Parmar, M.K.B. (1994). Bayesian approaches to randomized trials. *Journal of the Royal Statistical Society, Series A* 157: 357–416. https://www.jstor.org/stable/2983527.

Thompson, W.C. and Schumann, E.L. (1987). Interpretation of statistical evidence in criminal trials. *Law and Human Behavior* 11: 167–187.

Trafimow, D. (2014). Editorial. *Basic and Applied Social Psychology* 36: 1–2.

Trafimow, D. and Marks, M. (2015). Editorial. *Basic and Applied Social Psychology* 37: 1–2. https://doi.org/10.1080/01973533.2015.1012991.

Wasserstein, R.L. and Lazar, N.A. (2016). The ASA statement on *p*-values: context, process, and purpose. *The American Statistician* 70: 129–133. https://doi.org/10.1080/00031305.2016.1154108.

7

Alternative Specifications of the FDR

7.1 The Local and Non-Local FDR (LFDR and NFDR)

The BH criterion for controlling the FDR at a pre-specified rate q^* has been criticised on the basis that it gives equal status to all the p-values within the selected set. Having identified the set of test results that collectively meet the criterion q^*, the BH criterion makes no distinction between them. It has been likened to a procedure which selects applicants for a university course by replacing the failure probability of each applicant with the average failure probability of the applicant in question together with all better-qualified applicants (Bickel 2020, Section 6.1, Chapter 6). If interpreted uncritically, a value obtained in this way is unduly generous to the applicant under consideration (except for the best-qualified applicant in the whole set). It is argued that it would be preferable to have a decision-making criterion that reflected the fact that smaller p-values are less likely to be false-positives than larger ones, and that this pattern continues below whatever arbitrary significance threshold $p_{(k)}$ is specified. What we would ideally wish for is an estimate, for each individual ordered p-value, of the probability that it would be a false-positive discovery if it were announced to be significant – a *local* false discovery rate (LFDR). The prospects for obtaining an LFDR, or something approaching it, will be explored in this chapter.

Consider a population of hypotheses, each of which can be tested by calculation of a statistic Z, with distribution

$$Z \sim N(\mu, 1), \tag{7.1}$$

that is, with the probability density function

$$f(Z|\mu) = \frac{1}{\sigma\sqrt{2\pi}} e^{-\frac{1}{2}\left(\frac{Z-\mu}{\sigma}\right)^2},$$

where $\sigma = 1$. The null and alternative hypotheses are

$$H_0: \mu = 0,$$
$$H_1: \mu > 0,$$

that is, a one-sided significance test is to be conducted on each hypothesis. H_1 is true for a proportion π_1 of the hypotheses, and H_0 is true for the remaining proportion $\pi_0 = (1 - \pi_1)$.

The False Discovery Rate: Its Meaning, Interpretation and Application in Data Science, First Edition.
N.W. Galwey.
© 2025 John Wiley & Sons Ltd. Published 2025 by John Wiley & Sons Ltd.
Companion website: www.wiley.com/go/falsediscoveryrate

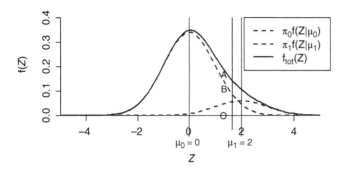

Figure 7.1 Probability density of the test statistic Z, and its components on H_0 and H_1.

For the sake of simplicity, we specify that in all cases in which H_1 is true, μ has a particular value, $\mu = \mu_1$. Thus, the total probability density of Z is

$$f_{tot}(Z) = (f(Z)|\mu = 0) \cdot \pi_0 + (f(Z)|\mu = \mu_1) \cdot \pi_1. \tag{7.2}$$

This model is illustrated in Figure 7.1, which shows the probability density, over a range of values of Z, of the two components of f(Z), and the total probability density, when $\pi_1 = 0.15$, and $\mu = 2$ in the cases where H_1 is true. What we would ideally like to know, at each value of Z, is the local false discovery rate,

$$fdr(Z) = \frac{f(Z|\mu = 0).\pi_0}{f_{tot}(Z)} = \frac{\text{length}(BO)}{\text{length}(AO)}. \tag{7.3}$$

We will now consider how this local FDR is related to the FDR as we have specified it so far.

If a one-sided significance test with significance threshold α is to be performed, the value Z_α is identified such that

$$P(Z > Z_\alpha|\mu = 0) = \alpha, \tag{7.4}$$

that is, Z_α cuts off a proportion α of the area of the distribution on H_0, and any Z-value greater than Z_α is considered significant. This criterion is marked on Figure 7.2 for the value

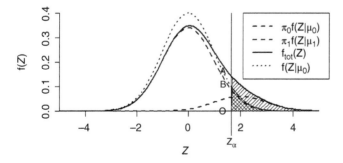

Figure 7.2 Probability density of Z and its components, with the region designated significant marked.

$\alpha = 0.05$, and the proportion of the observed (total) distribution that exceeds Z_α is represented by the hatched area, including the cross-hatched part. This observed proportion will be greater than α, provided that $\pi_1 > 0$ and $\mu_1 > 0$. The cross-hatched area represents the part of this significant proportion that is due to cases in which H_0 is nevertheless true. The proportion represented by this cross-hatched area will be less than α, unless $\pi_1 = 0$.

Now define the corresponding cumulative probability function,

$$F(Z|\mu) = \int_{-\infty}^{Z} f(w|\mu)dw, \tag{7.5}$$

that is, the area under the probability density curve from minus infinity up to the value under consideration, Z. Then the probability of obtaining a significant value of Z, conditional on a particular value μ, is $1 - F(Z_\alpha|\mu)$. The total probability of obtaining a *non-significant* value can then be specified as

$$F_{tot}(Z_\alpha) = (F(Z_\alpha)|\mu = 0) \cdot \pi_0 + (F(Z_\alpha)|\mu = \mu_1) \cdot \pi_1, \tag{7.6}$$

and the total probability of obtaining a significant value is

$$1 - F_{tot}(Z_\alpha) = (1 - F(Z_\alpha)|\mu = 0) \cdot \pi_0 + (1 - F(Z_\alpha)|\mu = \mu_1) \cdot \pi_1. \tag{7.7}$$

The average FDR among the tests judged to give a significant result (i.e., giving $Z > Z_\alpha$) is then

$$\begin{aligned}
Fdr(Z_\alpha) &= \frac{(1 - F(Z_\alpha|\mu = 0)) \cdot \pi_0}{(1 - F(Z_\alpha|\mu = 0)) \cdot \pi_0 + (1 - F(Z_\alpha|\mu = \mu_1)) \cdot \pi_1} \\
&= \frac{(1 - F(Z_\alpha|\mu = 0)) \cdot \pi_0}{1 - F_{tot}(Z_\alpha)}.
\end{aligned} \tag{7.8}$$

This quantity has been designated the *non-local false discovery rate* (NFDR) by Bickel (2020, Section 3.3, Chapter 3). It corresponds to the FDR as it was specified in Display (2.5) in Chapter 2, Section 2.3: that is,

$$\begin{aligned}
E\left(\frac{V}{V+S}|Z > Z_\alpha, \pi_0, \mu_1\right) &= \frac{(1 - F(Z_\alpha|\mu = 0)) \cdot \pi_0}{(1 - F(Z_\alpha|\mu = 0)) \cdot \pi_0 + (1 - F(Z_\alpha|\mu = \mu_1)) \cdot \pi_1} \\
&= Fdr(Z_\alpha),
\end{aligned} \tag{7.9}$$

where

V = number of false positive conclusions,
S = number of true positive conclusions.

However, this value cannot in general be estimated, because π_1 and μ_1 are unknown. A low FDR may occur either because $\pi_1 = (1 - \pi_0)$ is large, or because μ_1 is large, or both. The best that can be done is to substitute the limiting value $\pi_0 = 1$ into the numerator of Equation (7.8), giving the value at which the FDR is controlled:

$$Fdr(Z_\alpha) < \frac{(1 - F(Z_\alpha|\mu = 0))}{1 - F_{tot}(Z_\alpha)} = \lim(Fdr(Z_\alpha)). \tag{7.10}$$

lim(Fdr(Z_α)) is represented by the ratio of the cross-hatched area to the total hatched area under the probability-density curve in Figure 7.2. Note that the cross-hatched area extends beyond the curve representing $(f(Z)|\mu = 0) \cdot \pi_0)$, up to the curve representing $(f(Z)|\mu = 0)$, so that the ratio between the hatched areas corresponds to the upper bound of Fdr(Z_α). (But N.B. within the hatched region, the difference between these two curves is slight.)

Note the use of the function fdr(Z), with a lower-case 'f', to indicate the local FDR, and the function Fdr(Z), with an initial capital 'F', to indicate the corresponding non-local FDR. This is consistent with the use of the lower-case function f(Z) to indicate probability density, and the capital-letter function F(Z) to indicate the corresponding cumulative probability.

The trade-off between π_1 and μ_1 is illustrated in Figure 7.3, showing the situation for different values of μ in the cases where H_1 is true:

$$H_1: \mu = 1, 2 \text{ or } 3.$$

In each case a value of π_1 is specified such that lim(Fdr(Z_α)) has the same value, 0.364, when $\alpha = 0.05$ (though N.B. not for other values of α): the values required are found to be

$$\pi_1 = 0.423, 0.151, 0.105,$$

respectively. The smaller the proportion of tests for which there is a real effect, the larger that effect must be to attain a particular upper bound for Fdr(Z_α). But though the lim(Fdr(Z_α)) values for the three scenarios are the same, the average FDRs over the significant test results differ considerably:

$$\text{Fdr}(Z_\alpha) = 0.210, 0.308, 0.325,$$

respectively. lim(Fdr(Z_α)) is always based on the value $\pi_1 = 0$, whereas Fdr(Z_α) reflects the differing values of π_1 in the model.

Although this illustration is idealised, many test statistics follow essentially the pattern shown here: when H_0 is true, the statistic has a single maximum probability density at a particular value, and the probability density declines monotonically on either side of that maximum, towards a minimum or asymptote at probability density zero. When H_1 is true, the position of the maximum is shifted, usually to a larger value (i.e., to the right), to an extent that reflects the magnitude of the effect, i.e., the departure from H_0. In these circumstances, the population values of fdr(Z_α), Fdr(Z_α) and lim(Fdr(Z_α)), defined by the mathematical form of the distribution of the test statistic, are monotonically related to α and Z_α: these false discovery rates decrease as α is decreased and Z_α increased, as illustrated in Figures 7.4 and 7.5. Moreover, the local FDR is always larger than the corresponding non-local FDR, as intuition suggests it should be: the local FDR has the potential to indicate the value of each 'discovery' on its merits, uninfluenced by those of more significant 'discoveries'.

As a demonstration that the pattern explored in the previous two paragraphs is not specific to the Z statistic, consider the case in which hypotheses are tested by a χ^2 (chi-square) statistic with degrees of freedom (DF) = 5. When H_0 is true, this has the standard χ^2 distribution, with its mean equal to DF, but when H_1 is true, the distribution is shifted to the right, to an extent specified by a *non-centrality parameter* (NCP), so that

$$\text{mean}(\chi^2) = \text{DF} + \text{NCP}. \tag{7.11}$$

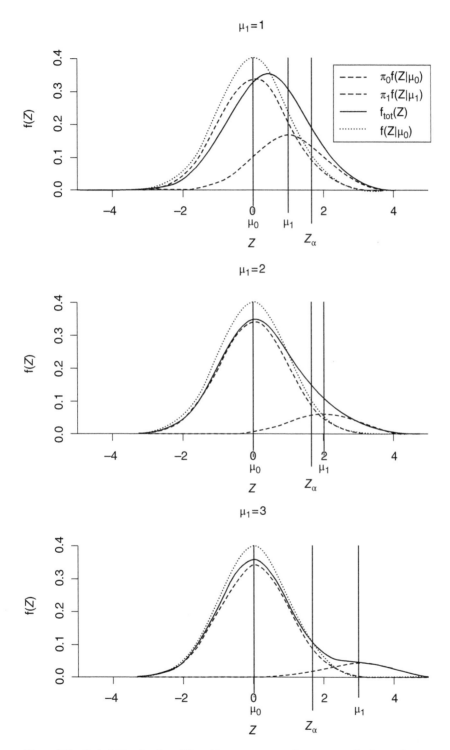

Figure 7.3 Probability density of Z and its components, for a range of values of μ_1.

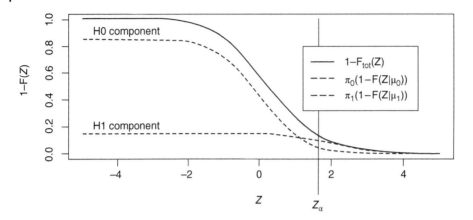

Figure 7.4 Cumulative probability distribution of Z, and its components, for $\mu_1 = 2$, $\pi_1 = 0.15$.

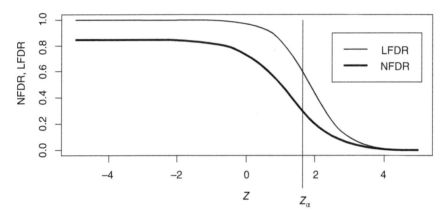

Figure 7.5 The non-local and local FDR as a function of Z, for $\mu_1 = 2$, $\pi_1 = 0.15$.

Hence, on H_0, NCP $= 0$, and we will also consider the alternative case in which on H_1, NCP $= 4$. The two distributions are then as shown in Figure 7.6.

The overall probability density of the test statistic χ^2 is then given by

$$f_{tot}(\chi^2) = \pi_0 \cdot f(\chi_5^2|\text{NCP} = 0) + \pi_1 \cdot f(\chi_5^2|\text{NCP} = 4). \tag{7.12}$$

This probability density function and its two components are shown in Figure 7.7, and the corresponding upper-tail cumulative distributions are shown in Figure 7.8. The local FDR obtained from the probability density functions when $\pi_1 = 0.15$ and the non-local FDR obtained from the corresponding cumulative distributions are shown in Figure 7.9. The basic pattern is the same as that obtained from the Z-statistic.

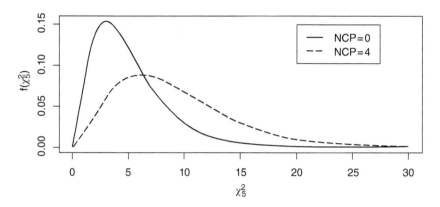

Figure 7.6 The probability density of the χ^2 statistic with DF = 5, on H_0 (non-centrality parameter (NCP) = 0) and H_1 (NCP = 4).

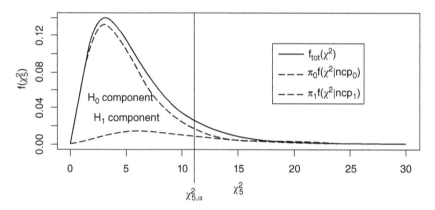

Figure 7.7 Probability density of the test statistic χ^2 (with DF = 5), and its components on H_0 and H_1, for NCP = 4, $\pi_1 = 0.15$.

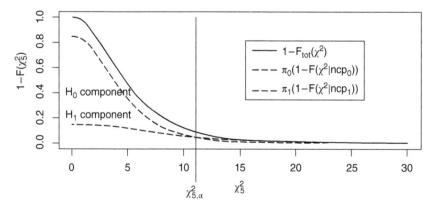

Figure 7.8 Cumulative probability distribution of χ^2 (with DF = 5), and its components, for NCP = 4, $\pi_1 = 0.15$.

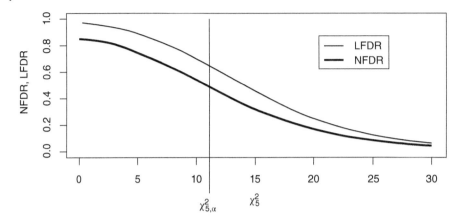

Figure 7.9 Non-local and local FDR as a function of χ^2 (with DF = 5), for NCP = 4, π_1 = 0.15.

7.2 Direct Estimation of the LFDR

To define the LFDR in theory is thus fairly straightforward, but to estimate it in practice is another matter: in a finite family of m p-values, the monotonic relationships described in Section 7.1 are not necessarily conserved. Specification of the numerator for the fraction in Equation (7.3) is achieved by strong theoretical assumptions, namely, the mathematical form of the probability density function $f(Z|\mu = 0)$, and the limiting assumption that π_0 is close to 1. But specification of the denominator, $f_{tot}(Z)$, requires an appropriate value for μ_1, and this is unknown – if indeed such a single value exists. It must be estimated from the data, but such an estimate will not be very precise unless m is very large. The problem is illustrated in Figure 7.10, which shows the distribution of Z-values in a

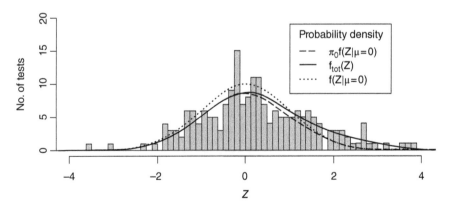

Figure 7.10 Expected and observed mixture distribution of Z in a sample of m = 200 tests from a population with μ_1 = 2, π_1 = 0.15.

sample of $m = 200$, from a 'mixture distribution' in which a proportion $\pi_0 = 0.85$ comes from the distribution

$$Z_0 \sim N(0,1), \tag{7.13}$$

and a proportion $\pi_1 = 1 - \pi_0 = 0.15$ from the distribution

$$Z_1 \sim N(2,1). \tag{7.14}$$

In this plot, each vertical bar represents the observed number of tests giving a Z-value in the corresponding range: the empirical distribution. The dashed, solid and dotted lines represent the corresponding expected (theory-based, population) distributions. For example, if Z follows Distribution (7.13), then, given $m = 200$ and a histogram constructed using 'bins' of width

$$w = 0.125,$$

the expected number of tests giving Z-values in the bin with range $0.250 \leq Z \leq 0.375$ and mid-point $Z = 0.3125$ is

$$
\begin{aligned}
\text{E(No. of tests)} &= \text{No. of tests} \times \text{proportion of distribution in bin,} \\
&\approx m \times \text{probability density} \times w, \\
&= 200 \times \text{f0}(0.3125 | \mu = 0) \times 0.125, \\
&= 200 \times 0.3799 \times 0.125 = 9.50,
\end{aligned}
\tag{7.15}
$$

as indicated by the dotted line. The corresponding vertical bar indicates that the observed number of Z-values in this bin is 11. The empirical distribution in this limited sample is very irregular compared to the population mixture distribution from which the sample was drawn.

An estimated upper bound for fdr(Z) (based on the assumption $\pi_0 = 1$) at the mid-point of each bin is given by

$$\widehat{\text{fdr}(Z)} = \frac{\text{E(count}(Z)|H_0)}{\text{count}(Z)} = \frac{m \cdot f(Z|\mu = 0)}{\text{count}(Z)}, \tag{7.16}$$

where count(Z) = number of Z-values in the bin containing Z, and this 'sample LFDR' is plotted in Figure 7.11. The corresponding 'true' upper-bound value of fdr(Z) in the mixture-distribution population from which the sample was drawn is obtained from Equation (7.3):

$$\text{fdr}(Z) = \frac{f(Z|\mu = 0) \cdot \pi_0}{f_{\text{tot}}(Z)} < \frac{f(Z|\mu = 0)}{f_{\text{tot}}(Z)} = \lim(\text{fdr}(Z)), \tag{7.17}$$

and this 'population LFDR' value ($\lim(\text{fdr}(Z))$) is also plotted. Due to the irregularity of the histogram, the sample gives poor estimates of the population values. Consequently, a larger Z-value (smaller p-value) is often associated with a larger value of $\widehat{\text{fdr}(Z)}$, which cannot occur for the population fdr(Z). Another unsatisfactory feature is that if the number of Z-values in a bin is less than E(count(Z)|H_0), then $\widehat{\text{fdr}(Z)} > 1$. If there are no Z-values in a

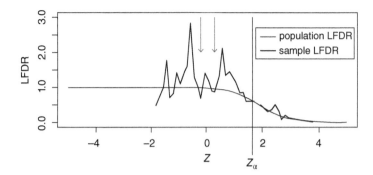

Figure 7.11 Population and estimated sample values of LFDR from $m = 200$ tests with $\mu_1 = 2$, $\pi_1 = 0.15$. Arrows indicate regions with many z-values: see Figure 7.10.

bin, then $\widehat{\text{fdr}(Z)}$ is infinite and is not plotted: this accounts for the gaps in the 'sample LFDR' line in the figure.

7.3 Estimation of the NFDR

In order to smooth out the irregularity of the direct estimate of the LFDR, $\widehat{\text{fdr}(Z_\alpha)}$, we can instead seek an estimate of the NFDR, $\text{Fdr}(Z_\alpha)$, the FDR for the p-value under consideration and all smaller p-values – that is, the average FDR over the range $Z \geq Z_\alpha$. The basis for this approach is the observation that from Equation (7.9) and Inequality (7.10),

$$E\left(\frac{V}{V+S} \middle| Z \geq Z_\alpha, \pi_0\right) = \text{Fdr}(Z_\alpha) < \lim(\text{Fdr}(Z_\alpha)). \tag{7.18}$$

This means that in a finite sample of m p-values, we can obtain a limiting value for the estimate of $\text{Fdr}(Z_\alpha)$ on the basis of the methods used to obtain the BH-FDR criterion. However, the choice of the largest p-value to be considered significant need not be based on controlling the FDR at a pre-specified rate as proposed by Benjamini and Hochberg (1995): the significance threshold may be defined on some other basis, and designated by the usual symbol α. Provided that the tests for which H_0 is true are mutually independent, the equations and inequality corresponding to the BH criterion (Chapter 2, Section 2.4, Equations and Inequalities (2.8)–(2.11)) are

$$E\left(\frac{V}{V+S}\right) = \frac{E(V)}{V+S} = \frac{m_0\alpha}{k} \leq \frac{m\alpha}{k}, \tag{7.19}$$

where

$V =$ number of false-positive conclusions,
$S =$ number of true-positive conclusions,
$m_0 =$ number of tests for which H_0 is true,
$m =$ total number of tests,

and k is the rank of the largest p-value smaller than α, designated $p_{(k)}$. It is important to remember that $\dfrac{m\alpha}{k}$ is not an estimate of $\dfrac{V}{V+S}$ in the usual sense, but an upper boundary on its expected value. An unbiased estimate would be provided by

$$\frac{m_0\alpha}{k} = \frac{m\pi_0\alpha}{k}, \tag{7.20}$$

but this cannot be calculated since π_0 is unknown. However, in situations where H_0 is thought to be true for all but a few of the tests performed, and hence where π_0 is close to 1, $\dfrac{m\alpha}{k}$ provides a useful upper-bound estimate, and we can write

$$\widehat{\text{NFDR}}_{(k)} = \frac{m\alpha}{k}. \tag{7.21}$$

By specifying a series of increasing values of α such that each successive p-value is the largest considered significant, the NFDR value can be estimated for each test, as

$$\widehat{\text{NFDR}}_k = \frac{mp_{(k)}}{k} = \frac{p_{(k)}}{k/m}. \tag{7.22}$$

The corresponding expected (population) value is obtained by substituting k/m for α in Display (7.10) to obtain

$$\lim\left(\text{Fdr}\left(Z_{k/m}\right)\right) = \frac{\left(1 - F\left(Z_{k/m}|\mu = 0\right)\right)}{k/m}. \tag{7.23}$$

These values are plotted for the sample of $m = 200$ tests in Figure 7.12. The line for $\widehat{\text{NFDR}}$ is much smoother than that for $\widehat{\text{LFDR}}$, and follows the corresponding line for the population more closely. It is also much more nearly monotonic, though not quite: there are short regions where a larger Z-value (smaller p-value) is associated with a slightly larger $\widehat{\text{NFDR}}$, indicated by arrows on the figure. These are regions where there are many Z-values (Figure 7.10), and consequently $\widehat{\text{LFDR}}$ is low. The stability of the $\widehat{\text{NFDR}}$–Z relationship,

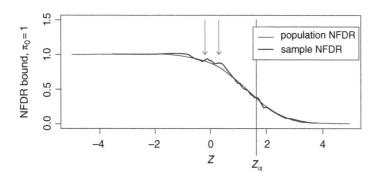

Figure 7.12 Population and estimated sample values of NFDR from $m = 200$ tests with $\mu_1 = 2$, $\pi_1 = 0.15$.

compared to the $\widehat{\text{LFDR}}$–Z relationship, occurs because each value of $\widehat{\text{NFDR}}_k$ draws on information from all the values $p_{(i)}$, $i = 1...k$, not just those in the immediate vicinity of $p_{(k)}$.

7.4 Estimation of the LFDR from the NFDR: Re-Ranking Approach

The desirable properties of the $\widehat{\text{NFDR}}$ suggest a question: Can the relationship between NFDR and LFDR, namely,

$$\text{LFDR}_{(k)} > \text{NFDR}_{(k)} \text{ for all } k, \tag{7.24}$$

be used to predict LFDR from $\widehat{\text{NFDR}}$, rather than seeking to estimate it directly? Bickel (2020, Section 3.3, Chapter 3) suggested a method for doing so, based on the relationship between $p_{(i)}$, $i = 1...m$, and i/m. This is presented for the p-values in the present example, and compared with the corresponding curve derived directly from the known probability distribution from which the p-values were sampled, in Figure 7.13. For the purpose of defining this 'true' curve, i is allowed to take non-integer values, and i/m, referred to as the *quantile rank*, is allowed to cover the whole range $i/m \in [0, m]$ (where the symbol '$\in$' means 'is an

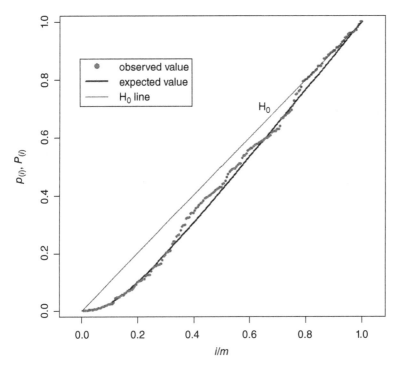

Figure 7.13 Untransformed Q–Q plot for expected and observed ordered p-values ($P_{(i)}$ and $p_{(i)}$) from $m = 200$ tests with $\mu_1 = 2$, $\pi_1 = 0.15$.

element of'). The p-value corresponding to i/m, based on the known distribution, is referred to here as $P_{(i)}$: its derivation is specified more formally in Section 7.5. $p_{(i)}$ and $P_{(i)}$ can be referred to as the sample and population p-values, respectively. (N.B. The meaning of $P_{(i)}$ here is distinct from its meaning in Chapter 2 and in Benjamini and Hochberg (1995). There, it was a random variable, conditional on (i). Here, it is the expected value of the observed or simulated value $p_{(i)}$.) The points on the 'true' curve are then given by the coordinates $\left(\dfrac{i}{m}, P_{(i)}\right)$.

We then have the results

$$\text{NFDR}_{(k)} = \frac{P_{(k)}}{k/m} \tag{7.25}$$

and

$$\text{LFDR}_{(k)} = \frac{dP_{(k)}}{d(k/m)}, \tag{7.26}$$

that is, the local FDR is the gradient of the curve, the rate at which the non-local FDR accumulates as $P_{(i)}$ increases. Since only small p-values are usually of individual interest, say values in the range $0 \le P_{(i)} \le \alpha$, attention can be focused on p-values in the range from 0 to a value *somewhat larger than* α. The task is then to estimate the curve over this range on the basis of the observed p-values, then use it to estimate NFDR and LFDR, rather than using the p-values directly.

Over a sufficiently small range, any smooth curve can be approximated by a quadratic function. In order to use this approach to estimate the local FDR corresponding to $p_{(i)}$ (LFDR$_i$), we need to consider the quadratic curve passing through the points $(0, 0)$ and $\left(\dfrac{2k}{m}, P_{(2k)}\right)$, with a gradient of zero at $(0, 0)$. The curve required is

$$P_{(i)} = \frac{P_{(2k)}}{(2k/m)^2}\left(\frac{i}{m}\right)^2. \tag{7.27}$$

Note that the vertical coordinate of the curve is the *expected* p-value $P_{(i)}$, but that one of the *sampled* p-values, $p_{(2k)}$, contributes to the curve's coefficient. In Figure 7.14, this curve is plotted, together with the true curve for the model specified, over the range

$$i/m \in [0, 2k],$$

where k is chosen so that $p_{(k)}$ is the largest value for which $p_{(k)} < \alpha = 0.05$. The two curves agree fairly well. This quadratic curve has the property that the ratio of its coordinates at the point $\left(\dfrac{2k}{m}, P_{(2k)}\right)$, that is, $\dfrac{P_{(2k)}}{2k/m}$, the gradient of the line OA, is equal to its gradient at the point where its horizontal coordinate is $\dfrac{k}{m}$, that is, the gradient of line BC. That is, the estimate of the *non-local* FDR for the $2k^{\text{th}}$ ranked p-value is also an estimate of the *local* FDR for the kth ranked value – and the non-local basis of this estimate gives it stability.

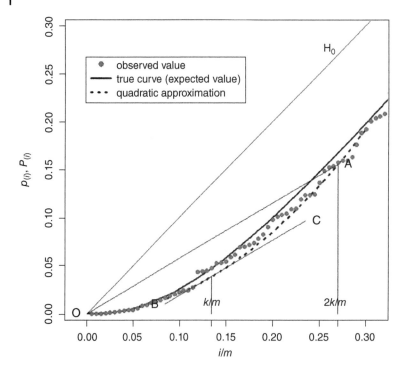

Figure 7.14 Region close to the origin in the Q–Q plot from *m* = 200 tests in Figure 7.13.

This is analogous to arguing that the LFDR for the test at rank i is expected to be the average of all LFDRs for tests from ranks 1 to $2i$, since i lies in the middle of this range. Similarly, one might argue that if an examination candidate's performance is *just* within the top 5%, that person is an *average* member of the set of candidates comprising the top 10%.

The LFDRs corresponding to the smaller half of the m p-values, $p_{(k)}$, $k = 1...m/2$, can be estimated by this method, and in this simulated dataset, in which the true values of μ_1 and π_1 are known, the true LFDR corresponding to each Z-value can also be calculated. The results for the largest and smallest values of m, and some values in the middle of the range, are presented in Table 7.1, and the LFDRs estimated from re-ranking are compared graphically with the corresponding true LFDRs in Figure 7.15. The figure shows that the agreement between the two is good in this particular set of hypothesis-test results: the concordance correlation coefficient between $\widehat{\text{LFDR}}$ from re-ranking and the true LFDR is 0.985. (The concordance correlation coefficient (Lin, 1989) is based on departures from equality between two variables (https://en.wikipedia.org/wiki/Concordance_correlation_coefficient, accessed 13 May 2024), and is therefore more stringent than the commonly used Pearson correlation coefficient, which is based on departures from a more general linear relationship.) However, it should not be assumed that the re-ranking

Table 7.1 Comparison of the true LFDR at rank k with an estimate based on the NFDR at rank $2k$. Arrows indicate the mapping of $\widehat{\text{NFDR}}$ to $\widehat{\text{LFDR}}$.

k	k/m	$p_{(k)}$	True LFDR$_{(k)}$	$2k$	$\widehat{\text{NFDR}}_{(k)}$	$\widehat{\text{LFDR}}_{(k)}$ from reranking
200	1.000	0.999802	1.0000	400	0.9998	—
199	0.995	0.998755	0.9999	398	1.0038	—
198	0.990	0.98842	0.9997	396	0.9984	—
197	0.985	0.980619	0.9996	394	0.9956	—
196	0.980	0.968217	0.9994	392	0.9880	—
⋮					⋮	
105	0.525	0.472657	0.9733	210	0.9003	—
104	0.520	0.461599	0.9719	208	0.8877	
103	0.515	0.447565	0.9699	206	0.8691	
102	0.510	0.440079	0.9687	204	0.8629	
101	0.505	0.437203	0.9683	202	0.8657	
100	0.500	0.426674	0.9666	200	0.8533	0.9998
99	0.495	0.426456	0.9666	198	0.8615	0.9984
98	0.490	0.421912	0.9658	196	0.8610	0.9880
97	0.485	0.421014	0.9656	194	0.8681	0.9923
96	0.480	0.415568	0.9647	192	0.8658	0.9994
⋮					⋮	
10	0.05	0.004077	0.1741	20	0.0815	0.2259
9	0.045	0.003781	0.1669	18	0.0840	0.2086
8	0.04	0.003025	0.1474	16	0.0756	0.1792
7	0.035	0.003007	0.1469	14	0.0859	0.1675
6	0.03	0.002023	0.1177	12	0.0674	0.1461
5	0.025	0.001568	0.1022	10	0.0627	0.0815
4	0.020	0.00076	0.0687	8	0.0380	0.0756
3	0.015	0.000187	0.0329	6	0.0125	0.0674
2	0.010	0.000102	0.0243	4	0.0102	0.0380
1	0.005	0.000068	0.0199	2	0.0136	0.0102

method would work equally well in other sets of hypotheses, with different values of μ_1 and π_1. Moreover, Figure 7.16 confirms that the relationship between LFDR estimated on this basis and $p_{(k)}$ is not quite monotonic, and it is surely undesirable that a hypothesis giving a larger p-value should be preferred over a hypothesis giving a smaller one, on the basis of their estimated LFDRs.

The fit of the relationship between $P_{(i)}$ and $\dfrac{i}{m}$ to a quadratic curve is only approximate, and Bickel (2020) indicated that a more appropriate re-ranking factor than 2 is 1.6. This choice is justified on the basis that $1/(1 - e^{-1}) \approx 1.6$ (D.R. Bickel, personal communication), but the mathematical reasoning that supports this choice is elaborate. Nevertheless, it is

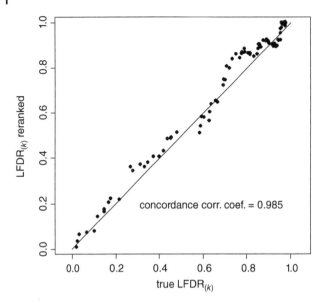

Figure 7.15 LFDR from re-ranking method versus true LFDR, re-ranking factor = 2.

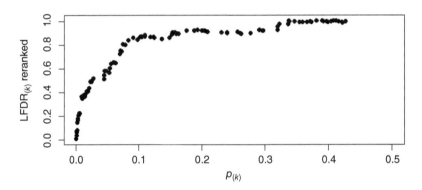

Figure 7.16 LFDR from re-ranking method versus $p_{(k)}$, re-ranking factor = 2.

straightforward to test the relationship proposed by Bickel in practice with simulated data such as the present example. Each value $LFDR_{(k)}$ is estimated by finding the smallest integer greater than $1.6k$, designated 'ceiling($1.6k$)', and using $\widehat{NFDR}_{ceiling(1.6k)}$ as the estimate. The process is illustrated in Table 7.2.

Figure 7.17 shows that the agreement between the estimated and true LFDR is as good as with re-ranking factor = 2, though very little better (concordance correlation coefficient = 0.986). However, Figure 7.18 suggests that the relationship between the LFDR from re-ranking and $p_{(k)}$ may be more nearly monotonic when re-ranking factor = 1.6.

Table 7.2 Comparison of the true LFDR at rank k with an estimate based on the NFDR at rank $1.6k$. Arrows indicate the mapping of $\widehat{\text{NFDR}}$ to $\widehat{\text{LFDR}}$.

k	k/m	$P_{(k)}$	True LFDR$_{(k)}$	$1.6k$	$\widehat{\text{NFDR}}_{(k)}$	$\widehat{\text{LFDR}}_{(k)}$ from reranking
200	1.000	0.999802	1.0000	320	0.9998	—
199	0.995	0.998755	0.9999	319	1.0038	—
198	0.990	0.988420	0.9997	317	0.9984	—
197	0.085	0.980619	0.9996	316	0.9956	—
196	0.980	0.968217	0.9994	314	0.9880	—
195	0.975	0.967463	0.9994	312	0.9923	—
⋮					⋮	
130	0.650	0.588588	0.9850	208	0.9055	—
129	0.645	0.586481	0.9848	207	0.9093	
128	0.640	0.582791	0.9845	205	0.9106	
127	0.635	0.581136	0.9844	204	0.9152	
126	0.630	0.577213	0.9841	202	0.9162	
125	0.625	0.575431	0.9839	200	0.9207	
124	0.620	0.571649	0.9836	199	0.9220	0.9998
123	0.615	0.568287	0.9834	197	0.9240	1.0038
122	0.610	0.561684	0.9828	196	0.9208	0.9956
121	0.605	0.560707	0.9827	194	0.9268	0.9880
						0.9923
⋮					⋮	
10	0.050	0.004077	0.1741	16	0.0815	0.1792
9	0.045	0.003781	0.1669	15	0.0840	0.1750
8	0.040	0.003025	0.1474	13	0.0756	0.1442
7	0.035	0.003007	0.1469	12	0.0859	0.1461
6	0.030	0.002023	0.1177	10	0.0674	0.0815
5	0.025	0.001568	0.1022	8	0.0627	0.0756
4	0.020	0.000760	0.0687	7	0.0380	0.0859
3	0.015	0.000187	0.0329	5	0.0125	0.0627
2	0.010	0.000102	0.0243	4	0.0102	0.0380
1	0.005	0.000068	0.0199	2	0.0136	0.0102

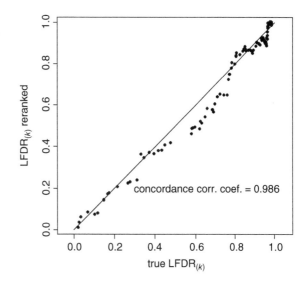

Figure 7.17 LFDR from re-ranking method versus true LFDR, re-ranking factor = 1.6.

concordance corr. coef. = 0.986

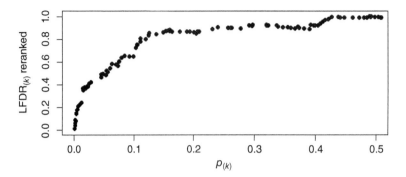

Figure 7.18 LFDR from re-ranking method versus $p_{(k)}$, re-ranking factor = 1.6.

7.5   Estimation of the LFDR from the NFDR: Power Parameter Approach

An alternative approach to relating the local FDR to the non-local FDR is:

- to seek a function that will connect the two at a particular point in the distribution of test-statistic values and *p*-values, rather than
- by re-ranking *p*-values so as to connect different points in the distribution.

An appropriate function (for small *p*-values) can be found if the cumulative distributions of the test statistic on the null and alternative hypothesis are connected by a *power parameter*, as follows.

We consider a test statistic Z, which on H_0 has probability density $f_0(Z)$. (N.B. This is a more concise and general notation than the expression '$(f(Z)|\mu = 0)$' used in Equation (7.2).) Hence, over the region below a specified value Z, its cumulative distribution function (CDF) is

$$F_0(Z) = \int_{-\infty}^{Z} f_0(w)dw. \tag{7.28}$$

$F_0(Z)$ is interpreted as a *p*-value: that is, *lower* values of Z (larger *negative* values if the distribution of Z extends below zero) are more highly significant. For example, if Z is the usual Z-statistic, with the standard normal distribution (7.13) on H_0, then a one-sided test with the alternative hypothesis H_1: $\mu_1 < 0$ is implied, with significant outcomes in the *lower* tail of the distribution. However, the method is quite general: it can be applied to a test statistic with significant values in its upper tail, such as χ^2 or F, by specifying $Z = -\chi^2$ or $Z = -F$, respectively.

Now suppose that on the alternative hypothesis H_1 the CDF is

$$F_1(Z) = F_0(Z)^{\alpha}, \tag{7.29}$$

where

$$\alpha < 1,$$

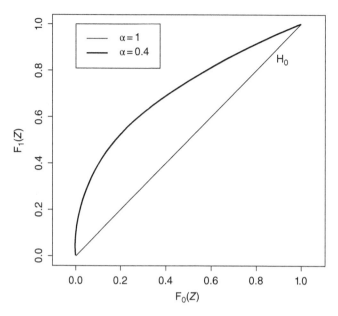

Figure 7.19 Cumulative probability distribution of a test statistic Z on H_1 (power parameter $\alpha = 0.4$) versus H_0 ($\alpha = 1$).

as illustrated in Figure 7.19. (N.B. In this context, the symbol 'α' does *not* represent a significance threshold: this parameter affects the shape of the function $F_1(Z)$ across its entire range. The symbol is used for consistency with the notation of Efron (2005).) The probability density on H_1 is then given by

$$f_1(Z) = \frac{dF_1(Z)}{dZ} = \frac{dF_0(Z)^\alpha}{dZ} = \frac{dF_0(Z)^\alpha}{dF_0(Z)} \cdot \frac{dF_0(Z)}{dZ} = \alpha F_0(Z)^{\alpha-1} f_0(Z). \tag{7.30}$$

This relationship between $f_1(Z)$ and $f_0(Z)$ has the effect of shifting the distribution of Z on H_1 to the left, relative to the distribution on H_0, as shown in Figure 7.20. It is analogous to the shift from $\mu = 0$ to $\mu > 0$ in Section 7.1 (Distribution (7.1)), though in that case the shift was to the right, as H_1 increased the frequency of large values of Z, and values in the upper tail of the distribution of Z were classified as significant in the one-sided test.

These relationships between $F_0(Z)$, $F_1(Z)$, $f_0(Z)$ and $f_1(Z)$, as a function of α, provide the basis for finding a relationship between the non-local and local FDR at Z, also as a function of α (Efron 2005). This relationship is obtained as follows (G.Q. Cai, personal communication), referring to the non-local and local FDR at Z as Fdr(Z) and fdr(Z), respectively.

By the definition of Fdr(Z) and from Equation (7.29),

$$\frac{\text{Fdr}(Z)}{1 - \text{Fdr}(Z)} = \frac{\pi_0 F_0(Z)}{\pi_1 F_1(Z)} = \frac{\pi_0 F_0(Z)}{\pi_1 F_0(Z)^\alpha}, \tag{7.31}$$

and similarly by the definition of fdr(Z),

$$\frac{\text{fdr}(Z)}{1 - \text{fdr}(Z)} = \frac{\pi_0 f_0(Z)}{\pi_1 f_1(Z)}. \tag{7.32}$$

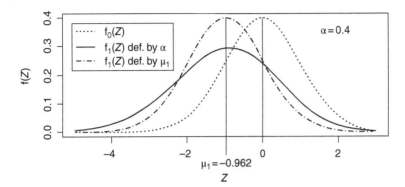

Figure 7.20 Probability density of a test statistic Z on H_0 and on H_1. The H_0 probability density ($f_0(Z)$) is $Z \sim N(0, 1)$. The H_1 probability density ($f_1(Z)$) is related to ($f_0(Z)$) either by the power parameter α or by the corresponding value of μ_1 (i.e., the distributions on H_1 obtained by the two specifications have the same mean value, μ_1).

Substituting Equation (7.30) into Equation (7.32),

$$\frac{\text{fdr}(Z)}{1-\text{fdr}(Z)} = \frac{\pi_0 f_0(Z)}{\pi_1 \alpha F_0(Z)^{\alpha-1} f_0(Z)} = \frac{\pi_0 F_0(Z)}{\pi_1 F_0(Z)^\alpha} \cdot \frac{1}{\alpha}, \tag{7.33}$$

and substituting Equation (7.31) into Equation (7.33),

$$\frac{\text{fdr}(Z)}{1-\text{fdr}(Z)} = \frac{\text{Fdr}(Z)}{1-\text{Fdr}(Z)} \cdot \frac{1}{\alpha}. \tag{7.34}$$

In the extreme left-hand tail of the distribution of Z, in the limit, as $\text{Fdr}(Z) \to 0$, $\text{fdr}(Z) \to 0$, and Equation (7.34) approaches

$$\text{fdr}(Z) = \text{Fdr}(Z) \cdot \frac{1}{\alpha}, \tag{7.35}$$

giving a simple relationship between the local and non-local FDRs. If we are uneasy about applying the limits $\text{Fdr}(Z) \to 0$ and $\text{fdr}(Z) \to 0$ simultaneously, Equation (7.34) can be rearranged to give

$$\text{fdr}(Z) = \frac{\text{Fdr}(Z)}{\alpha + (1-\alpha)\text{Fdr}(Z)}. \tag{7.36}$$

Then applying $\text{Fdr}(Z) \to 0$ only, we obtain Equation (7.35).

To explore these relationships empirically, we can consider the case where Z is the standard Z-statistic, with values in the *left-hand* tail considered significant, $\pi_1 = 0.3$ (a rather large value, chosen to give a clear visual illustration of the concepts) and hence $\pi_0 = 0.7$, and $\alpha = 0.4$. The values of $\pi_0 f_0(Z)$, $\pi_1 f_1(Z)$ and

$$f_{\text{tot}}(Z) = \pi_0 f_0(Z) + \pi_1 f_1(Z) \tag{7.37}$$

are then as shown in Figure 7.21.

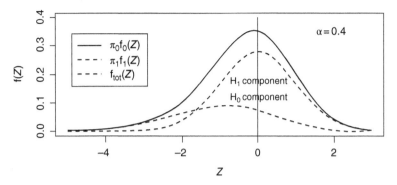

Figure 7.21 Probability density of the test statistic Z, and its components on H_0 and H_1, connected by the power parameter α, with $\pi_1 = 0.3$.

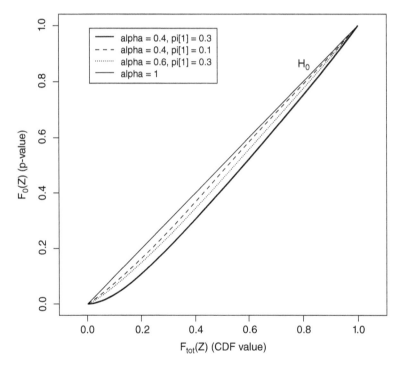

Figure 7.22 Untransformed Q–Q plot for the test statistic Z with its distribution on H_0 and H_1 connected by the power parameter α, for a range of values of α and π_1.

We can now obtain the corresponding untransformed Q–Q plot, by plotting $F_0(Z)$ versus $F_{tot}(Z)$, giving a curve of the familiar shape shown in Figure 7.22. As before, the local FDR (fdr(Z)) at any p-value is the gradient at the corresponding point on this curve, and the non-local FDR (Fdr(Z)) is the slope of a line connecting the corresponding point on the curve to the origin. A larger value of α, or a smaller value of π_1, brings the curve closer to the H_0 line, that is, brings the distribution of p-values closer to that expected on the null hypothesis.

A few more technical points about the relationship between $F_0(Z)$ and $F_{tot}(Z)$ are worth noting. For any given realisation of Z, taken from the mixture distribution with probability density $f_{tot}(Z)$ specified in Equation (7.37), $F_0(Z)$ is the p-value, that is, the observed quantile of the Uniform(0, 1) distribution, while $F_{tot}(Z)$ is the CDF value, which is the expected quantile of the Uniform(0, 1) distribution on H_0. If $F_{tot}(Z) = i/m$ in a finite family of m tests, then $F_0(Z) = P_{(i)}$, the expected ordered p-value at the quantile rank i/m.

On this basis, we can explore the values of fdr(Z) and Fdr(Z), and the relationship between them, over the whole range of the CDF of Z, $F_{tot}(Z)$, from 0 to 1: this is done in Figure 7.23. As expected, fdr(Z) and Fdr(Z) both increase monotonically at larger CDF values, and fdr(Z) is always larger than Fdr(Z), so that the ratio Fdr(Z)/fdr(Z) is always less than 1. This figure also shows that

$$\mathrm{Fdr}(Z)/\mathrm{fdr}(Z) \approx \alpha$$

at very small quantiles (small p-values), and

$$\mathrm{Fdr}(Z) = \pi_0 = 1 - \pi_1,$$

not a function of α, at very large quantiles (p-values close to 1). However, there is no simple, near-constant proportional relationship between fdr(Z) and Fdr(Z) on the basis of α or π: The ratio Fdr(Z)/fdr(Z) varies widely over the range of quantiles.

It is instructive to compare this plot with that obtained when $f_1(z)$ is defined, not by the relationship in Equation (7.29), but by the relationship

$$Z|H_0 \sim N(0, 1), \tag{7.38}$$

$$Z|H_1 \sim N(\mu_1, 1), \tag{7.39}$$

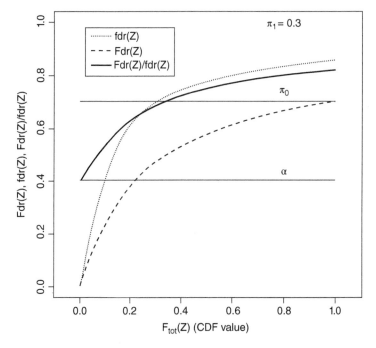

Figure 7.23 LFDR and NFDR values, and the NFDR/LFDR ratio, for the power-parameter-based test statistic Z, versus the cumulative probability of Z, when $\alpha = 0.4$, $\pi_1 = 0.3$.

which was considered (using slightly different notation) in Section 7.1 (Distribution (7.1)), with the specification $\mu_1 = -0.962$, which is the value of mean(Z) when $\alpha = 0.4$. This function is shown, together with that given in Equation (7.29), in Figure 7.20. Although the distributions $f_{tot}(Z)$ with $f_1(Z)$ defined by α and μ_1 have the same mean value, the distribution with $f_1(Z)$ defined by α is broader and flatter, with a longer *lower* tail, that is, a larger proportion of highly significant values. The effect of this difference on fdr(Z), Fdr(Z) and the Fdr(Z)/fdr(Z) ratio is seen by comparing Figure 7.23 and Figure 7.24. The ratio again varies widely over the quantiles, but in a very different range, from close to 1 for very small quantiles (small p-values), to values approaching $(1 - \pi_1) = \pi_0 = 0.7$ for very large quantiles (p-values close to 1). Once again there is no simple, near-constant proportional relationship between fdr(Z) and Fdr(Z).

The success of the re-ranking approach for estimating the local FDR on the basis of the non-local FDR is assessed for the case in which the distributions on H_0 and H_1 are related by the power parameter α (Equation (7.29)), for different combinations of values of α and π_1, in Figure 7.25a, and for the case in which the distributions are related by μ_1 (Distributions (7.38) and (7.39)) in Figure 7.25b. In both cases, estimation of fdr(Z) by Fdr(Z) at $2 \times$ the quantile gives a good approximation, particularly at small p-values. However, all the scenarios explored in panels (a) and (b) of Figure 7.25 relate to moderate values of α and μ_1. If the value of α is close to zero, so that extreme negative values of Z are common on H_1, then the re-ranking method works less well, especially if π_1 is large (Figure 7.26a,b).

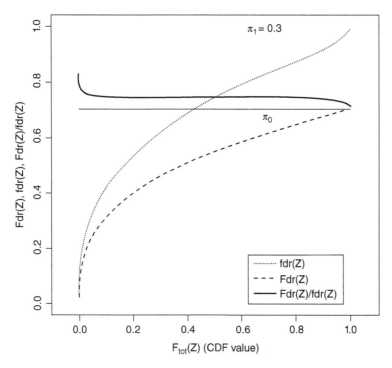

Figure 7.24 LFDR and NFDR values, and the NFDR/LFDR ratio, for the normal-distribution-based test statistic Z, versus the cumulative probability of Z, when $\mu_1 = -0.962$, $\pi_1 = 0.3$.

(a)

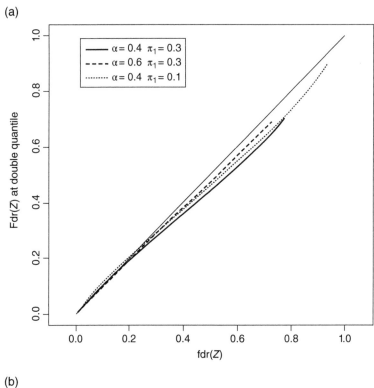

(b)

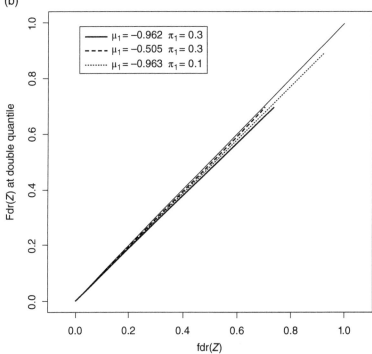

Figure 7.25 LFDR obtained from re-ranking (Fdr(Z) at double quantile) versus true LFDR (fdr(Z)), non-extreme values of α. (a) Distribution defined by α. (b) Distribution defined by corresponding μ_1.

(a)

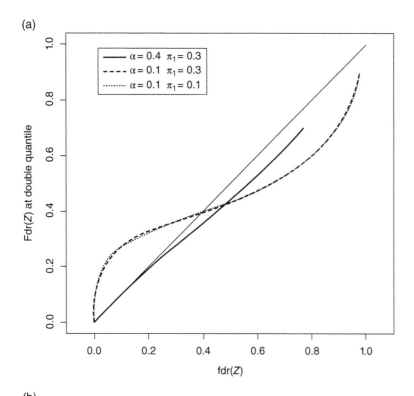

(b)

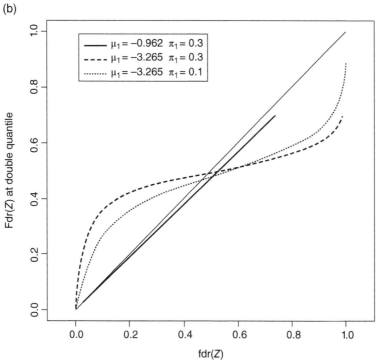

Figure 7.26 LFDR obtained from re-ranking (Fdr(Z) at double quantile) versus true LFDR (fdr(Z)), extreme values of α. (a) Distribution defined by α. (b) Distribution defined by corresponding μ_1

7.6 Review of Methods for Estimation of the LFDR

Direct estimates of the LFDR, as described in Section 7.2, are too unstable to be of practical use except in very large families of significance tests (i.e., very large values of m), and in such cases they will be vulnerable to concerns about mis-specification of the null distribution, as explored in Chapter 8. As regards methods for estimation of the LFDR based on the NFDR, the re-ranking approach, with the ranks related by a factor of 2, works better in the explorations presented here than does the power-parameter approach based on relationships at the same rank (same value of the CDF). However, the re-ranking approach is found not to be reliable in all circumstances, and it must not be forgotten that in practice its accuracy will be reduced by random variation, and that this may introduce non-monotonicity into the LFDR versus p-value relationship.

A more robust approach to eliminating the stochastic variation in estimates of the LFDR is simply to use the NFDR directly, accepting that it gives only a relative measure of the strength of the evidence from each p-value. However, even this does not eliminate the stochastic variation altogether. Therefore, the relationship between $\widehat{\text{NFDR}}_k$ and $p_{(k)}$ is not necessarily monotonic: that is, there may still be regions of the distribution of the p-values in which smaller p-values are associated with larger NFDR estimates. Such a relationship should not occur for the true NFDR values associated with any well-behaved significance test statistic, provided that the distribution of the test statistic, within the family of m tests under consideration, is unimodal on H_1 as well as on H_0. (It is possible to construct cases in which there are local minima and maxima in the LFDR, for example, if the test statistic is bimodal on H_1, but such a scenario seems unrealistic.)

Avoidance of such non-monotonic patterns is surely a key consideration when choosing between hypotheses for further investigation, so for this purpose it is perhaps best to stick to the BH criterion. The fact that this criterion gives only a relative indication of the local FDR may not matter, and the relationship between $p_{(i)}$ and $q_{(i)}$ is always at least non-negative (as illustrated in Chapter 3, Section 3.2), if not always strictly monotonically positive. And the BH-FDR does give an absolute measure of the strength of the evidence from the *set of* p-values to which it relates. If an estimate of the absolute value of the local FDR is called for – but only in this situation – one may then turn to the re-ranked FDR.

7.7 Summary

The BH criterion for controlling the FDR has been criticised on the basis that it gives equal status to all the p-values within the selected set.

Alternative criteria are introduced, namely, the local and non-local FDR (LFDR and NFDR).

The LFDR is the FDR relating to an individual value of a test statistic Z.

The NFDR is the FDR relating to the set of p-values that meet a specified significance criterion, such as $Z > Z_\alpha$, where α is the significance threshold.

A connection is made between the specification of LFDR and NFDR in relation to the distribution of Z (fdr(Z) and Fdr(Z), respectively), and the FDR as specified in relation to the confusion matrix (Display (2.5) in Chapter 2, Section 2.3).

For a test statistic with distribution $Z \sim N(\mu, 1)$ (where $\mu = 0$ on H_0), the relationship between π_1 (the proportion of tests for which H_1 is true), μ_1 (the value of μ on H_1) and Fdr(Z) is explored. Small values of Fdr(Z) can be due to large values of π_1, large values of μ_1, or both. Combinations of π_1 and μ_1 that control the FDR at the same value, lim(Fdr(Z_a)), for a given value of α, are identified.

However, it is noted that although lim(Fdr(Z_a)) is the same for the scenarios presented, Fdr(Z_a), the actual average FDR over the significant range of Z, differs considerably depending on the value of π_1.

The relationships between Z, fdr(Z) and Fdr(Z), explored for $Z \sim N(\mu, 1)$, are common to other test statistics that have a similar distribution, namely, a single maximum on H_0, the location of which is shifted, usually to a larger value, on H_1.

For such a test statistic:

- fdr(Z_a), Fdr(Z_a) and lim(Fdr(Z_a)) decrease as α is decreased and Z_a increased.
- fdr(Z_a) is always larger than the corresponding value of Fdr(Z_a).

The χ^2 distribution with DF $= 5$ is used to illustrate the generality of these relationships.

The method for estimating the LFDR directly from a family of m p-values is illustrated, with simulated data from $m = 200$ tests using the test statistic $Z \sim N(\mu, 1)$.

The method depends on counting the Z-values in each of a large number of narrow histogram 'bins', so is highly vulnerable to stochastic variation. Specifically:

- a smaller p-value is often associated with a larger value of $\widehat{fdr}(Z)$,

- if the number of Z-values in a bin is less than E(count(Z)|H_0), then $\widehat{fdr}(Z) > 1$, and

- if there are no Z-values in a bin, then $\widehat{fdr}(Z)$ is infinite and is not plotted.

The NFDR is estimated using the same approach as for the BH-FDR criterion. However, the choice of the largest p-value to be considered significant need not be based on control of the FDR at a pre-specified rate.

In the simulated data, the estimate of NFDR varies much more smoothly over the range of Z than does the estimate of LFDR, and follows the true value more closely.

A more stable estimate of LFDR is sought by a re-ranking approach. It is argued that for small values of i, corresponding to $0 \leq P_{(i)} \leq \alpha$ (where $P_{(i)}$ is the expected value of $p_{(i)}$), it can be expected that LFDR$_{(i)} \approx$ NFDR$_{(2i)}$.

The re-ranking approach can be justified by arguing that in the region $i/m \in [0, 2k]$, where k is chosen so that $p_{(k)}$ is the largest value for which $p_{(k)} < \alpha$, the relationship between $P_{(i)}$ and i/m is approximately a quadratic curve passing through the points $(0, 0)$ and $\left(\dfrac{2k}{m}, P_{(2k)}\right)$. LFDR$_{(k)}$ is then estimated by the gradient of this curve at the point where its horizontal coordinate is $\dfrac{k}{m}$, which is $\dfrac{P_{(2k)}}{2k/m}$, that is, the estimate of NFDR$_{(2k)}$.

This is analogous to arguing that the LFDR for the test at rank i is expected to be the average of all LFDRs for tests from ranks 1 to $2i$, since i lies in the middle of this range.

Empirical exploration of the re-ranking approach in the sample of simulated p-values, with the re-ranking factor 2, indicates that it performs fairly well in this case. The concordance correlation coefficient between $\widehat{\text{LFDR}}$ and true LFDR is 0.985, and the relationship between $\widehat{\text{LFDR}}_{(k)}$ and $p_{(k)}$ is nearly, though not quite, monotonic.

Bickel (2020) indicated that a more appropriate re-ranking factor than 2 is 1.6. Empirical exploration with this factor gives a marginally higher concordance correlation coefficient (0.986) and a slightly more nearly monotonic $\widehat{\text{LFDR}}_{(k)}$ versus $p_{(k)}$ relationship.

An alternative approach to relating the LFDR to the NFDR is to assume that the distributions of the test statistic on H_0 and H_1 are related by a power parameter α. The test statistic is represented by Z, its distribution on H_0 unspecified, but the cumulative distribution function (CDF) on H_0 represented by $F_0(Z)$. The CDF on H_1 is then specified as $F_1(Z) = F_0(Z)^\alpha$, $\alpha < 1$. $F_0(Z)$ is interpreted as a p-value: that is, *small* values of Z (larger *negative* values if the distribution of Z extends below zero) are considered significant.

It can then be shown that as $\text{Fdr}(Z) \rightarrow 0$, $\text{fdr}(Z) \rightarrow \text{Fdr}(Z) \cdot \dfrac{1}{\alpha}$.

This relationship is explored empirically for the case in which on H_0, $Z \sim N(0, 1)$, $\pi_1 = 0.3$ $\alpha = 0.4$. The untransformed Q–Q plot is presented, and it is confirmed that a larger value of α, or a smaller value of π_1, brings the curve representing the expected observations closer to the H_0 line.

The relationship between $\text{fdr}(Z)$ and $\text{Fdr}(Z)$ is explored graphically over the range of the CDF of Z $(0 \leq F_{\text{tot}}(Z) \leq 1)$. $\dfrac{\text{Fdr}(Z)}{\text{fdr}(Z)}$ is found to vary greatly, and to approach α only at very small values of $F_{\text{tot}}(Z)$.

When $F_1(Z)$ is defined as indicated earlier in this summary, the mean value of $Z|H_1$ is -0.962. The relationships between $\text{fdr}(Z)$, $\text{Fdr}(Z)$ and $F_{\text{tot}}(Z)$ are therefore explored with the specification $Z|H_1 \sim N(\mu_1, 1)$, where $\mu_1 = -0.962$, for comparison with the specification $F_1(Z) = F_0(Z)^\alpha$, where $\alpha = 0.4$. Once again $\dfrac{\text{Fdr}(Z)}{\text{fdr}(Z)}$ varies greatly, and with this specification, it does not approach α when $F_{\text{tot}}(Z)$ is small. It seems that the power-parameter approach is unlikely to be reliable for the practical estimation of $\text{fdr}(Z)$.

The success of the re-ranking approach, with re-ranking factor 2, is assessed graphically when the distributions of the test statistic on H_0 and H_1 are related by the power parameter α or by μ_1, for different values of these parameters and of π_1. The approach works well with moderate values of α, μ_1 and π_1. However, for values of α close to zero and values of μ_1 far from zero, especially with large values of π_1, the method works less well.

None of the methods for estimating the LFDR is entirely satisfactory. It may therefore be better simply to use the NFDR directly, accepting that it gives only a relative measure of the strength of the evidence from each p-value.

However, $\widehat{\text{NFDR}}_{(k)}$ is susceptible to stochastic variation (though less so than $\widehat{\text{LFDR}}_{(k)}$), and there may still be regions of the distribution of the p-values in which smaller p-values are associated with larger NFDR estimates.

It is therefore perhaps best to stick to the BH criterion when choosing between hypotheses for further investigation. The fact that this criterion gives only a relative indication of the local FDR may not matter, and the relationship between $p_{(i)}$ and $q_{(i)}$ is always at least non-negative, if not always strictly monotonically positive.

If an estimate of the absolute value of the local FDR is called for – but only in this situation – one may then turn to the re-ranked FDR.

References

Benjamini, Y. and Hochberg, Y. (1995). Controlling the false discovery rate: a practical and powerful approach to multiple testing. *Journal of the Royal Statistical Society B* 57: 289–300.

Bickel, D.R. (2020). *Genomic Data Analysis. False Discovery Rates and Empirical Bayes Methods.* Boca Raton, Florida: CRC Press 121 pp.

Efron, B. (2005). *Local False Discovery Rates.* Document not formally published but available from https://www.efron.ckirby.su.domains/papers/2005LocalFDR.pdf (accessed 13 May 2024).

Lin, L.I. (1989). A concordance correlation coefficient to evaluate reproducibility. *Biometrics* 45: 255–268. https://doi.org/10.2307/2532051. JSTOR 2532051. PMID 2720055.

8

The FDR in Relation to an 'Uninteresting' Rather Than a Null Hypothesis

8.1 The Vulnerability of the FDR to Mis-Specification of the Statistical Model

In considering the problems that occur when significance tests are applied to the very large datasets produced by high-throughput technology, we have so far focused on the inevitable production of large numbers of false-positive results if p-values are interpreted using a conventional significance criterion (typically the threshold level $\alpha = 0.05$), and the excessive number of false-negative results obtained if a Bonferroni-type correction is applied (i.e., a threshold such as α/m, where m is the number of tests). However, significant p-values obtained from 'big data' can be an inappropriate guide to conclusions and further investigation, even when they are, formally speaking, true-positives. This can occur in two ways:

- When a single significance test is performed on a very large number of observations (large n), even a slight departure from the H_0 statistical model, of no practical interest, can lead to a highly significant result.
- When a very large number of significance tests are performed (large m), but each is based on a small number of observations from the same set of sampling units (small n), a slight departure in the distribution of the p-values on H_0 from that assumed in the statistical model – a departure too small to be noticed in the result of a single test – can cause a clear perturbation in the distribution of the large set of p-values to be considered.

The causes that can give rise to either type of phenomenon include:

- a weak association between the explanatory variable and the response, perhaps not related to any causal connection between them, or
- a distribution of residual variation that departs slightly from the formal distribution on H_0 for the statistical model fitted (here referred to as the formal null distribution), for example, slight departure from a normal distribution with constant variance.

It may seem perverse to test many hypotheses on a small set of sampling units, but this situation commonly occurs in genomics and other biological disciplines using high-throughput automated technology, when samples are obtained from a small number of

The False Discovery Rate: Its Meaning, Interpretation and Application in Data Science, First Edition.
N.W. Galwey.
© 2025 John Wiley & Sons Ltd. Published 2025 by John Wiley & Sons Ltd.
Companion website: www.wiley.com/go/falsediscoveryrate

valuable donors, and many gene-expression or biomarker variables can readily be measured in each sample.

8.2 'Uninteresting' and 'Interesting' Distributions of Test Results Versus Distributions on H_0 and H_1: A Defence Against Model Mis-Specification

The problem of small departures from the formal null distribution, which become important because n is small and m is large, was considered by Efron (2004), who proposed a modification of the FDR approach in which the distinction between the distributions of test results on H_0 and H_1 is replaced by a distinction between *Uninteresting* and *Interesting* distributions of test results. If an appropriate 'Uninteresting' distribution of test results can be identified, it can be used in place of the formal null distribution on H_0, and the rest of the methods relating to local and non-local FDRs can be used as before. The problem, then, is to identify such a distribution. Efron argued that the large-scale hypothesis testing situation that creates the problem of numerous false or uninteresting 'discoveries' also offers its solution, because an appropriate distribution can be identified from the data themselves:

> In classic situations involving only a single hypothesis test, one must, out of necessity, use the theoretical null hypothesis [which in the case under consideration is] $Z \sim N(0, 1)$. [However,]... large-scale testing situations permit empirical estimation of the null distribution.

Efron explored this approach in the context of two observational studies:

- A study of more than a thousand patients with human immunodeficiency virus (HIV) infection, testing association between exposure to six protease inhibitor (PI) drugs and frequency of mutation at 74 sites on the viral genome, giving $6 \times 74 = 444$ tests.
- A study using microarrays to assay the expression of more than 3000 genes in 15 breast cancer patients, seven of whom carried a harmful mutation in the gene BRCA1, and eight of whom carried a harmful mutation in BRCA2. (Both mutations increase breast-cancer risk.)

In both studies, there is reason to doubt that the standard null hypothesis is precisely appropriate. In the HIV study, a separate univariate logistic model was fitted to each PI drug–genome site combination, meaning that when exposure to each drug was considered, the possible effects of the others on the mutation-frequency response were not taken into account. If exposure to another drug is associated with exposure to the drug under consideration, either because patients who take one tend also to take the other, or because they tend to avoid it, this may cause unmeasured confounding, and a spurious association between the drug in question and mutation frequency at one of the sites (the first type of phenomenon noted in Section 8.1). Even if exposure to the other drug is unassociated with exposure to the drug under consideration, it may nevertheless cause the patients who take it to have a similar mutation-frequency response to each other, effectively reducing the number of independent observations contributing to the model fit (the second type of phenomenon).

In the breast cancer study there was evidence, from the data, of non-independence of gene expression levels between the microarrays in the BRCA2 patient group, again effectively reducing the number of independent observations. Efron observed that 'the microarray experiment, for all its impressive technology, is still an observational study, with a wide range of unobserved covariates possibly distorting the BRCA1–BRCA2 comparison.' Fifteen individuals is a small number on which to conduct a statistical test, particularly when the levels of the explanatory variable under consideration have not been assigned by a formal randomisation process but have been determined by nature: the testing of a large number of hypotheses may distract a researcher from this constraint, but does not alter it.

8.3 An 'Uninteresting' Distribution to Account for Unrecognised Pseudoreplication: Fewer Discoveries Announced

Efron (2004) used the results from these large sets of tests to seek to identify appropriate 'Uninteresting' distributions of test statistics. Here, the complementary approach will be taken: statistical models that correspond to the 'Uninteresting' and 'Interesting' hypotheses will be specified, and simulated data will be produced from these models. The success of different methods of analysis in identifying those tests for which the 'Interesting' hypothesis is true will then be assessed and compared.

We start by considering 16 sampling units (e.g., human individuals, biological cell cultures or manufactured items in a quality control process), of which eight have been exposed to some influence (e.g., a disease or experimental treatment) and the other eight are unexposed. Many continuous numerical response variables have been measured on each sampling unit, and each variable may or may not be influenced by the exposure. Thus, the structure of the data for a single response variable (the ith response) is as shown in Table 8.1.

For each response variable, the sample size is too small to support an elaborate statistical model, and the possible effect of the exposure will be explored by a simple t test, with an assumption that the variance of the response is homogeneous in the two exposure groups, perhaps after a suitable transformation, for example, from the original scale to a logarithmic scale.

Table 8.1 Structure of data in an experiment comprising 16 sampling units, to determine the effect of an exposure of interest on each of m response variables.

	Sampling unit															
	1	2	3	4	5	6	7	8	9	10	11	12	13	14	15	16
Exposure (U = unexposed E = exposed)	U	U	U	U	U	U	U	U	E	E	E	E	E	E	E	E
Value of ith response variable	y_{i1}	y_{i2}	y_{i3}	y_{i4}	y_{i5}	y_{i6}	y_{i7}	y_{i8}	y_{i9}	y_{i10}	y_{i11}	y_{i12}	y_{i13}	y_{i14}	y_{i15}	y_{i16}

Our simple initial null-hypothesis model is that the 16 observations of each individual response variable are sampled from the same normal distribution: that is, y_{ij}, the observation of the ith response variable on the jth sampling unit, comes from the distribution

$$Y_{ij} \sim N(\mu_i, \sigma_i).$$

This model can also be written as

$$Y_{ij} = \mu_i + E_{ij},$$

where

$$E_{ij} \sim N(0, \sigma_i).$$

It indicates that the responses of the sampling units are not influenced by the exposure, or by any other factor that some of them have in common. However, note that the different response variables (different values of i) do not necessarily have the same mean or variance over the sampling units.

Simulated observations are here generated from this model for $m = 2000$ response variables, for which μ_i, $i = 1...m$, is a realisation of a variable with distribution N(20, 1), and

$$\sigma_i = \sqrt{\frac{\chi^2_{3,i}}{3}},$$

where $\chi^2_{3,i}$ is a realisation of a variable with a chi-square distribution with three degrees of freedom. This ensures that for large values of m, the average value of σ_i^2 over the m variables approaches 1. The data for the first and last few response variables are presented in Table 8.2.

The t test is used to test the null hypothesis,

H_0: no effect of exposure,

against the one-sided alternative,

H_1: exposure increases the response,

for each response variable. A Q–Q plot of the p-values obtained (Figure 8.1) confirms that their distribution is approximately Uniform(0, 1), as is expected in the present case, when H_0 is true for every test. An alternative method for comparing the observed and expected distributions of the p-values is given by transforming them to the corresponding values of the standard normal variable,

$$Z \sim N(0, 1). \tag{8.1}$$

If

$$\Phi(z_{ij}) = P(Z < z_{ij}) = 1 - p_{ij},$$

then z_{ij}, the value of Z corresponding to p_{ij}, is obtained using the inverse of the function Φ: that is,

$$z_{ij} = \Phi^{-1}(1 - p_{ij}). \tag{8.2}$$

Table 8.2 Simulated data for $m = 2000$ normally distributed response variables, to compare 16 sampling units, of which eight are exposed to a stimulus and eight unexposed. In these simulated data, H_0 (no effect of exposure) is true for every variable. The exact simulated values have 5 places of decimals: they are presented here to one place, for conciseness.

	Sampling unit															
	1	2	3	4	5	6	7	8	9	10	11	12	13	14	15	16
Exposure	U	U	U	U	U	U	U	U	E	E	E	E	E	E	E	E
Response variable																
1	21.4	22.0	21.3	22.0	21.7	21.9	22.4	21.1	21.7	22.2	22.0	21.6	21.0	21.6	21.6	21.6
2	20.1	22.1	21.7	21.9	22.7	21.0	19.3	22.7	21.6	22.0	22.6	21.1	20.9	22.2	20.5	21.5
3	20.5	17.1	19.5	17.4	19.3	19.5	20.1	18.9	17.9	18.4	19.2	17.6	19.6	19.6	19.2	18.3
4	19.9	20.1	20.1	19.9	18.9	19.6	19.4	19.5	20.0	19.8	19.3	19.1	20.2	20.2	19.2	19.3
5	18.4	19.6	18.2	19.7	17.6	18.8	19.4	19.5	20.2	17.6	17.8	19.1	19.0	17.9	19.8	17.4
⋮																⋮
1996	21.5	20.2	18.8	17.8	19.1	20.6	20.0	19.9	19.1	16.7	20.4	24.1	22.1	21.5	22.8	19.2
1997	20.5	18.8	21.2	21.0	22.2	20.6	19.1	18.2	20.1	22.1	21.1	21.9	22.1	18.9	21.0	20.7
1998	19.6	21.5	21.0	20.8	22.0	21.6	22.4	22.9	19.3	22.8	22.0	20.6	22.2	20.8	18.6	21.7
1999	21.2	21.6	20.4	21.7	22.5	19.3	22.8	20.7	20.9	23.4	21.0	24.0	21.4	21.6	22.3	20.7
2000	20.9	23.2	21.7	21.3	22.1	21.9	22.4	22.4	22.8	21.1	24.1	22.4	22.2	20.8	22.3	21.7

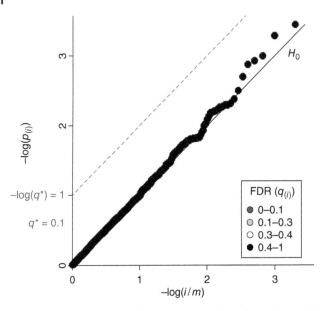

Figure 8.1 Q–Q plot, on the $-\log_{10}$ scale, of p-values obtained from $m = 2000$ tests when H_0 is true for every test and the assumptions of the model are correct.

In the present case, with p-values obtained from a t test with $16 - 2 = 14$ degrees of freedom (DF), this is nearly the same thing as transforming the p-values back to the t-values from which they were derived, but not quite: the standard normal distribution (Distribution (8.1)) is different from the t distribution unless the DF are infinite. Distribution (8.1) is used in preference to the t distribution to remove this dependence on DF, and for the sake of familiarity. The distribution of Z-values can then be presented in a histogram, and compared with the distribution expected on H_0, namely, Distribution (8.1), scaled to take account of the $m = 2000$ tests. In the present case (Figure 8.2), the fit is good, as expected.

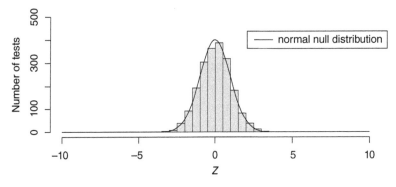

Figure 8.2 Histogram of Z-values obtained from $m = 2000$ tests when H_0 is true for every test and the assumptions of the model are correct. The solid line indicates the expected distribution on H_0, namely, Distribution (8.1) scaled to m.

Our choice of H_1 indicates that we anticipate only that exposure may increase each response, not that it may decrease it. But now suppose that there is some other influence, affecting some of the sampling units but not others, which may increase some responses but decrease others. For example, it may have been necessary to process the sampling units in four batches. Suppose also that – perhaps unwisely, perhaps unavoidably – all the unexposed units were allocated to Batches 1 and 2, and all the exposed units to Batches 3 and 4.

Such batch effects are here simulated by specifying dummy variables, X_1... X_4:

- X_1 with the value 1 for each sampling unit in Batch 1 and value 0 for all other units,
- X_2 with the value 1 for each sampling unit in Batch 2 and value 0 for all other units,

etc., as shown in Table 8.3.

The m response variables are now assumed to be a random sample from an infinite population of possible response variables, and the effect of batch is zero on average over all response variables, but varies from one response variable to another, and from batch to batch within each response variable. Its distribution is modelled as

$$\theta_{ik} \sim N(0, \sigma_\theta), \tag{8.3}$$

where θ_{ik} is the effect of being in the kth batch, $k = 1...4$, on the ith response variable, and σ_θ indicates how widely the batch effects vary. The model that generates the simulated data is then

$$Y_{ij} = \mu_i + \theta_{i1}X_{1j} + \theta_{i2}X_{2j} + \theta_{i3}X_{3j} + \theta_{i4}X_{4j} + E_{ij}$$

Data from this model are here simulated with the specification $\sigma_\theta = 2.4$.

Now suppose that the data are analysed by a researcher who is unaware of the distribution of the sampling units among processing batches (a situation that is not as rare in practice as it should be – for a discussion of the issue of avoidable and often unrecognised confounding, in the context of genome-wide association studies (GWAS), see Lambert and Black (2012)). When the same t test as before is performed on each response variable, the resulting Q–Q plot (Figure 8.3) indicates many more significant results, at whatever threshold α is chosen, than are expected on H_0. However, note that as well as the departure

Table 8.3 Specification of dummy variables to indicate the allocation of sampling units to batches.

	Sampling unit															
	1	2	3	4	5	6	7	8	9	10	11	12	13	14	15	16
Exposure	U	U	U	U	U	U	U	U	E	E	E	E	E	E	E	E
Batch	1	1	1	1	2	2	2	2	3	3	3	3	4	4	4	4
X_1	1	1	1	1	0	0	0	0	0	0	0	0	0	0	0	0
X_2	0	0	0	0	1	1	1	1	0	0	0	0	0	0	0	0
X_3	0	0	0	0	0	0	0	0	1	1	1	1	0	0	0	0
X_4	0	0	0	0	0	0	0	0	0	0	0	0	1	1	1	1

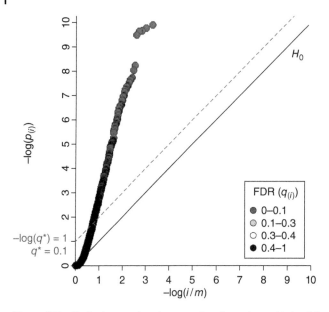

Figure 8.3 Q–Q plot, on the $-\log_{10}$ scale, of p-values obtained from m = 2000 tests when H_0 is true for every test but unrecognised pseudoreplication is present.

of the plotted points from the H_0 line at large values of $-\log(p)$, there is also a slight twist in the distribution of the plotted points at small values of $-\log(p)$, close to the origin. Comparison of the histogram of Z-values with the standard normal distribution (Distribution (8.1)) (Figure 8.4) offers further insight into the distribution of these test results. Large positive *and negative* values of Z are much more common than expected by chance. This is because the t test is based on the assumption that the data for each response comprise 16 *independent* observations of a normal variable, whereas in fact they comprise four groups of observations, the observations within each group being similar to each other. Consequently, large mean differences between the exposed and unexposed groups occur more often than

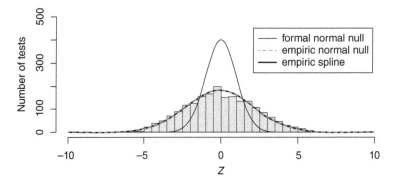

Figure 8.4 Histogram of Z-values obtained from m = 2000 tests when H_0 is true for every test but unrecognised pseudoreplication is present.

expected, because there is less opportunity for large positive and negative values to cancel out. In the limiting case, if the four observations of the same response variable within each batch were always identical (i.e., $E_{ij} \sim N(0, 0)$), the observations from the 16 samples would be equivalent to four independent observations, two from exposed and two from unexposed units. (See Chapter 2, Section 2.8 for a fuller exploration of this situation.) Therefore, the test for the effect of exposure produces many large t-values, positive or negative, depending on the directions of the batch effects for the response variable in question, and the histogram of Z-values is wider and flatter than the standard normal distribution. But because a one-sided test was conducted, only the large positive t-values result in a significant p-value: the large negative t-values produce unexpectedly *large* p-values, and it is these that produce the twist close to the origin in the Q–Q plot.

This situation is referred to as *pseudoreplication*. Its defining features are:

- the sampling units are treated as if they were independent, but
- in fact they belong to groups, within each of which there is a positive correlation between the observations, unrelated to the exposure or treatment of interest, and
- the members of each group share the same value of the exposure or treatment;
- hence, the n units are equivalent to a smaller number of independent units.

If only one or a few response variables were studied (small m), it would probably not be possible to detect the batch effects from the response-variable data themselves, and they could only be incorporated into the statistical analysis if external information about the allocation of units to batches was available. However, in the large-scale testing situation, examination of the pattern of correlations between the n units, over the $m = 2000$ response variables, can reveal such patterns. If these correlations are calculated between the uncentred variables, that is, the variables $Y_j, j = 1...n$, as recorded, they are heavily influenced by the variation in $\mu_i, i = 1...m$, and are all positive (Table 8.4). However, if they are *centred* by subtracting the mean value in each row, $\bar{y}_{i.}$, from every value in the row, $y_{ij}, j = 1...n$, a different pattern emerges (Table 8.5). The values from sampling units 1...4 are strongly positively correlated with each other: likewise those from units 5...8, 9...12 and 13...16. That is, there are strong positive correlations among units allocated to the same batch. Note that there are also moderate *negative* correlations between the values from sampling units in different batches (the correlations in the off-diagonal 4×4 blocks in the table: for example, between Units 1 and 5, or Units 10 and 15), even though the batch effects contributing to these values were specified to be independent in the simulation process. This is because the correlation coefficients are determined not by the *true* batch effects for the four batches, which may all be positive for a particular response variable, but by their *estimates*, which are required to sum to zero: if the estimate for one batch is positive, then that for at least one other batch must be negative.

Such a pattern indicates that even if H_0 is true in every case with regard to the exposure under investigation, it cannot be expected that the p-values from t tests will be uniformly distributed. There *are* real differences between the exposure groups, relative to the formal distribution of the t statistic on H_0, but they are not necessarily due to the exposure – nor should this be expected, if the data are not obtained from a formally randomised experiment. Exposure to the influence of interest may be related to the pattern of other influences on the sampling units. The pattern in the correlation matrix suggests that it would be

Table 8.4 Correlations between sampling units over $m = 2000$ response variables, uncentred, when H_0 is true for all tests and pseudoreplication is present. Correlations between units in the same batch are highlighted.

Batch	Unit	1	2	3	4	5	6	7	8	9	10	11	12	13	14	15	16
1	1	1.000															
	2	0.856	1.000														
	3	0.857	0.862	1.000													
	4	0.862	0.868	0.862	1.000												
2	5	0.082	0.096	0.090	0.091	1.000											
	6	0.079	0.094	0.083	0.089	0.871	1.000										
	7	0.082	0.097	0.079	0.093	0.866	0.869	1.000									
	8	0.092	0.108	0.100	0.092	0.871	0.878	0.883	1.000								
3	9	0.115	0.124	0.111	0.113	0.124	0.134	0.130	0.123	1.000							
	10	0.118	0.119	0.115	0.110	0.123	0.124	0.125	0.118	0.884	1.000						
	11	0.124	0.129	0.123	0.125	0.121	0.122	0.126	0.121	0.881	0.886	1.000					
	12	0.120	0.121	0.114	0.117	0.131	0.138	0.141	0.135	0.879	0.877	0.876	1.000				
4	13	0.128	0.136	0.127	0.135	0.145	0.151	0.134	0.144	0.084	0.080	0.070	0.088	1.000			
	14	0.114	0.131	0.131	0.144	0.130	0.134	0.119	0.132	0.096	0.087	0.086	0.089	0.866	1.000		
	15	0.119	0.134	0.124	0.135	0.131	0.135	0.125	0.125	0.091	0.082	0.076	0.085	0.858	0.863	1.000	
	16	0.131	0.134	0.136	0.149	0.151	0.153	0.143	0.157	0.096	0.091	0.082	0.093	0.871	0.867	0.863	1.000
Batch		1				2				3				4			
Unit		1	2	3	4	5	6	7	8	9	10	11	12	13	14	15	16

Table 8.5 Correlations between sampling units over $m = 2000$ response variables, each variable centred over the sampling units, when H_0 is true for all tests and pseudoreplication is present. Correlations between units in the same batch are highlighted.

Batch	Unit	1	2	3	4	5	6	7	8	9	10	11	12	13	14	15	16
1	1	1.000															
	2	0.796	1.000														
	3	0.800	0.804	1.000													
	4	0.805	0.811	0.804	1.000												
2	5	-0.317	-0.313	-0.310	-0.318	1.000											
	6	-0.326	-0.320	-0.324	-0.324	0.809	1.000										
	7	-0.317	-0.310	-0.325	-0.313	0.803	0.807	1.000									
	8	-0.311	-0.302	-0.303	-0.322	0.809	0.819	0.828	1.000								
3	9	-0.272	-0.273	-0.281	-0.286	-0.288	-0.278	-0.279	-0.297	1.000							
	10	-0.263	-0.276	-0.271	-0.286	-0.285	-0.287	-0.281	-0.299	0.829	1.000						
	11	-0.255	-0.261	-0.259	-0.265	-0.289	-0.292	-0.281	-0.296	0.825	0.833	1.000					
	12	-0.268	-0.281	-0.280	-0.284	-0.281	-0.274	-0.266	-0.281	0.821	0.819	0.818	1.000				
4	13	-0.244	-0.246	-0.248	-0.246	-0.249	-0.244	-0.265	-0.257	-0.340	-0.340	-0.356	-0.336	1.000			
	14	-0.260	-0.250	-0.239	-0.229	-0.268	-0.267	-0.283	-0.272	-0.319	-0.326	-0.328	-0.332	0.805	1.000		
	15	-0.248	-0.242	-0.244	-0.238	-0.262	-0.261	-0.270	-0.274	-0.322	-0.329	-0.337	-0.333	0.794	0.802	1.000	
	16	-0.250	-0.261	-0.247	-0.236	-0.253	-0.253	-0.263	-0.251	-0.334	-0.336	-0.350	-0.341	0.810	0.805	0.800	1.000
Batch		1				2				3				4			
Unit		1	2	3	4	5	6	7	8	9	10	11	12	13	14	15	16

appropriate to replace the formal null distribution (Distribution (8.1)) with an empirically identified 'Uninteresting' distribution of Z-values, as proposed by Efron.

The next step towards doing so is to fit a smooth curve to the histogram of Z-values. The curve used is a *spline*, consisting of a series of polynomial functions, estimated piecewise from the data over a series of adjacent ranges of the Z-values, and joined at *knot-points* at the boundaries of the ranges (see, for example, Perperoglou et al. 2019. In addition, 'A Very Gentle Introduction to Splines' is available at https://joshua-nugent.github.io/splines/, accessed 14 May 2024). Efron (2004) fitted a spline to the histogram counts using Poisson regression, but here, an appropriate spline is obtained directly from the Z-values, using the statistical software R (R Core Team 2020), the R package 'logspline' and the function logspline(). The curve obtained is very sensitive to the maximum number of knot-points specified: specification of the argument value 'maxknots = 4' (i.e., five knot-points, defining four adjacent regions between knot-points) is found to give a reasonable fit in the present case, following the shape of the histogram fairly closely, without overfitting (i.e., without following every local variation in the height of the histogram bars).

This smoothing spline is then used as a tool to identify more appropriate values of the mean (δ_0) and standard deviation (σ_0) of the 'Uninteresting' distribution than the values $\delta_0 = 0$ and $\sigma_0 = 1$ in Distribution (8.1), while retaining the normal-distribution form. This spline function is defined as f(Z), and the mean of the 'Uninteresting' distribution is estimated by the value of Z at which f(Z) reaches its maximum,

$$\delta_0 = \text{argmax}(f(Z)).$$

In the present case, the fitted spline gives

$$\delta_0 = -0.10.$$

To obtain the estimate of σ_0, use is made of the relationship between the standard deviation of a normally distributed variable and its second differential at its maximum, namely, that if

$$Z \sim N(\delta_0, \sigma_0), \tag{8.4}$$

then

$$\left(\frac{d^2 \log(f(Z))}{dZ^2}\right)_{\delta_0} = \frac{-1}{\sigma_0^2}. \tag{8.5}$$

The smoothing spline is too irregular for its second differential to be reliably estimated directly from the second differences (differences of differences) of the values around its maximum, for substitution into this equation. However, $\log(f(Z))$ can be approximated by a quadratic curve in the region around the maximum (say, in the range $\delta_0 - 1.5 \leq Z \leq \delta_0 + 1.5$), and the parameters of this curve can be estimated by fitting the ordinary least squares regression model

$$\log(f(z_i)) = a_0 + a_1 z_i + a_2 z_i^2 + e_i$$

in this range. The second differential of this curve is $2a_2$, and substituting this into Equation (8.5) and rearranging, we obtain

$$\sigma_0 = \frac{1}{\sqrt{-2a_2}}.$$

(Note that, provided the quadratic curve has a maximum, a_2 will be negative and hence $-2a_2$ will be positive.) Applied to the present data, this process yields

$$\log(f(z_i)) = -1.71174828 - 0.01987111z_i - 0.10429790z_i^2 + e_i,$$

whence

$$\sigma_0 = \frac{1}{\sqrt{2 \times 0.10429790}} = 2.189511.$$

The variable

$$Z \sim N(-0.10, 2.190)$$

is converted to the scale of the histogram bars, namely,

$$\text{vertical coordinate} = mw \cdot f(Z), \tag{8.6}$$

where

$$w = \text{width of histogram bin}$$

and

$$f(Z) = \text{probability density of } Z \text{ as defined in Distribution (8.4).}$$

If superimposed on the histogram, Distribution (8.4) agrees closely with the empirical spline from which it was obtained (the heavy solid curve in Figure 8.4), and therefore is not separately displayed. It fits the histogram much better than does the formal null distribution.

If information about the allocation of sampling units to batches is available, and the presence of batch effects is suspected, there is an alternative to this empirical, 'Uninteresting'-distribution approach: the statistical analysis can be extended from a simple t test to a 'correct' regression model that takes batch effects into account. If at least one batch contains both exposed and unexposed units, then the model

$$\text{response} \sim \text{batch} + \text{exposure} \tag{8.7}$$

(expressed in the notation of Wilkinson and Rogers 1973) can be fitted. However, when only one level of exposure occurs within each batch, this model is overparameterised: when all the differences between the four batches have been accounted for, there is no variation left for the 'exposure' term to explain. Batch and exposure effects are then said to be *partially aliased* (see NIST/SEMATECH 2012, Chapter 5, Section 5.7, A Glossary of DOE Terminology, for further information on this concept). In order to estimate both batch and exposure effects in this situation, it is necessary to specify 'batch' as a random-effect model term in a *mixed model*: that is, a model containing both fixed- and random-effect terms. This is expressed by the following extension of the notation:

$$\text{response} \sim \text{exposure} + (1 \mid \text{batch}) \tag{8.8}$$

(For an explanation of the distinction between fixed- and random-effect model terms, see, for example, Galwey (2014, Chapters 1 and 2), and for the notation used here to distinguish between these types of term, see Galwey (2014, Section 3.16).)

This model is now fitted to each response variable. When a regression model contains a fixed-effect term with only two levels, the significance of this term can be tested by a

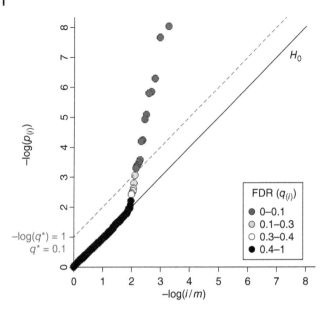

Figure 8.5 Q–Q plot, on the $-\log_{10}$ scale, of p-values obtained from $m = 2000$ tests when H_0 is true for every test and pseudoreplication is accounted for in the fitted model.

t statistic, which is used in the same way as that from a simple t test. In the present case, the one-sided p-value corresponding to the t statistic for each response variable is obtained, and these p-values are used to produce a Q–Q plot and a histogram of Z-values, as before (Figures 8.5 and 8.6). These show that the results now agree closely with H_0, except for a relatively small number of tests giving very small p-values, which are conspicuous on the Q–Q plot but barely detectable on the histogram. More detailed exploration of the numerical results (not presented here) shows that these are an artefact, resulting from the way in which the function lmer(), in the R package 'lme4', fits the mixed model. In cases where the batch effects are by chance very small, relative to the residual within-batch variation, the standard calculations to estimate the batch variance component would result in a negative value. But lmer() does not allow this, and sets the estimate to zero, and

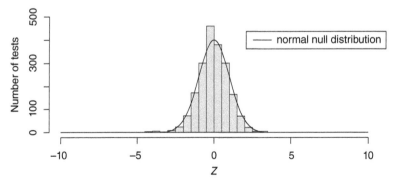

Figure 8.6 Histogram of Z-values obtained from $m = 2000$ tests when H_0 is true for every test and pseudoreplication is accounted for in the fitted model.

reduces the estimate of the residual variance correspondingly. The standard error of the exposure effect ($SE_{Exposure}$) normally includes a component due to the batch variance component, which is recognised as being estimated with some uncertainty. In the absence of this component, $SE_{Exposure}$ is based solely on the reduced residual variance. This biases the t statistic upwards (when the estimated exposure effect is positive), and biases the p-value downwards. In these cases, it can be argued that the p-values in relation to the 'Uninteresting' distribution are preferable to those from the 'correct' model. Taking this artefact into account, the apparent effects of exposure are entirely explained by the batch effects.

When this empirical approach to the identification of an 'Uinteresting' distribution is applied to data from real experiments or observational studies, causal effects of the exposure variable are usually expected or hoped to be present. Indeed, the reason for limiting the quadratic curve-fitting step to the region around the maximum is to minimise the influence of such effects on the estimated 'Uninteresting' distribution. The next step is to explore the results of the empirical approach when such effects are present.

8.4 Unrecognised Pseudoreplication: Results When Real Effects Are Present

We now extend the data-simulation process, specifying that the exposure has a causal effect on some of the response variables, and that in most cases this effect increases the response in each exposed sampling unit. We simulate such effects by specifying that they occur in 10% of the response variables (that is, $\pi_1 = 0.1$), and that for each of these variables, the causal exposure effect (specified as θ_{iExp} for the ith variable) is a realisation of a random variable with the distribution

$$\theta_{iExp} \sim N\left(\theta_{Exp}, \sigma_{Exp}\right). \tag{8.9}$$

We specify $\theta_{Exp} = 7$, $\sigma_{Exp} = 2.4$: that is, the effect of exposure on nearly every response variable is positive, though there may be a few extreme cases (a few values of i) in which it is negative. We specify an additional dummy variable, X_{Exp}, to indicate whether each sampling unit is unexposed or exposed, as shown in Table 8.6. The model from which the data are simulated is then

$$Y_{ij} = \mu_i + \theta_{iExp}X_{Expj} + \theta_{i1}X_{1j} + \theta_{i2}X_{2j} + \theta_{i3}X_{3j} + \theta_{i4}X_{4j} + E_{ij}.$$

When the simple t test is performed on each response variable in these data, the Q–Q and histogram obtained (Figures 8.7 and 8.8) clearly indicate the presence of these exposure effects. The points in the Q–Q plot lie even further above the H_0 line than before (in

Table 8.6 Specification of a dummy variable to indicate the exposure status of each sampling unit.

	Sampling unit															
	1	2	3	4	5	6	7	8	9	10	11	12	13	14	15	16
Exposure	U	U	U	U	U	U	U	U	E	E	E	E	E	E	E	E
X_{Exp}	0	0	0	0	0	0	0	0	+1	+1	+1	+1	+1	+1	+1	+1

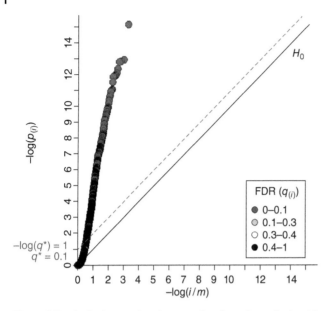

Figure 8.7 Q–Q plot, on the $-\log_{10}$ scale, of p-values obtained from $m = 2000$ tests when H_1 is true for a proportion $\pi_1 = 0.1$ of tests and unrecognised pseudoreplication is present.

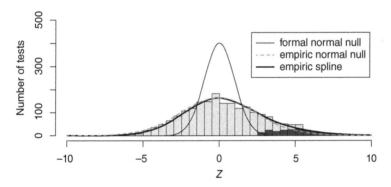

Figure 8.8 Histogram of Z-values obtained from $m = 2000$ tests when H_1 is true for a proportion $\pi_1 = 0.1$ of tests and unrecognised pseudoreplication is present.

Figure 8.3), and the histogram has a long upper tail, comprising the Z-values from those response variables that have large positive estimated exposure effects. The sampling units for which H_1 is true are now represented by a dark grey component in each histogram bar, while those for which H_0 is true are represented by light grey as before, confirming that former are mostly in the upper tail. (However, note that this information would not be available in a real study: it can only be shown because the results come from simulated data, generated by a known mechanism.) But it is clear that besides this directional effect of exposure, there is something else going on: the histogram is much wider, in both directions, and flatter, than is expected from the formal null distribution. The batch effects are still at work.

Again, inspection of the correlations between the n units, over the $m = 2000$ response variables, after centring, is revealing (Table 8.7). The positive correlations between variables

Table 8.7 Correlations between sampling units over $m = 2000$ response variables, each variable centred over the sampling units, when H_1 is true for a proportion $\pi_1 = 0.1$ of the tests and pseudoreplication is present. Correlations between units in different batches but at the same exposure level are highlighted.

Batch	Unit	1	2	3	4	5	6	7	8	9	10	11	12	13	14	15	16
1	1	1.000															
	2	0.836	1.000														
	3	0.840	0.843	1.000													
	4	0.843	0.848	0.843	1.000												
2	5	−0.053	−0.050	−0.039	−0.050	1.000											
	6	−0.064	−0.061	−0.054	−0.059	0.848	1.000										
	7	−0.061	−0.056	−0.059	−0.054	0.843	0.846	1.000									
	8	−0.053	−0.048	−0.039	−0.059	0.848	0.856	0.862	1.000								
3	9	−0.406	−0.407	−0.418	−0.420	−0.426	−0.415	−0.413	−0.429	1.000							
	10	−0.397	−0.407	−0.408	−0.417	−0.420	−0.420	−0.413	−0.429	0.859	1.000						
	11	−0.392	−0.396	−0.399	−0.402	−0.425	−0.425	−0.414	−0.428	0.856	0.861	1.000					
	12	−0.398	−0.409	−0.413	−0.414	−0.415	−0.407	−0.398	−0.412	0.851	0.850	0.849	1.000				
4	13	−0.398	−0.400	−0.407	−0.402	−0.408	−0.402	−0.416	−0.412	−0.077	−0.081	−0.092	−0.082	1.000			
	14	−0.415	−0.407	−0.403	−0.393	−0.426	−0.423	−0.434	−0.427	−0.054	−0.064	−0.063	−0.072	0.848	1.000		
	15	−0.402	−0.397	−0.404	−0.396	−0.419	−0.416	−0.421	−0.425	−0.061	−0.072	−0.076	−0.079	0.839	0.846	1.000	
	16	−0.404	−0.413	−0.407	−0.395	−0.412	−0.409	−0.416	−0.407	−0.071	−0.077	−0.086	−0.084	0.852	0.848	0.844	1.000
Batch		1				2				3				4			
Unit		1	2	3	4	5	6	7	8	9	10	11	12	13	14	15	16

representing units in the same batch are stronger than ever. The pattern of the negative correlations is somewhat changed: those between units in different batches, but at the same exposure level (the correlations in the off-diagonal 4 × 4 blocks in the top-left and bottom-right quarters of the table, that is, of Units 1...4 with Units 5...8 and of Units 9...12 with Units 13...16), are weakened, whereas those between units in different batches and at different exposure levels (the off-diagonal 8 × 8 block in the bottom-left quarter of the table, that is, of Units 1...8 with Units 9...16) are stronger than ever. Nevertheless, though weaker, the negative correlations between batches within the same exposure level are still present: the batch effects are still detectable, and empirical identification of an 'Uninteresting' distribution may be helpful.

An empirical spline is therefore fitted to the histogram as before, giving the heavy solid line in Figure 8.8, and this spline clearly reflects the long upper tail in the data. An 'Uninteresting' normal distribution is identified by the same process as before, giving the dashed line in Figure 8.8, and this line, now distinguishable from the empirical spline, is also wider than the formal null distribution. However, like the formal null distribution, it is symmetrical: it is derived from the central portion of the histogram, excluding the long upper tail, and is required to be symmetrical by its normal (Gaussian) form.

The next step is to estimate the local FDR for the Z-value at the mid-point of each bin in the histogram, by comparing the null- or 'Uninteresting'-distribution probability density with the observed count for the bin, using Equation (8.6) to relate the probability density to the height of the corresponding histogram bar. Figure 8.9 presents the relationship between the estimated LFDR and Z based on the formal null distribution of Z derived from theory, the 'Uninteresting' distribution, and the true distribution in the cases in which H_0 is true in this particular family of m tests. Note that in regions where the vertical coordinate of

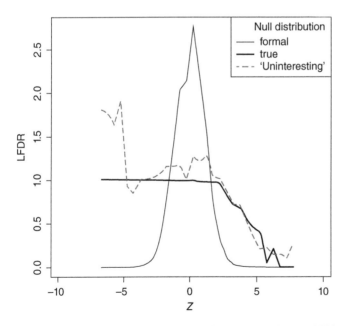

Figure 8.9 LFDR values, estimated on different bases, for m = 2000 tests when H_1 is true for a proportion π_1 = 0.1 of tests and pseudoreplication is present.

the null or 'Uninteresting' probability density is above that of the histogram bar, the estimated LFDR is greater than one. Although the true LFDR cannot exceed one, such estimates are presented unchanged, so as to make clear their contribution to the calculation of the estimated NFDR (to be considered shortly).

There is considerable irregularity in the LFDR estimates due to stochastic variation, but some patterns are clear. The LFDR estimate based on the formal null distribution has a strong maximum around $Z = 0$, corresponding to the tall peak of the formal null distribution in this region: the observed number of Z-values is here much lower than expected. Perversely, on the left-hand side of this peak, smaller one-sided p-values are associated with larger values of LFDR. The LFDR estimate based on the 'Uninteresting' distribution also has a peak around $Z = 0$, but also has high values at large negative values of Z. This is because the long upper tail of the histogram forces this symmetrical distribution also to be wider on the left-hand side. Some Z-values are predicted by the 'Uninteresting' distribution in this region, but few occur. The true LFDR is of course never greater than 1, and is close to this value around $Z = 0$ and at all negative values of Z. Only at large positive values of Z does the true LFDR fall much below 1, and this is expected, because the mean exposure effect is positive in those cases in which H_1 is true.

The key finding is that overall, the estimated LFDR based on the 'Uninteresting' distribution follows the pattern of the true LFDR much more closely than does the estimated LFDR based on the formal null distribution.

The non-local FDR is then obtained for mid-point Z-value of each histogram bin, as the average of the local FDRs for all mid-point Z-values greater than or equal to the one in question, for each method of calculating the LFDR (Figure 8.10). It is important to remember that the estimates of NFDR are based on the expected count in each histogram column

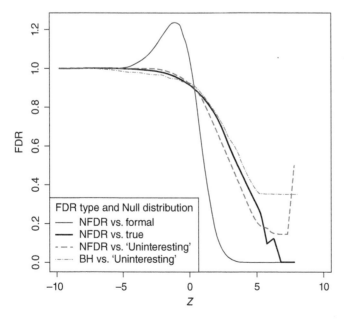

Figure 8.10 NFDR values, estimated on different bases, for m = 2000 tests when H_1 is true for a proportion π_1 = 0.1 of tests and pseudoreplication is present.

when $\pi_1 = 0$, whereas in fact $\pi_1 = 0.1$. Therefore, the true values of NFDR are multiplied by $(1 - 0)/(1 - 0.1) = 1.11$ for plotting in Figure 8.10, to obtain values directly comparable with the corresponding estimates. (If this adjustment were not made, true and estimated NFDR values would not converge to the same asymptote of 1 at extreme negative values of Z.) As expected, the NFDRs are much less irregular than the LFDRs, the stochastic variation being smoothed out by the summation. The NFDR estimate based on the formal null distribution has a strong maximum around $Z = 0$, like the corresponding LFDR. However, this is eliminated in the NFDR estimate based on the 'Uninteresting' distribution, which fits more nearly to the broader peak of the histogram (Figure 8.8). At and above $Z = 0.75$, the 'Uninteresting' distribution gives consistently higher NFDR values than the formal null distribution: because the 'Uninteresting' distribution is wider, it indicates that more of the 'discoveries' reported in this range are false-positives. At large values of Z, the NFDR on either basis falls towards zero: nearly all the 'discoveries' reported in this range are true-positives.

As in the case of the LFDR, the NFDR based on the 'Uninteresting' distribution follows the pattern of the true NFDR much more closely than does the NFDR based on the formal null distribution.

As noted in Chapter 7, Sections 7.1 and 7.4, the LFDR of a given test, unlike the NFDR, is not biased downwards, and made anti-conservative, by dependence on information from other, more significant test results. This is an attractive feature, but it comes at a high price in irregularity due to stochastic variation, and also in non-monotonicity. The NFDR is more stable, but can also have regions of non-monotonicity, where the data are scarce (in the present example, where Z is very large) or where the test results are in the 'wrong' direction (in the present example, where Z is negative). This leads one back to the BH-FDR, which, if it does not always get smaller as p-values get smaller, at least never gets larger. It is then natural to ask whether the BH-FDR can be calculated on the basis of the 'Uninteresting' distribution rather than the formal null distribution, and the answer is that it can.

To obtain BH-FDR values on the basis of the 'Uninteresting' distribution, this distribution is used in the same way that the formal null distribution is routinely used in the calculation of a p-value. That is, the value of the test statistic Z is noted for each hypothesis, and the corresponding cumulative distribution function (CDF) value of the 'Uninteresting' distribution, $F_{\text{Uninteresting}}(Z)$, is obtained. (See Chapter 7, Section 7.5, for an introduction to the CDF.) The value $(1 - F_{\text{Uninteresting}}(Z))$ is then taken as a 'p-value', just as the equivalent proportion of the formal null distribution would be. The set of 'p-values' obtained in this way from the full set of hypotheses is then used as input for the calculation of BH-FDR values in the usual way (Chapter 3, Section 3.2). The BH-FDR values obtained in this way are also presented in Figure 8.10. They generally agree well with the true NFDR, and the NFDR estimated relative to the 'Uninteresting' distribution, over most of the range of Z, though they substantially overestimate the true value at large values of Z where the data are sparse.

The Q–Q plot produced by the BH-FDR values obtained using the 'Uninteresting' distribution is presented in Figure 8.11. It shows that many tests give FDR values above the H_0 line – but not nearly so far above it as when the BH-FDRs were obtained using the formal null distribution (Figure 8.7). In the present example, use of the 'Uninteresting' distribution would not allow any test results to be announced as significant while controlling the FDR at $q^* = 0.1$.

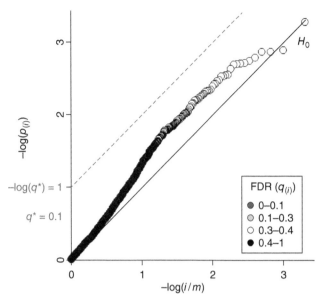

Figure 8.11 Q–Q plot, on the $-\log_{10}$ scale, of p-values obtained from the m = 2000 tests presented in Figure 8.7, on the basis of the 'Uninteresting' distribution instead of the formal null distribution. H_1 is true for a proportion π_1 = 0.1 of tests and unrecognised pseudoreplication is present.

It is important to keep in mind that the empirical 'Uninteresting' distribution is only able to improve the estimation of the FDR because all real exposure effects are specified to be in the same direction, whereas the batch effects of a particular batch are sometimes positive, sometimes negative. This leads to asymmetry in the observed histogram, and hence a clear distinction between the observed histogram and the 'Uninteresting' distribution, which is required to be symmetrical.

How well does the use of the 'Uninteresting' distribution compensate for the lack of information external to the data concerning the batch effects? This question can be explored by fitting the mixed model including batch effects (Model (8.8)), known to be correct in relation to the simulated data, and comparing the p-values obtained with those obtained relative to the 'Uninteresting' distribution. The results (Figure 8.12) show that in this case, the 'Uninteresting' distribution has performed reasonably well – certainly well enough to be useful in a situation where external information is not available. The values of $-\log_{10}(p)$ from the 'Uninteresting' distribution are generally fairly similar to those from the correct model, both for cases in which H_0 is true and for cases in which there is a true exposure effect. However, there is a small subset of cases in which the 'correct' statistical model produces much smaller p-values than the 'Uninteresting' distribution – the line of points extending to the lower-right part of the plot. Examination of the numerical results reveals that these are cases in which, by chance, the batch effects are small, so that the variance estimate for this term, obtained from fitting the correct model, is zero. In these cases, it can be argued that the 'correct' statistical model is *incorrectly* implemented for the purpose of calculating p-values, and that the p-values obtained in relation to the 'Uninteresting' distribution should be preferred. (This subset of cases extends beyond the right-hand margin of the plot: the smallest

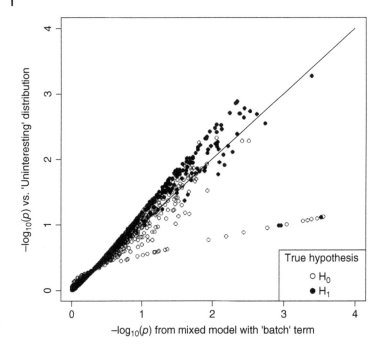

Figure 8.12 Comparison of $-\log_{10}(p)$ values obtained relative to the 'Uninteresting' distribution and from the correct model, when H_1 is true for a proportion $\pi_1 = 0.1$ of tests and unrecognised pseudoreplication is present.

p-value obtained from the correct model is $p = 9.3675 \times 10^{-12}$ ($-\log_{10}(p) = 11.028$)! Such extreme values are excluded from the plot so as to present the rest more clearly.)

8.5 An 'Uninteresting' Distribution to Account for Unrecognised Balanced-Block Effects: More Discoveries Announced

The use of an 'Uninteresting' distribution obtained empirically from the data, in place of the formal null distribution, does not always reduce the proportion of tests giving significant results and low FDRs, as it did in the preceding example where pseudoreplication was present. Other types of departure from the model assumed for the analysis of each response variable are possible, causing other patterns of correlation between the variables. In particular, if each group of sampling units that share a common influence (e.g., members of the same batch) comprises both exposed and unexposed units – for example, in a randomised block design – the consequences are very different from those of pseudoreplication. This can be illustrated with another simulated dataset, in which each batch of sampling units comprises equal numbers at each exposure level, as illustrated in Table 8.8. Such batches will be referred to as *balanced blocks*.

Table 8.8 Specification of dummy variables to indicate the allocation of sampling units to batches, with sampling units at both exposure levels occurring in each batch.

	Sampling unit															
	1	2	3	4	5	6	7	8	9	10	11	12	13	14	15	16
Exposure	U	U	U	U	U	U	U	U	E	E	E	E	E	E	E	E
Batch	1	1	2	2	3	3	4	4	1	1	2	2	3	3	4	4
X_{Exp}	0	0	0	0	0	0	0	0	+1	+1	+1	+1	+1	+1	+1	+1
X_1	1	1	0	0	0	0	0	0	1	1	0	0	0	0	0	0
X_2	0	0	1	1	0	0	0	0	0	0	1	1	0	0	0	0
X_3	0	0	0	0	1	1	0	0	0	0	0	0	1	1	0	0
X_4	0	0	0	0	0	0	1	1	0	0	0	0	0	0	1	1

All other specifications of the structure of the simulated data are unchanged from the specification in Tables 8.3 and 8.6, in which each batch comprised a single exposure level. Now, the points on the Q–Q plot, in the absence of any real exposure effects, lie consistently *below* the H_0 line (Figure 8.13): that is, there are *fewer* significant results, at whatever threshold α is chosen, than are expected on H_0. Correspondingly, the histogram of Z-values is narrower and more sharply pointed than the formal null distribution (Distribution (8.1))

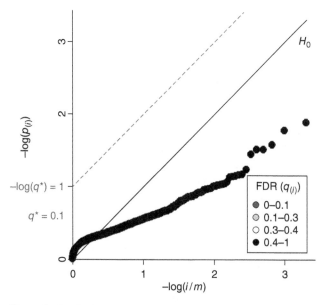

Figure 8.13 Q–Q plot, on the $-\log_{10}$ scale, of p-values obtained from $m = 2000$ tests when H_0 is true for every test but unrecognised balanced-block effects are present.

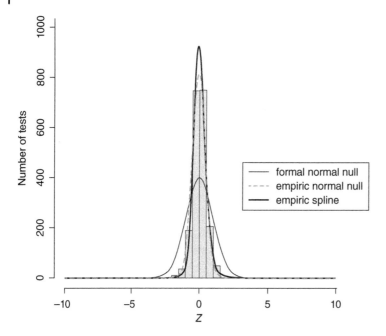

Figure 8.14 Histogram of Z-values obtained from m = 2000 tests when H_0 is true for every test but unrecognised balanced-block effects are present.

(Figure 8.14). The batch effects now do not lead to pseudoreplication, because the exposure effect is estimated *within* each batch. On the contrary, if their presence is not recognised, they will lead to overestimation of the amount of random variation that contributes to apparent exposure effects, and will tend to conceal any real exposure effects that are present. Using the terminology of experimental design, in the previous case the batch effects were *nested within* each level of exposure; in this case, they are *orthogonal to* the levels of exposure.

As in the previous case, the large-scale testing situation makes it possible to detect the batch effects from the data themselves, even in the absence of external information. The correlations between the n units, over the $m = 2000$ response variables, after centring, again show a clear pattern (Table 8.9): as before, there are four groups of four positively correlated sampling units, but now each group contains two units at each exposure level. For example, unexposed units 1 and 2 and exposed units 9 and 10 (which all belong to Batch 1) are strongly positively correlated with each other but moderately negatively correlated with all the other units.

As before, the departure from the formal null distribution can be taken into account by obtaining an empirically derived 'Uninteresting' distribution. Once again, a smoothing spline is first fitted to the histogram of Z-values, then a quadratic curve is fitted to the log-transformed spline in the region around the maximum, then the location of the maximum and the second differential of the quadratic curve are used to specify the

Table 8.9 Correlations between sampling units over $m = 2000$ response variables, each variable centred over the sampling units, when H_0 is true for all tests and batches are balanced blocks. Correlations between units in the same batch are highlighted.

Batch	Unit	1	2	3	4	5	6	7	8	9	10	11	12	13	14	15	16
1	1	1.000															
	2	0.796	1.000														
2	3	-0.321	-0.321	1.000													
	4	-0.309	-0.306	0.809	1.000												
3	5	-0.271	-0.278	-0.280	-0.298	1.000											
	6	-0.284	-0.289	-0.275	-0.286	0.819	1.000										
4	7	-0.262	-0.256	-0.252	-0.227	-0.339	-0.333	1.000									
	8	-0.250	-0.242	-0.245	-0.251	-0.341	-0.329	0.820	1.000								
1	9	0.803	0.817	-0.325	-0.310	-0.292	-0.293	-0.256	-0.250	1.000							
	10	0.806	0.808	-0.334	-0.329	-0.254	-0.268	-0.263	-0.256	0.816	1.000						
2	11	-0.300	-0.294	0.814	0.817	-0.294	-0.287	-0.254	-0.265	-0.294	-0.305	1.000					
	12	-0.311	-0.313	0.807	0.812	-0.287	-0.270	-0.247	-0.257	-0.312	-0.332	0.809	1.000				
3	13	-0.263	-0.277	-0.279	-0.304	0.821	0.817	-0.334	-0.340	-0.292	-0.266	-0.300	-0.274	1.000			
	14	-0.273	-0.275	-0.284	-0.303	0.814	0.807	-0.337	-0.339	-0.275	-0.256	-0.296	-0.294	0.819	1.000		
4	15	-0.248	-0.242	-0.263	-0.262	-0.327	-0.330	0.812	0.806	-0.225	-0.244	-0.269	-0.265	-0.344	-0.329	1.000	
	16	-0.250	-0.261	-0.240	-0.234	-0.338	-0.342	0.800	0.811	-0.244	-0.258	-0.262	-0.253	-0.329	-0.327	0.800	1.000
Batch		1	1	2	2	3	3	4	4	1	1	2	2	3	3	4	4
Unit		1	2	3	4	5	6	7	8	9	10	11	12	13	14	15	16

mean and standard deviation of an empirical 'Uninteresting' normal distribution. The smoothing spline and the empirical normal distribution are represented in Figure 8.14 by a heavy solid line and a dashed line, respectively: they do not agree with each other quite as well as the corresponding curves in the example with pseudoreplication (Figure 8.4).

As in the previous example (Section 8.4), we now simulate data that include causal effects of exposure, and apply the same methods to these. However, we choose a different distribution of exposure effects for demonstration purposes, specifying $\theta_{Exp} = 1$, $\sigma_{Exp} = 1$ in Distribution (8.9). When the simple t test is performed on each response variable in these data, the Q–Q plot and histogram obtained (Figures 8.15 and 8.16) do indicate the presence of these exposure effects: the points in the Q–Q plot corresponding to the smallest p-values now lie above the H_0 line, and the histogram has a long upper tail, comprising the Z-values from those response variables with large positive estimated exposure effects. As before, the sampling units for which H_1 is true are represented by dark grey, and again it is important to note that this information would not be available in a real study. The true-positive results are not readily distinguished by the simple t test, being largely masked by the width of the formal null distribution, which will tend to cause false-negative results. The true-positive effects have pushed the smallest p-values in the Q–Q plot and the largest Z-values in the histogram beyond the regions expected on the formal null distribution, but not by much. The correlations between units in the same

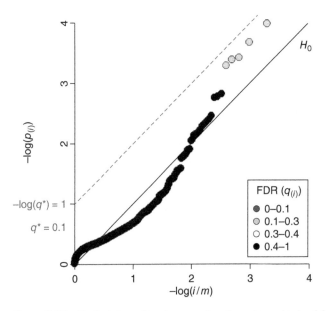

Figure 8.15 Q–Q plot, on the $-\log_{10}$ scale, of p-values obtained from $m = 2000$ tests when H_1 is true for a proportion $\pi_1 = 0.1$ of tests and unrecognised balanced-block effects are present.

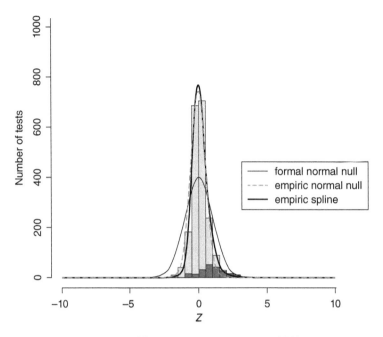

Figure 8.16 Histogram of Z-values obtained from $m = 2000$ tests when H_1 is true for a proportion $\pi_1 = 0.1$ of tests and unrecognised balanced-block effects are present.

batch are again strong (Table 8.10), though those between units in the same batch but at different exposure levels are slightly weaker than when true exposure effects are absent (Table 8.11).

The use of the empirical 'Uninteresting' distribution (the dashed line in Figure 8.16) goes a long way towards overcoming the problem of false-negative results due to unrecognised batch effects. It is much narrower than the formal null distribution, with the result that many more of the large Z-values give small p-values and low FDR values, leading to true discoveries.

The relationship between the LFDRs and Z in this dataset, calculated on the basis of the same three distributions as before (the formal null distribution derived from theory, the 'Uninteresting' distribution and the true distribution of the cases in which H_0 is true), are presented in Figure 8.17. It is instructive to compare this figure with Figure 8.9, which showed that when all sampling units in the same batch shared the same level of exposure there was a strong maximum of the LFDR, calculated on the basis of the formal null distribution, around $Z = 0$. Conversely, in the present case, when exposed and unexposed units occur in the same batch, there is a strong *minimum* around $Z = 0$, with maxima either side of it, corresponding to the narrower spread of the observed distribution. The maximum at negative values of Z, where there are few true-positives, is particularly high. The LFDR calculated on the basis of the empirical 'Uninteresting' distribution does a much better job of tracking the true false discovery rate.

The NFDR and the BH-FDR calculated on the basis of the empirical 'Uninteresting' distribution likewise do a much better job of representing the true NFDR than do the

Table 8.10 Correlations between sampling units over $m = 2000$ response variables, each variable centred over the sampling units, when H_1 is true for a proportion $\pi_1 = 0.1$ of tests and batches are balanced blocks. Correlations between units in the same batch are highlighted.

Batch	Unit	1	2	3	4	5	6	7	8	9	10	11	12	13	14	15	16
1	1	1.000															
1	2	0.798	1.000														
2	3	−0.307	−0.307	1.000													
2	4	−0.297	−0.294	0.811	1.000												
3	5	−0.255	−0.263	−0.262	−0.282	1.000											
3	6	−0.268	−0.274	−0.258	−0.271	0.821	1.000										
4	7	−0.257	−0.251	−0.244	−0.221	−0.329	−0.323	1.000									
4	8	−0.244	−0.237	−0.237	−0.245	−0.330	−0.319	0.820	1.000								
1	9	0.787	0.802	−0.332	−0.315	−0.301	−0.302	−0.259	−0.253	1.000							
1	10	0.791	0.793	−0.340	−0.335	−0.263	−0.277	−0.265	−0.259	0.817	1.000						
2	11	−0.306	−0.300	0.796	0.802	−0.302	−0.295	−0.256	−0.267	−0.284	−0.296	1.000					
2	12	−0.317	−0.318	0.791	0.798	−0.295	−0.278	−0.249	−0.260	−0.302	−0.323	0.810	1.000				
3	13	−0.266	−0.280	−0.283	−0.308	0.805	0.802	−0.334	−0.340	−0.287	−0.260	−0.295	−0.269	1.000			
3	14	−0.278	−0.280	−0.291	−0.308	0.795	0.788	−0.339	−0.341	−0.266	−0.247	−0.288	−0.286	0.820	1.000		
4	15	−0.259	−0.252	−0.274	−0.273	−0.339	−0.342	0.796	0.790	−0.209	−0.228	−0.253	−0.249	−0.331	−0.313	1.000	
4	16	−0.260	−0.271	−0.251	−0.244	−0.349	−0.352	0.785	0.795	−0.229	−0.242	−0.247	−0.239	−0.318	−0.312	0.804	1.000
Batch		1	2	3	4	3	4	1	2	3	4						
Unit		1	2	3	4	5	6	7	8	9	10	11	12	13	14	15	16

Table 8.11 Correlation coefficients between sampling units in the same batch, when H_1 is true for a proportion $\pi_1 = 0.1$ of tests and batches are balanced blocks.

Units compared		True exposure effect = 0	True exposure effect > 0	Difference
Units at same level of exposure				
1	2	0.796	0.798	0.002
3	4	0.809	0.811	0.002
5	6	0.819	0.821	0.002
7	8	0.820	0.820	0.000
9	10	0.816	0.817	0.001
11	12	0.809	0.810	0.001
13	14	0.819	0.820	0.001
15	16	0.800	0.804	0.004
Units at different levels of exposure				
1	9	0.803	0.787	−0.016
1	10	0.806	0.791	−0.015
2	9	0.817	0.802	−0.015
2	10	0.808	0.793	−0.015
3	11	0.814	0.796	−0.018
3	12	0.807	0.791	−0.016
4	11	0.817	0.802	−0.015
4	12	0.812	0.798	−0.014
5	13	0.821	0.805	−0.016
5	14	0.814	0.795	−0.019
6	13	0.817	0.802	−0.015
6	14	0.807	0.788	−0.019
7	15	0.812	0.796	−0.016
7	16	0.800	0.785	−0.015
8	15	0.806	0.790	−0.016
8	16	0.811	0.795	−0.016

corresponding variables calculated on the basis of the formal null distribution (Figure 8.18). Which of them should be preferred depends on the importance attached to avoiding association of larger values of Z with larger FDR values, which does happen to a very slight extent (barely detectable in the plot) around $Z = -2$ in the present case, if NFDR is chosen.

The Q–Q plot produced by the BH-FDR values obtained using the 'Uninteresting' distribution is presented in Figure 8.19. It shows a spectacular increase in the number of tests giving $-\log_{10}(p)$ values above the H_0 line, and in their distance above the line, relative to the results when the BH-FDRs are obtained using the formal null distribution

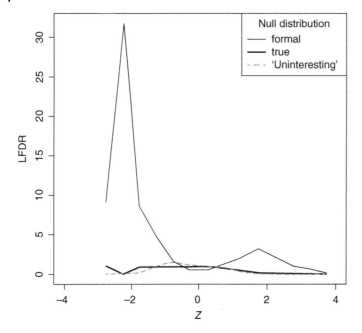

Figure 8.17 LFDR values, estimated on different bases, for m = 2000 tests when H_1 is true for a proportion π_1 = 0.1 of tests and batches are balanced blocks.

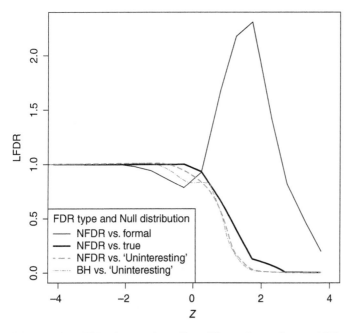

Figure 8.18 NFDR values, estimated on different bases, for m = 2000 tests when H_1 is true for a proportion π_1 = 0.1 of tests and batches are balanced blocks.

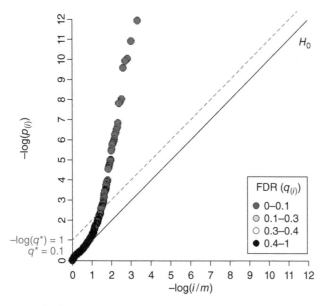

Figure 8.19 Q–Q plot, on the $-\log_{10}$ scale, of p-values obtained from the $m = 2000$ tests presented in Figure 8.15, on the basis of the 'Uninteresting' distribution instead of the formal distribution. H_1 is true for a proportion $\pi_1 = 0.1$ of tests and unrecognised balanced-block effects are present.

(Figure 8.15). That is, the estimated FDRs are greatly reduced, because of the much narrower distribution of 'Uninteresting' results, and hence the greater proportion of test results that are recognised as potentially true discoveries.

Thus, when unrecognised balanced-block effects are present, p-values obtained relative to an 'Uninteresting' distribution may enable many true discoveries (cases in which H_1 is true) that would have been missed on the basis of a simple t test. However, the agreement of these p-values with those obtained from the correct model is much less good when batches of experimental units comprise balanced blocks (Figure 8.20) than when they are a source of pseudoreplication (Figure 8.12). These two scenarios are compared further in the following section.

8.6 The Relative Merits of the Correct Model and an 'Uninteresting' Distribution as a Basis for Testing

Which is the better basis for multiple significance testing: p-values obtained by fitting a statistical model known to be correct on the basis of external information, or those obtained in relation to an empirically identified 'Uninteresting' distribution? It might be thought that the former approach was more rigorous and powerful, but when simulated data are analysed, neither constitutes a 'gold standard': the 'gold standard' is provided by the true hypothesis in each of the m tests, known from the process by which the data were simulated. From inspection of Figure 8.12 (batch effects causing pseudoreplication) and Figure 8.20

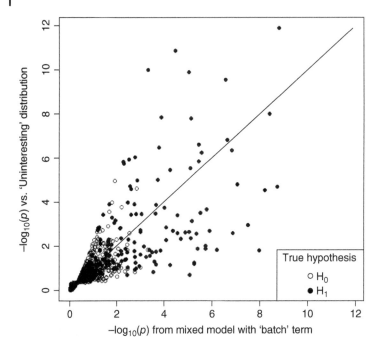

Figure 8.20 Comparison of *p*-values obtained relative to the 'Uninteresting' distribution and from the correct model, when H_1 is true for a proportion $\pi_1 = 0.1$ of tests and unrecognised balanced-block effects are present.

(batches comprise balanced blocks), it is not clear which approach is preferable: both are of some value, but both will give some false-positives and false-negatives, particularly when the batches are balanced blocks.

In the discussion that follows, it should be remembered that the comparison between the pseudoreplication and balanced-block scenarios is not strictly a comparison of like with like, because different values were specified for the mean and standard deviation of the exposure effect (in the pseudoreplication scenario, $\theta_{Exp} = 7$, $\sigma_{Exp} = 2.4$, and in the balanced-block scenario, $\theta_{Exp} = 1$, $\sigma_{Exp} = 1$). However, in each case the values were chosen to give a clear distinction between the results from the formal H_0 distribution and the 'Uninteresting' distribution.

The confusion matrix can be used to assess each approach (correct statistical model and 'Uninteresting' distribution) more formally against the gold standard of the true hypotheses, setting a threshold such as $\alpha = 0.05$ for *p*-values to be considered significant. The performance of each approach can then be summarised from the counts in the matrix (Chapter 2, Table 2.2) in a single value:

$$OR = (S/T)/(V/U) = (U \times S)/(V \times T). \tag{8.10}$$

In the context of diagnostic testing (see Chapter 2, Section 2.9), this is known as the Diagnostic Odds Ratio (OR) (Glas et al. 2003), a higher OR indicating better test performance. The two approaches are assessed in this way, for the two types of batch effect, in Table 8.12. This table suggests that the approach based on the 'Uninteresting' distribution performs better than that based on the correct model when the batch effects cause pseudoreplication,

Table 8.12 Confusion matrices to assess the performance of multiple testing in the presence of different batch-effect patterns, using p-values calculated on different bases.

Type of batch effect	Basis of p-value					OR
Pseudoreplication	Correct model	True hypothesis	Hypothesis accepted			
			H_0	H_1	Total	
		H_0	1721	78	1799	
		H_1	87	114	201	
		Total	1808	192	2000	28.9
	'Uninteresting' distribution	True hypothesis	Hypothesis accepted			
			H_0	H_1	Total	
		H_0	1727	72	1799	
		H_1	70	131	201	
		Total	1797	203	2000	44.9
Balanced blocks	Correct model	True hypothesis	Hypothesis accepted			
			H_0	H_1	Total	
		H_0	1712	87	1799	
		H_1	75	126	201	
		Total	1787	213	2000	33.1
	'Uninteresting' distribution	True hypothesis	Hypothesis accepted			
			H_0	H_1	Total	
		H_0	1726	73	1799	
		H_1	93	108	201	
		Total	1819	181	2000	27.5

and that there is little to choose between the two approaches when the batches comprise balanced blocks.

But the choice of the significance threshold $\alpha = 0.05$ is of course arbitrary, and a fuller picture, covering the whole range of possible significance thresholds from 0 to 1, is given by the Receiver Operating Characteristic (ROC) curve for each combination of significance-testing approach and batch pattern. This tool for the assessment of a diagnostic test criterion is produced by obtaining the sensitivity ($1 -$ False Negative Rate) and specificity ($1 -$ False Positive Rate) of the test for values of α over the full range $\alpha \leq 0 \leq 1$, for the set of m p-values under consideration, then plotting the sensitivity versus the specificity. The area under the curve (AUC) gives an indication of the performance of the test criterion: a perfect diagnostic test connects the points (0, 0), (0, 1) and (1, 1), whence AUC $= 1$. (A fuller introduction to the ROC curve is given by Fawcett (2006).)

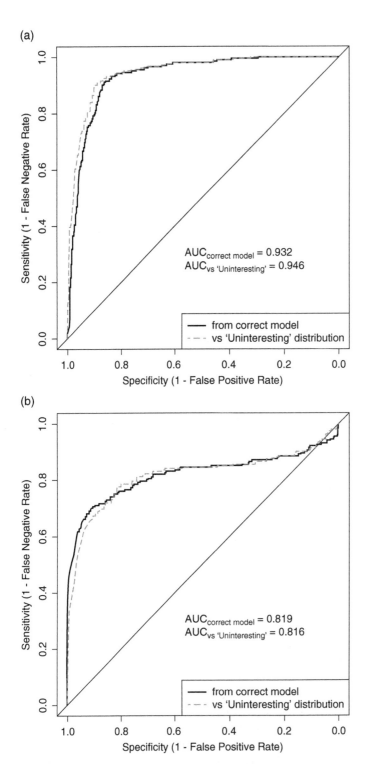

Figure 8.21 Receiver Operating Characteristic (ROC) curves to assess the performance of multiple testing in the presence of different batch-effect patterns, using p-values calculated on different bases. False-positive rate = $P(H_1 \text{ accepted}|H_0)$. False-negative rate = $P(H_0 \text{ accepted}|H_1)$. Note that for an ROC curve it is conventional to plot the horizontal axis from right to left. (a) Batch effects causing pseudoreplication. (b) Batches are balanced blocks.

In the present case, the ROC curves obtained (Figure 8.21) confirm the pattern observed in the confusion matrices. When batch effects cause pseudoreplication, the p-value obtained on the basis of the 'Uninteresting' distribution performs slightly better (gives a slightly higher AUC) than that obtained from the correct model, and when batches are balanced blocks, there is almost nothing to choose between the two approaches.

It may be counter-intuitive that an approach to multiple significance testing based on an empirical null distribution obtained from the data (the 'Uninteresting' distribution) can perform as well as, or even slightly better than, the approach based on the known, correct statistical model and the corresponding formal null distribution. The reason why this can occur is because, even after centring, the responses of any two units in the same batch are positively correlated, over the m response variables. The approach based on the 'Uninteresting' distribution takes advantage of these correlations, being influenced by the batch effects on *all* response variables when evaluating the significance of the exposure effect on *each* response variable, and this to some extent compensates for the small sample size n. In contrast, the approach based on the correct model uses only the information about the response variable under consideration.

Besides the method for seeking to identify an empirical 'Uninteresting' distribution presented here, other approaches have been developed that seek to compensate for a small value of n by 'borrowing' information from all the m tests under consideration, when specifying the null distribution to be used for each test. Some of these approaches have been implemented in the widely used R package `'limma'`, developed for the analysis of gene-expression microarrays to identify differentially expressed genes. Within this package, the function `eBayes()` implements an 'empirical Bayes' approach, which is 'equivalent to shrinkage of the estimated sample variances towards a pooled estimate, resulting in far more stable inference when the number of arrays is small' (Smyth 2004). Another function, `voom()`, estimates the relationship between the mean and the variance of the response variable over the m tests (with special features to take account of the structure of RNA-seq gene-expression data), fitting an empirically determined smooth curve (a LOWESS curve) to this relationship (Law et al. 2014).

Of course, if, on the null hypothesis, the distribution of the response-variable values for each test is unrelated to the distribution for all the other tests, then no improvement to the outcome of multiple testing is to be expected from these information-'borrowing' methods.

8.7 Summary

When 'big data' are analysed, results that are formally true-positives may nevertheless not be good candidates for further investigation.

This can occur when there is a slight departure from the H_0 statistical model and either a single significance test is performed with large n, or a very large number of tests are performed with small n.

It can be due either to a weak association between the explanatory variable and the response, or to a departure of the H_0 distribution from the formal distribution specified.

Testing of many hypotheses with a small value of n, though not ideal, is often practiced, and sometimes justified.

To address the problem of non-useful true-positives, the formal distributions on H_0 and H_1 indicated by theory may be replaced by empirically identified 'Uninteresting' and 'Interesting' distributions.

The application of this approach is explored here using simulated data, complementing previous studies using real data.

A study with $n = 16$ sampling units is simulated, with equal numbers unexposed and exposed to an influence of interest (e.g., disease, experimental treatment), and with $m = 2000$ response variables recorded. Batch effects are simulated, with all units in the same batch receiving the same exposure level.

The data are analysed using a simple t test, that is, without recognition of the batch effects. Even when no real exposure effect is present, a Q–Q plot and a histogram show that the significance test against the corresponding formal null distribution gives many more small p-values than are expected on H_0. This situation is referred to as *pseudoreplication*.

The pattern of correlations among the n units, over the m response variables, reveals the presence of possible batch effects, in a way that could not be achieved if only a few response variables were studied. This indicates that the formal null distribution, derived from the statistical model assumed for the significance test, may be inappropriate.

If it is assumed that the real exposure effects on the m response variables are mostly in the same direction, it is possible to specify an empirical 'Uninteresting' distribution which takes account of the possible presence of batch effects. A method for doing so is presented.

When the significance tests are performed against the 'Uninteresting' distribution instead of the formal null distribution, the spurious small p-values are eliminated.

Real exposure effects are now introduced into the model, in the same direction for most of the response variables. Their effect on the Q–Q plot, the histogram and the pattern of correlations among the n units over the m response variables is examined.

A symmetrical 'Uninteresting' distribution is obtained, in relation to the m p-values obtained from the formal null distribution when real exposure effects are present. New p-values are obtained, in relation to this 'Uninteresting' distribution.

The estimated LFDR, NFDR and BH-FDR obtained in relation to the formal null distribution and the 'Uninteresting' distribution are compared with the true LFDR and NFDR. The 'Uninteresting' distribution gives much better estimates than the formal null distribution.

The Q–Q plot of the p-values obtained in relation to the 'Uninteresting' distribution gives some indication that real exposure effects are present, but much more weakly than when the Q–Q plot is based on the formal null distribution.

p-values are also obtained from the correct statistical model for the simulated data, which includes batch as a random-effect term.

These p-values are compared with those obtained in relation to the 'Uninteresting' distribution. They agree fairly well, except for a small subset of the m tests in which the batch effects are very small and hence the estimate of the 'batch' component of variance is zero. In these cases, the p-values from the correct statistical model are much smaller, and it can be argued that the p-values in relation to the 'Uninteresting' distribution are preferable.

Another set of p-values from $m = 2000$ tests is simulated, this time from a study in which each batch contains equal numbers of unexposed and exposed units. Such batches are referred to as *balanced blocks*.

Now, a Q–Q plot shows that when no real exposure effect is present, a significance test without recognition of the batch effects, against the corresponding formal null distribution, gives many *fewer* small p-values than are expected on H_0.

Once again, the pattern of correlations among the n units, over the m response variables, reveals the presence of possible batch effects.

Once again, real exposure effects are introduced into the model, in the same direction for most of the response variables. Again, their effect on the Q–Q plot, the histogram and the pattern of correlations among the response variables is examined.

Again, a symmetrical 'Uninteresting' distribution is obtained, and new p-values are obtained in relation to this 'Uninteresting' distribution.

The estimated LFDR, NFDR and BH-FDR obtained in relation to the formal null distribution and the 'Uninteresting' distribution are compared with the true LFDR and NFDR. The 'Uninteresting' distribution again gives much better estimates than the formal null distribution.

Now that the batches are balanced blocks, and do not cause pseudoreplication, the Q–Q plot of the p-values obtained in relation to the 'Uninteresting' distribution shows a spectacular *increase* in the number of small p-values, relative to the results from the formal null distribution.

Again, p-values are also obtained from the correct statistical model for the simulated data, including batch as a random-effect term, and these are compared with the p-values obtained in relation to the 'Uninteresting' distribution. The agreement is less good now that batches comprise balanced blocks than it was when all units in each batch received the same exposure level (causing pseudoreplication when not recognised).

The relative merits of p-values obtained from the correct statistical model, and those obtained from an 'Uninteresting' distribution, as a basis for multiple testing, are assessed by comparing each approach with the 'gold standard' provided by the true hypothesis in each test, known from the data-simulation process.

Each approach is assessed in the case where batch effects potentially cause pseudoreplication, and the case where batches are balanced blocks. The approaches are assessed on the basis of the Odds Ratio (OR) from the corresponding confusion matrix, with the significance threshold specified as $\alpha = 0.05$.

To get beyond this arbitrary threshold, the two approaches and two cases are also assessed by the areas under their Receiver Operating Characteristic (ROC) curves.

ORs and ROC curves both indicate that in the case of batches causing pseudoreplication the 'Uninteresting' distribution performs slightly better than the correct statistical model, and in the case of batches that comprise balanced blocks, just as well.

The apparent paradox that the empirical 'Uninteresting' distribution can perform as well as the correct statistical model is explained by noting that even after centring, the responses of any two units in the same batch are positively correlated, over the m response variables.

The approach based on the 'Uninteresting' distribution takes advantage of these correlations, whereas the approach based on the correct model uses, for each test, only the information about the response variable under consideration.

Other approaches have been developed that seek to compensate for a small value of n by 'borrowing' information from all the m tests under consideration, when specifying the null distribution to be used for each test. Those implemented in the R package `'limma'` are briefly outlined.

References

Efron, B. (2004). Large-scale simultaneous hypothesis testing: the choice of a null hypothesis. *Journal of the American Statistical Association* 99: 96–104. https://doi.org/10.1198/016214504000000089.

Fawcett, T. (2006). An introduction to ROC analysis. *Pattern Recognition Letters* 27: 861–874. https://doi.org/10.1016/j.patrec.2005.10.010.

Galwey, N.W. (2014). *Introduction to Mixed Modelling: Beyond Regression and Analysis of Variance*, 2e. Chichester, U.K.: Wiley 487 pp.

Glas, A.S., Lijmer, J.G., Prins, M.H. et al. (2003). The diagnostic odds ratio: a single indicator of test performance. *Journal of Clinical Epidemiology* 56: 1129–1135. https://doi.org/10.1016/S0895-4356(03)00177-X. PMID 14615004.

Lambert, C.G. and Black, L.J. (2012). Learning from our GWAS mistakes: from experimental design to scientific method. *Biostatistics* 13: 195–203.

Law, C.W., Chen, Y., Shi, W., and Smyth, G.K. (2014). voom: precision weights unlock linear model analysis tools for RNA-seq read counts. *Genome Biology* 15: R29. https://doi.org/10.1186/gb-2014-15-2-r29.

NIST/SEMATECH (2012). *e-Handbook of Statistical Methods*. http://www.itl.nist.gov/div898/handbook/

Perperoglou, A., Sauerbrei, W., Abrahamowicz, M., and Schmid, M. (2019). A review of spline function procedures in R. *BMC Medical Research Methodology* 19: article 46. https://doi.org/10.1186/s12874-019-0666-3.

R Core Team (2020). *R: A Language and Environment for Statistical Computing*. Vienna, Austria: R Foundation for Statistical Computing https://www.R-project.org/.

Smyth, G. (2004). Linear models and empirical Bayes methods for assessing differential expression in microarray experiments. *Statistical Applications in Genetics and Molecular Biology* 3 (1): 3. https://doi.org/10.2202/1544-6115.1027.

Wilkinson, G.N. and Rogers, C.E. (1973). Symbolic description of factorial models for analysis of variance. *Journal of the Royal Statistical Society, Series C* 22: 392–399. https://www.jstor.org/stable/2346786.

9

Supplementation of p-Values with an Auxiliary Covariate: The Conditional FDR (cFDR)

9.1 Extension of the Relationship Between FDR and p to Take Account of an Additional Relevant Variable q

In a situation where multiple testing methods are to be applied to a set of p-values, information is often also available on 'relevant auxiliary covariates' (Hutchinson et al. 2021), which are expected to give additional guidance as to which null hypotheses should be rejected. For example, in a study of the effect of an environmental stress on the expression level of each of a large number of genes in an unusual plant genotype, information might also be available on the effects in a more standard genotype, and it might be expected that those genes strongly affected by the stress in the standard genotype would be the most likely also to be affected in the unusual genotype. In such a situation it is natural to ask whether such supplementary information can be taken into account when seeking to control the FDR at a specified low level. In order to combine auxiliary-covariate and p-value information in this way, it is helpful to define the FDR associated with a particular observed p-value (p) in Bayesian terms, as

$$\text{FDR}(p) = P(H_0^p | P \leq p), \tag{9.1}$$

where p is a realisation of the random variable P, and H_0^p is the null hypothesis relating to p (see Chapter 6, Section 6.1, Equation (6.2)). It is assumed that on H_0^p,

$$P \sim \text{Uniform}(0, 1). \tag{9.2}$$

When a relevant auxiliary covariate q is available, the observations of q being considered as realisations of a random variable Q, this formula can be extended to give the FDR conditional on q, namely,

$$\text{cFDR}(p, q) = P(H_0^p | P \leq p, Q \leq q). \tag{9.3}$$

Note that the symbols Q and q for the auxiliary covariate are used here for consistency with the literature on this topic. This usage is not to be confused with the use of q as a symbol for the FDR itself in Chapter 2, Section 2.4 and elsewhere. Note also that the notation '$P(A, B)$' is

The False Discovery Rate: Its Meaning, Interpretation and Application in Data Science, First Edition.
N.W. Galwey.
© 2025 John Wiley & Sons Ltd. Published 2025 by John Wiley & Sons Ltd.
Companion website: www.wiley.com/go/falsediscoveryrate

used in this chapter as shorthand for the more formal notation 'P($A \cap B$)', to indicate 'the probability that both Event A and Event B occur'. The conditional probability rule,

$$P(A \cap B) = P(A|B) \cdot P(B), \tag{9.4}$$

will also be used. (See Chapter 5, Section 5.3 concerning the notation and laws of probability.)

Methods for estimation of the conditional FDR (cFDR), and for identifying appropriate subsets of null hypotheses for rejection on the basis of the cFDR, have been developed in the context of genetic association studies, in relation to various types of auxiliary covariate (e.g., a parallel set of p-values relating to a different response variable; a binary, categorical or normally distributed variable; a non-normally distributed continuous variable), and this work is well summarised by Hutchinson et al. In outline, the approach is as follows.

Applying Bayes' theorem to Equation (9.1) gives

$$\text{FDR}(p) = \frac{P(P \le p|H_0^p) \cdot P(H_0^p)}{P(P \le p)} \tag{9.5}$$

(see Chapter 6, Section 6.1, Equations (6.1) and (6.2)). Examining the terms on the right-hand side of Equation (9.5), we note that:

- if a set of m ordered p-values, $p_{(i)}$, $i = 1...m$, are assumed to be a random sample from an infinite population, *not* assumed to have the null distribution in Display (9.2), then an unbiased estimate of $P(P_{(i)} \le p_{(i)})$, is given by i/m,
- $P(P \le p|H_0^p) = p$, and
- $P(H_0^p) \le 1$.

This leads to our usual formula

$$E\left(\text{FDR}\left(p_{(i)}\right)\right) \le \frac{p_{(i)}}{i/m}, \tag{9.6}$$

whence we obtain the usual conservative estimator of the FDR,

$$\widehat{\text{FDR}}\left(p_{(i)}\right) = \frac{p_{(i)}}{i/m}. \tag{9.7}$$

This relationship is represented graphically in Chapter 2, Figure 2.5. The numerator and denominator of the fraction on the right-hand side of Equation (9.7) correspond to the vertical and horizontal coordinates of the point representing $p_{(i)}$, respectively, and the conservatively estimated FDR is the slope of the line connecting this point to the origin.

The corresponding application of Bayes' theorem to Equation (9.3) gives

$$\text{cFDR}(p, q) = \frac{P(P \le p|H_0^p, Q \le q) \cdot P(H_0^p|Q \le q)}{P(P \le p|Q \le q)}. \tag{9.8}$$

The condition $Q \le q$ is simply added to each term on the right-hand side of Equation (9.5). As before, we need to compare the probability in the numerator, conditional on the null hypothesis, with the unconditional probability in the denominator. However, we are now working with two variables, P and Q, so we can no longer simply order the values of P and think in terms of lengths on two axes, both relating to P, one for the numerator (the p-values themselves) and one for the denominator (the quantile ranks of the p-values – see Chapter 7, Section 7.4). We must live without a single natural ordering of the values of P and Q, and think in terms of areas in the P–Q plane. In developing methods for dealing with this situation, Hutchinson et al. made a simplifying assumption that any relationship between P and Q is due to the effects we are trying to discover: that is, the relationship is present only in the cases in which H_0^p is false, and hence

$$P \perp\!\!\!\perp Q | H_0^p, \tag{9.9}$$

where the symbol '$\perp\!\!\!\perp$' means 'is independent of'. Hutchinson et al. further note that

> The cFDR framework implicitly assumes that there is a 'positive stochastic mono-tonic relationship' between p and q, meaning that on average [hypotheses that give smaller values of the conditional-trait variable q] are enriched for smaller p-values in the principal trait [p].

We proceed as follows. From Bayes' theorem,

$$P(H_0^p | Q \leq q) = \frac{P(Q \leq q | H_0^p) \cdot P(H_0^p)}{P(Q \leq q)}. \tag{9.10}$$

Substituting Equation (9.10) into Equation (9.8), we obtain

$$\text{cFDR}(p, q) = \frac{P(P \leq p | H_0^p, Q \leq q) \cdot P(Q \leq q | H_0^p) \cdot P(H_0^p)}{P(P \leq p | Q \leq q) \cdot P(Q \leq q)}. \tag{9.11}$$

Further, from the conditional probability rule (Equation (9.4)),

$$P(P \leq p | Q \leq q) \cdot P(Q \leq q) = P(P \leq p, Q \leq q), \tag{9.12}$$

and substituting Equation (9.12) into Equation (9.11),

$$\text{cFDR}(p, q) = \frac{P(P \leq p | H_0^p, Q \leq q) \cdot P(Q \leq q | H_0^p) \cdot P(H_0^p)}{P(P \leq p, Q \leq q)}. \tag{9.13}$$

We note that given the independence condition (9.9),

$$P(P \leq p | H_0^p, Q \leq q) = P(P \leq p | H_0^p) = p. \tag{9.14}$$

We also note that

$$P(H_0^p) \leq 1. \tag{9.15}$$

Substituting Equation (9.14) and Inequality (9.15) into Equation (9.13) leads to the inequality

$$E(\text{cFDR}(p, q)) \leq \frac{p \cdot P(Q \leq q | H_0^p)}{P(P \leq p, Q \leq q)}, \tag{9.16}$$

and hence to the conservative estimator

$$\widehat{\mathrm{cFDR}}(p,q) = \frac{p \cdot \mathrm{P}(Q \le q | H_0^p)}{\mathrm{P}(P \le p, Q \le q)}. \tag{9.17}$$

We now have formulae (9.13), (9.16) and (9.17) relating to cFDR(p, q), analogous to (9.5), (9.6) and (9.7), respectively, relating to FDR(p). Equation (9.17) can be applied to any pair of observations (p_i, q_i): it relates to the probability mass in the rectangular area $(P \le p_i, Q \le q_i)$, as illustrated in Figure 9.1. The numerator of the right-hand side of Equation (9.17) is the probability mass conditional on H_0^p, and the denominator is the corresponding unconditional value, estimated by the proportion of observed (p, q) pairs in this region.

Note that in this schematic illustration, using simulated data, q, like p, is plotted on a $[0, 1]$ scale. This is appropriate if the auxiliary variable q itself comprises a second set of m p-values, forming natural pairs with the principal set, but testing a different but related set of hypotheses (e.g., hypotheses related to the same m response variables but in different circumstances). When developing methods related to the cFDR, it is helpful to focus on this case in which the auxiliary covariate comprises a second set of p-values. This is because, regardless of the underlying form of the additional variable, the information it provides can often be summarised in the p-value obtained from an appropriate significance test.

9.2 Method for the Evaluation of the cFDR from Data

In order to obtain values for the numerator and denominator of Equation (9.17) from data, we need to consider how the observations that lie within the rectangle $(P \le p_i, Q \le q_i)$ are related to the overall distribution of observations in the P–Q plane. The simulation process used to produce Figure 9.1 specifies that small p-values are more common than large ones, representing a situation in which H_1 is true for at least some of the tests. The process further specifies that along any boundary in the bivariate space specified by the relationship

$$q = 1/(kp) \tag{9.18}$$

where

$$k > 1,$$

the density of observations is constant. In this special case, the probability mass within the rectangle $(P \le p_i, Q \le q_i)$ is constant for all points that lie on the same boundary: that is, if

$$q_i = 1/(kp_i), \tag{9.19}$$

then

$$\mathrm{P}(P \le p, Q \le q) = \mathrm{P}(P \le p_i, Q \le q_i) \tag{9.20}$$

for all points (p, q) that satisfy Equation (9.18), and the probability mass within the two hatched rectangles in Figure 9.1 is the same. Such a region of high probability density, adjacent to the P and Q axes and with its boundary defined in this way, has been called an 'L-region' by Liley and Wallace (2021), and its boundary has been called an 'L-curve'.

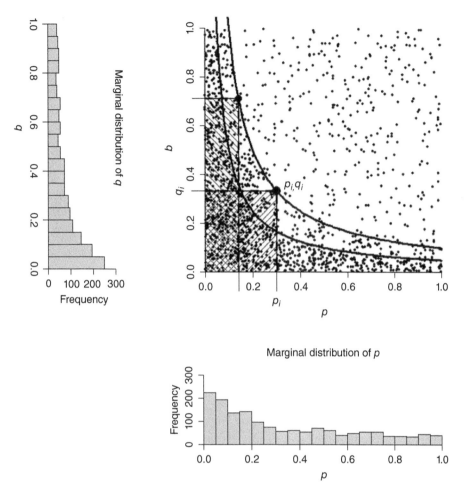

Figure 9.1 Bivariate distribution of a set of *p*-values and parallel values of a relevant auxiliary covariate (*q*-values). For explanation of the conventions, see the text.

Such L-curves are identified on the basis of cFDR values, as will be shown shortly, and not directly on the basis of the bivariate density of *p*- and *q*-values.

A series of non-intersecting L-curves (like the two shown in Figure 9.1) defines a series of smaller and smaller regions of increasing probability density towards the origin at ($P = 0$, $Q = 0$). As one moves from the top right-hand corner of the figure towards the axes and the origin, these concentric regions are analogous to increasingly stringent significance criteria in the univariate distribution of *P* when there is no auxiliary covariate: they provide a way of combining *P* and *Q* into a single measure of the strength of evidence.

The *q*-value on the [0, 1] scale can be back-transformed to obtain the corresponding *Z*-score, which can be thought of as the test statistic that might have produced this *q*-value as its *p*-value. That is, if *q* is the *p*-value obtained from a two-sided test with the test-statistic *Z*, and if on the null hypothesis *Z* is a standard normal variable with distribution

$$Z \sim N(0, 1), \tag{9.21}$$

and if the function Φ gives the cumulative probability of Z, that is,

$$q = 2 \times P(Z \geq |z|) = 2 \times P(Z \leq -|z|) = 2 \times \Phi(-|z|), \tag{9.22}$$

then, rearranging Equation (9.22),

$$z = -\Phi^{-1}(q/2) \tag{9.23}$$

is the Z-score corresponding to q. If the q-values were obtained from some significance test relating to a continuous variable, for example, the effect of an experimental treatment on some measurement, then transforming the q-values to the corresponding Z-scores produces a graphical representation that comes closer to the original data, and this is shown in Figure 9.2. Note that the region in which the test results on both the principal trait and the auxiliary covariate are significant (the angle of the L-region) has now moved from the bottom-left to the top-left corner of the bivariate plot.

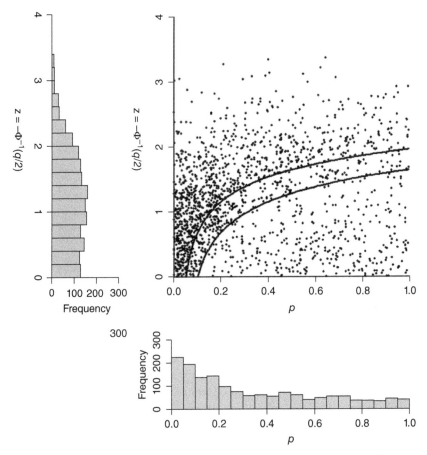

Figure 9.2 Bivariate distribution of a set of p-values and parallel Z-scores ($-\Phi^{-1}(q/2)$), obtained from the q-values presented in Figure 9.1.

Of course, real data will rarely if ever conform to the ideal relationship in Equation (9.20), but many datasets conform approximately to this pattern. Empirical, numerical methods for the identification of L-regions that have a constant value of cFDR along the boundary have been extensively explored by Liley and Wallace (2021) and by Hutchinson et al. (2021). In outline, their method is as follows.

The requirement is to obtain estimates of the terms (other than p) in $\widehat{\mathrm{cFDR}}(p,q)$ (Equation (9.17)), namely, the term $P(Q \leq q | H_0^p)$ in the numerator and the term $P(P \leq p, Q \leq q)$ in the denominator. To obtain these estimates, a smooth mathematical function is fitted to the data. The first step is to transform both the p-values and the q-values to the corresponding quantiles of the standard normal distribution. A smooth function is then fitted to these values over the whole P–Q plane by the method of kernel density estimation (KDE). Such 'kernel smoothing' methods are reviewed by, for example, Hastie et al. (2001, Chapter 6). KDE is fairly mathematically elaborate, but can be envisaged as a blurring of each data point to produce a probability density function, covering the whole bivariate space but with its maximum at the observed value, from which the observed value is imagined to be sampled. The probability densities corresponding to all the data points are then summed at every position in the bivariate space, to give the value of the smooth function at that position. The greater the degree of blurring, the smoother the KDE function, but the less accurately it represents the data.

The estimate of $P(P \leq p, Q \leq q)$ is then obtained by integration over the relevant rectangular region of the bivariate space:

$$P(\widehat{P \leq p, Q} \leq q) = \text{integral of } P(P = p, \widehat{Q = q}) \text{ over } P \leq p, Q \leq q. \tag{9.24}$$

The process required to estimate $P(Q \leq q | H_0^p)$ is somewhat more elaborate. The steps are as follows. We first consider the composite event '$P = p$, $Q = q$ and H_0^p is true'. From the conditional probability rule (Equation (9.4)), the probability of this event is

$$P(P = p, Q = q, H_0^p) = P(H_0^p | P = p, Q = q) \cdot P(P = p, Q = q). \tag{9.25}$$

From the assumption that P is independent of Q conditional on H_0^p (Display 9.9), it is concluded that if H_0^p is true for most tests, the majority of information about H_0^p is contained in P, little additional information being contributed by Q, so that

$$P(H_0^p | P = p, Q = q) \approx P(H_0^p | P = p). \tag{9.26}$$

Substituting the approximate equality (9.26) into Equation (9.25), we obtain

$$P(P = p, Q = q, H_0^p) \approx P(H_0^p | P = p) \cdot P(P = p, Q = q). \tag{9.27}$$

For each value of P, the term $P(H_0^p | P = p)$ can then be estimated from the local false discovery rate, considering P alone (i.e., taking no account of Q), using the methods introduced in Chapter 7, Sections 7.1 and 7.2. The term $P(P = p, Q = q)$ can be estimated from the KDE function.

Having obtained estimates of the terms on the right-hand side of the approximate equality (9.27), we are in a position to integrate this function over P and/or Q. Integrating over P, we obtain an estimate of the probability of the combined event '$Q = q$ and H_0^p is true', which we designate by $P(\widehat{Q = q}, H_0^p)$. Integrating over p and q, we obtain an estimate of the probability that H_0^p is true, which we designate by $\widehat{P(H_0^p)}$. Then, again using the conditional probability rule, we obtain

$$P(\widehat{Q = q}, H_0^p) = \widehat{P(Q = q|H_0^p)} \cdot \widehat{P(H_0^p)},$$

which we rearrange to obtain

$$\widehat{P(Q = q|H_0^p)} = \frac{P(\widehat{Q = q}, H_0^p)}{\widehat{P(H_0^p)}},$$

whence, integrating over q,

$$\widehat{P(Q \leq q|H_0^p)} = \frac{P(\widehat{Q \leq q}, H_0^p)}{\widehat{P(H_0^p)}}. \tag{9.28}$$

Substituting Equation (9.28) into the numerator of Equation (9.17), and Equation (9.24) into the denominator, the value of the required conservative estimator $\widehat{cFDR}(p, q)$ is obtained.

However, a further step is required in order to obtain a set of probabilities and FDR values that can be used in the same ways as the p-values and BH-FDR values that are obtained when a set of m principal-trait p-values is considered in isolation, without a relevant auxiliary covariate. In this final step, the whole probability mass within the L-region on H_0^p is calculated – not just the mass within the rectangle $(P \leq p_i, Q \leq q_i)$. This is done by numerical integration of the bivariate probability density function of P and Q on H_0^p, over the L-region.

For this purpose, the non-intersecting boundaries of a set of concentric L-regions must first be defined. The true value of cFDR should be constant along the boundary of each L-region, so to obtain an estimated boundary passing through the point (p_i, q_i), a smooth contour curve is fitted using all the estimated values, $\widehat{cFDR}(p_i, q_i)$, $i = 1...m$, over the whole P–Q plane. The probability mass required is then the integral of the probability density within this boundary, conditional on H_0^p: that is,

$$v(p_i, q_i) = \int_{L(p_i, q_i)} f_0(p, q) dp dq, \tag{9.29}$$

where the symbol $\int_{L(p_i, q_i)}$ indicates integration over the L-region with the point (p_i, q_i) on its boundary, and $f_0(p, q)$ indicates the probability density, conditional on H_0^p, at any point (p, q), namely,

$$f_0(p, q) = p \cdot \widehat{P(Q = q|H_0^p)}. \tag{9.30}$$

The rationale for defining the boundary of the L-region in relation to cFDR, and $v(p, q)$ as the probability mass within the L-region on H_0^p, may be clarified by relating it to the

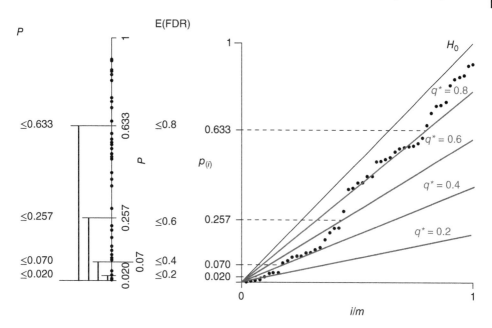

Figure 9.3 Untransformed Q–Q plot of principal-trait p-values from m = 50 hypothesis tests, and their distribution on the P axis.

corresponding argument when only the p-values for the principal trait are considered, and this is done for a set of $m = 50$ p-values (a representative subset of those considered in the following section) in Figure 9.3. In the plot of $p_{(i)}$ versus i/m in this figure, the thresholds for control of the FDR at $q^* = 0.2, 0.4, 0.6$ and 0.8 are indicated by sloping lines passing through the origin, as in Figure 2.5 (Chapter 2), and the p-value significance thresholds that control the FDR at these levels are projected onto the $p_{(i)}$ axis. To the left of this plot, the p-values are plotted along the P axis, and the significance thresholds that control the FDR at the specified levels are marked, with the corresponding q^* values noted on their right. This corresponds to the plot of (p, q) observation pairs in the P–Q space when cFDR is to be controlled (Figure 9.1), but because only the principal-trait p-values are considered, the plot occupies only one dimension. The FDR thresholds are points on this dimension, each corresponding to an L-curve in the P–Q space. To obtain the value of $v(p, q)$ corresponding to each cFDR threshold, the probability density on H_0^P must be integrated over the L-region within the L-curve. The corresponding process on the P-axis is integration of the probability density from 0 to the significance threshold that corresponds to the q^* threshold, and this is indicated by a heavy vertical bar for each threshold. Because P on H_0^P has uniform density over the range [0, 1] (Distribution 9.2), the numerical value of this integral is simply that of the significance threshold itself. However, the auxiliary trait Q does not follow any formal distribution, even on H_0^P, and certainly not Distribution (9.2). Therefore, in order to perform the corresponding integration on H_0^P within the P–Q space to obtain the $v(p, q)$, the required probability density must be estimated from the data, using the smooth function in Equation (9.30), at each point within the L-region.

Thus, the probability mass $v(p, q)$ represents an extreme region of the bivariate distribution on H_0^p, and is analogous to a *p*-value in the univariate case. Hutchinson et al. (2021) refer to it as a *v*-value, and note that:

> Deriving *v*-values, which are analogous to *p*-values, means that the output from Flexible cFDR can be used directly in any conventional error rate controlling procedure, such as the BH method. The derivation of *v*-values also allow[s] for iterative usage, whereby the *v*-values from the previous iteration are used as the 'principal trait' *p*-values in the current iteration. This allows users to incorporate additional layers of auxiliary data into the analysis at each iteration, akin to leveraging multi-dimensional covariates...

9.3 Application of the cFDR to Non-Genetic Data

These potential applications of *v*-values are very attractive, and they raise the question of whether the cFDR can be used outside the context of genetic association in which it has been developed. Although in many contexts correlations between *P* and *Q* and between tests will compromise the assumptions made in the methods outlined in Sections 9.1 and 9.2, there is no numerical obstacle to the wider application of these methods, and it is worth exploring the results obtained when this is done. Even if the *v*-values and BH-FDR values so obtained cannot be taken literally, the correlations present are likely to make them conservative, and they may thus still provide useful guidance on the relative merits of the *m* hypotheses under consideration for further investigation.

These methods are therefore now applied to the *Arabidopsis thaliana* gene-expression data introduced in Chapter 4. It is important to note that such 'genomics' data are distinct from strictly genetic data, in the following way:

- data on genetic association relate to the spatial position of genetic variants in an organism's genome, and correlations between variants are generally weak when the variants are far apart, whereas
- the expression levels of different genes may be positively or negatively correlated over a range of environmental (or other) conditions, regardless of the degree of separation between the genes in the genome.

The gene-expression data considered here will thus illustrate problems and opportunities likely to be encountered in a wide range of other contexts.

Two of the comparisons made in Chapter 4 will be considered: the NaCl versus untreated contrast in the Col(gl) genotype will provide the principal-trait *p*-values, and the same contrast in the Col(WT) genotype will be the related auxiliary covariate that provides the *q*-values. Expression values from every fourth probeset (gene) on the Affymetrix array ATH1-121501 will be used, giving $m = 5702 \approx 22{,}810/4$ tests. That is, a representative subset of the probesets will be considered: there is no obstacle to using the entire set, but limitation to this subset avoids overcrowding of the graphical displays. The results required for each probeset, as input for the cFDR analysis, are the effect estimate for the comparison in

Table 9.1 Results from the NaCl versus untreated contrast in each of two *Arabidopsis thaliana* genotypes, for the expression level of each of $m = 5702$ representative probesets (genes).

Row No.	Probeset ID	NaCl versus untreated, Col(gl)				NaCl versus untreated, Col(WT)			
		Estimate	t^a	Two-sided p	One-sided p	Estimate	t^a	Two-sided p	One-sided p
4	266600_at	−0.113	−0.796	0.4562	0.7719	−0.902	−6.351	0.0007	0.9996
8	245079_at	0.802	4.767	0.0031	0.0016	0.491	2.919	0.0267	0.0133
12	265978_at	0.134	0.624	0.5555	0.2777	−0.180	−0.843	0.4316	0.7842
16	266930_at	0.329	1.057	0.3310	0.1655	0.007	0.024	0.9817	0.4909
20	266583_at	0.292	2.352	0.0569	0.0284	−0.246	−1.980	0.0950	0.9525
⋮									⋮
22792	246664_at	0.047	0.238	0.8199	0.4099	−0.176	−0.892	0.4066	0.7967
22796	252610_x_at	−0.222	−1.576	0.1660	0.9170	−0.120	−0.851	0.4274	0.7863
22800	254315_at	−0.388	−1.714	0.1374	0.9313	−0.785	−3.466	0.0134	0.9933
22804	263340_at	0.034	0.244	0.8151	0.4075	−0.033	−0.236	0.8214	0.5893
22808	263644_at	−0.023	−0.322	0.7585	0.6208	−0.173	−2.461	0.0490	0.9755

[a] Degrees of freedom (DF) = 6.

question, the corresponding t-statistic with degrees of freedom (DF) = 6, and the two-sided and one-sided p-values. These results, from the first and last few probesets, are presented in Table 9.1.

The p-values for the principal trait indicate the strength of evidence that each probeset is differentially expressed between NaCl treated and untreated plants in the mutant genotype Col(gl). For the two-sided test, the alternative hypothesis is

$$\text{mean}(\text{NaCl treated}) \neq \text{mean}(\text{untreated}), \tag{9.31}$$

and for the one-sided test, it is

$$\text{mean}(\text{NaCl treated}) > \text{mean}(\text{untreated}). \tag{9.32}$$

Note that in some cases the one-sided p-value is larger than the two-sided value. This occurs when the observed effect is in the 'wrong' direction: the alternative hypothesis for the one-sided test is that the effect of NaCl on gene expression is positive, so when the estimated effect is negative, the one-sided p-value is greater than 0.5. The p-values for the relevant auxiliary covariate indicate the strength of the corresponding evidence in the wild-type genotype Col(WT). Combined analysis of the two parallel sets of test results is motivated by the argument that if there is evidence of differential expression in the wild-type genotype, it may increase the strength of one's belief in differential expression in the mutant genotype.

There is a weak but highly significant positive correlation between the t-statistics for the two comparisons considered, over the probesets (Figure 9.4; $r = 0.220$, $p < 0.001$). Histograms of the one-sided p-values for the principal trait and the auxiliary covariate (Figure 9.5) show that for both traits, p-values closes to both 0 and 1 are more common than values in the middle of the range: that is, in both genotypes, some genes are more strongly expressed in NaCl-treated plants, whereas others are more strongly expressed in untreated plants. If differential gene expression in either direction is of interest, then it is more relevant to interpret the results from two-sided tests. Interpretation of two-sided p-values is consistent with the application of cFDR presented by Hutchinson et al. (2021), and is standard practice in studies of the association of a phenotypic trait with each of m genetic loci.

The distribution of two-sided p-values for the principal trait is presented in the horizontal marginal histogram in Figure 9.6. Differential gene expression in either direction is now represented by p-values close to zero. The null distribution, represented by a solid line superimposed on the histogram, confirms that differentially expressed genes are more common than is expected on H_0^p.

The method of Hutchinson et al. does not restrict the observations of the auxiliary covariate to a set of p-values distributed over the range $[0, 1]$, but allows them to be sampled from an arbitrary distribution. To illustrate this, we convert the two-sided p-values for the auxiliary covariate to Z-scores using Equation (9.23). The distribution of these Z-scores is presented in the vertical marginal histogram in Figure 9.6. The corresponding null distribution, namely, the positive half of the standard normal distribution, is again represented by a solid line superimposed on the histogram, and again confirms that there are more extreme values than are expected on the null hypothesis. These Z-scores will be used in

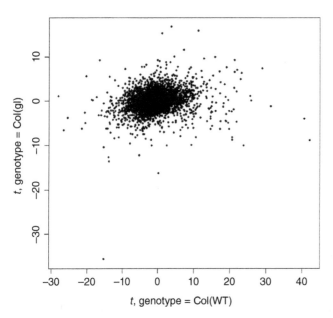

Figure 9.4 t-statistic for the NaCl versus untreated contrast in the *A. thaliana* genotype Col(gl) versus the corresponding statistic for Col(WT), in each probeset.

(a) principal trait

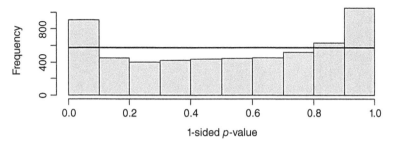

(b) auxiliary covariate

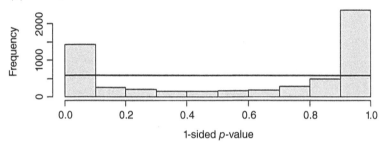

Figure 9.5 (a) and (b) Distributions, over probesets, of one-sided *p*-values for the principal trait and the auxiliary covariate, from the NaCl versus untreated contrast in *A. thaliana* genotypes.

the analysis presented here, but N.B. they will continue to be referred to as *q*-values, consistent with the usage of Hutchinson et al. The bivariate plot in Figure 9.6 shows the combined distribution of the observed values of *p* and *q*.

The excess of large values of *q* (large absolute *Z*-scores) relative to the expectation on the null hypothesis, and the positive correlation between the *t*-statistics for the principal trait and the auxiliary covariate, indicate that the *q*-values may be effective in supplementing the information from the principal-trait *p*-values.

The analysis proposed by Hutchinson et al. has been implemented in the software R (R Core Team 2021), in the package "fcfdr" (Hutchinson et al. 2022). Having loaded this package, the next step is to execute the following R command:

```
corr_plot(p = p, q = z.q),
```

'z.q' is the name of the numeric vector that holds the values of *q*, chosen to remind us that these have been transformed to *Z*-scores. This command produces a 'violin plot' (Figure 9.7), which represents the distribution of $-\log_{10}(p)$ within each of five ranges of *q*, arranged in ascending order on the horizontal axis and referred to as 'strata'. For each stratum, the width of the 'violin' indicates the density of principal-trait *p*-values at the corresponding value of $-\log_{10}(p)$. This plot shows that overall the required monotonic relationship between *p* and *q* is present, though it is not perfect: the median value of $-\log_{10}(p)$ is slightly higher in the lowest stratum of *q* than in the second-lowest.

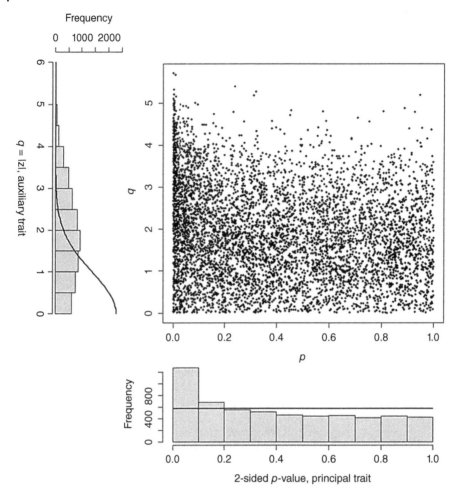

Figure 9.6 Bivariate distribution, over probesets, of p for the principal trait and q for the auxiliary covariate, from the NaCl versus untreated contrast in *A. thaliana* genotypes. The solid black line indicates the distribution expected on the null hypothesis.

A further check on the monotonic relationship is given by executing the following command:

```
stratified_qqplot(data_frame = data.frame(p, z.q),
  prin_value_label = "p", cond_value_label = "z.q",
  thresholds = quantile(z.q)[-1])
```

This produces the Q–Q plot of p, on the $-\log_{10}$ scale and stratified by q, shown in Figure 9.8. (N.B. The unmodified function `stratified_qqplot()` provided in the package "fcfdr" produces a colour-coded plot unsuitable for monochrome reproduction, so a slightly modified version has been used to produce the plot presented here.) The three lower strata of q are associated with a very similar range of values of $-\log_{10}(p)$, but the highest stratum (Stratum 4) is associated with consistently larger values, so that overall the required positive correlation is present.

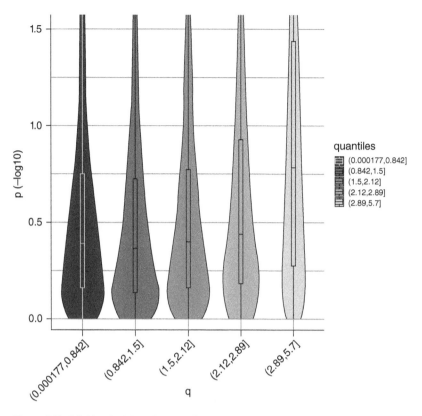

Figure 9.7 'Violin plot' showing the distribution of $-\log_{10}(p)$ stratified by q, from the NaCl versus untreated contrast in *A. thaliana* genotypes.

Next, the following commands are executed:

```
res <- flexible_cfdr(p = p, q = z.q,
   indep_index = seq(1, n, 1), enforce_p_q_cor = TRUE,
   plot = TRUE)
p <- res[[1]]$p
z.q <- res[[1]]$q
v <- res[[1]]$v
```

In the function-call `flexible_cfdr()`, the argument 'enforce_p_q_cor = TRUE' ensures that the correlation between p and q is positive, as the cFDR estimation method requires, by 'flipping' the sign of each value of q if the correlation is negative. (The argument-setting 'enforce_p_q_cor = FALSE' is not generally recommended.)

The function `flexible_cfdr()` produces further diagnostic plots, obtained from the values of p and q, shown in Figure 9.9. The top-left panel shows the distribution of absolute Z-scores obtained from the values of p for the principal trait. By definition, these are all non-negative, and this boundary effect could interfere with the KDE estimation process: to prevent this, the empirical Z-scores are 'mirrored' by a corresponding set of simulated negative values, which are also represented in the plot, creating a symmetrical distribution. The corresponding estimated density function is indicated by a solid line (grey in the monochrome

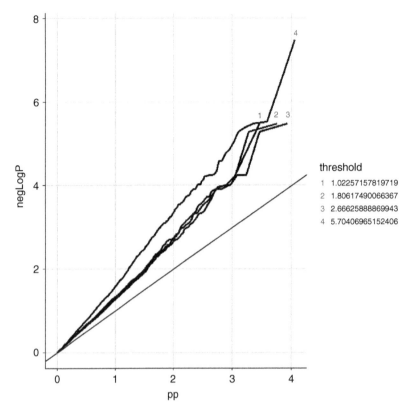

Figure 9.8   Q–Q plot of $-\log_{10}(p)$, stratified by q, from the NaCl versus untreated contrast in *A. thaliana* genotypes.

version of the plot, green in the colour version). This diagnostic plot also has the capability of presenting information concerning the proportion of the area of the distribution that is estimated to be attributed to the distribution on H_0^p (the 'null subdensity'), and regions of the Z-score in which the local FDR is low. However, in the present example, these features are not distinguishable because this proportion is small: further information on this capability is given by Efron et al. (2015).

The lower-left panel shows the marginal distribution of q, that is, the same information as in the vertical marginal histogram in Figure 9.6, but now:

- with q 'flipped' to negative values, because large positive Z-scores for q were associated with small values of p for the principal trait (whereas the correlation between p and q is required to be positive, as noted earlier in this section), and
- accompanied by a solid line that represents an empirical estimate of the corresponding density function, not the theory-based null-distribution function shown in the earlier figure.

The lower-right panel shows the estimated bivariate probability density of q versus p, that is, a smoothed representation of the bivariate plot of observed values in Figure 9.6, with the

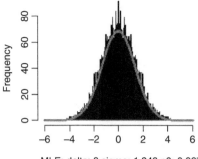

MLE: delta: 0 sigma: 1.342 p0: 0.997
CME: delta: 0 sigma: 1.378 p0: 1.02

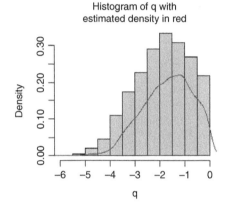

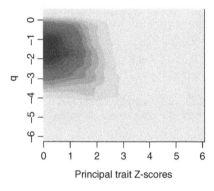

Figure 9.9 Diagnostic plots obtained from the values of *p* and *q* from *m* = 5702 probesets, for the NaCl versus untreated contrast in *A. thaliana* genotypes.

vertical scale reversed due to 'flipping' of *q*. In order to obtain a viable L-region for the combination of principal-trait *p* values and *q*-values into a single measure of the strength of evidence, it is necessary that the bivariate distribution of *p* and *q* should be approximately unimodal, with a maximum close to the origin, and these diagnostic plots show that this is the case.

The preceding series of commands also produces parallel vectors holding the values of *p* and *q* for each probeset (in the same order as in the input file), and the corresponding *v*-values. A plot of these values is next produced, by the following commands:

```
plot(p, z.q, pch = NA)
points(p[v < 0.1], z.q[v < 0.1],
  pch = 16, cex = 0.5, col = "black")
points(p[v >= 0.1 & v < 0.15], z.q[v >= 0.1 & v < 0.15],
  pch = 16, cex = 0.5, col = "grey")
points(p[v >= 0.15], z.q[v >= 0.15],
  pch = 1, cex = 0.5, col = "black")
```

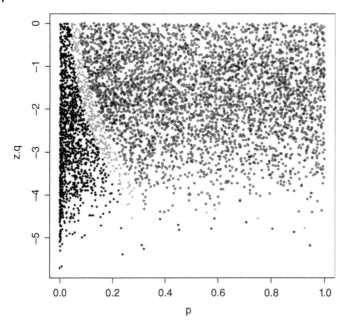

Figure 9.10 Bivariate plot of q versus p, with points in different L-regions identified by plotting symbol, from the NaCl versus untreated contrast in *A. thaliana* genotypes.

This plot is shown in Figure 9.10. It corresponds to the schematic plot of p versus z in Figure 9.2, with the L-region corresponding to $v < 0.15$ indicated by (p, q) pairs plotted with solid grey symbols, and the subset of this region corresponding to $v < 0.1$ by pairs plotted with solid black symbols. (An L-region is defined in terms of its cFDR threshold, but it can also be identified in terms of its v-value threshold. This is because the relationship between the cFDR and the v-value, like the relationship between the BH-FDR and the p-value, is (non-strictly) monotonic.) Pairs corresponding to larger values of v are indicated by open symbols. Note that the variable plotted on the vertical axis (relating to the auxiliary covariate) is *minus* the Z-score rather than the 'unflipped' Z-score, so that the region of interest is restored to an L-region, with those tests that give significant results for both variables in the bottom-left corner.

In order to compare the v-values with the 'raw' p-values for the principal trait, the following commands are executed:

```
pv_plot(p = p, q = z.q, v = v)
log10pv_plot(p = p, q = z.q, v = v,
    axis_lim = c(0, 10))
```

These produce the plots shown in Figure 9.11. Figure 9.11a shows that while there is of course a clear positive relationship between the raw p-values and the v-values (because the value of v is partly driven by the value of p) incorporation of information from the auxiliary covariate has had a substantial effect on the values of v, and on their ranking: if it had no effect, all the points would lie on the diagonal line $v = p$. 'Zooming in' on the region of

(a) **Flexible cFDR results**

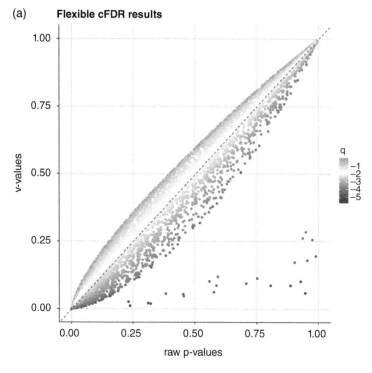

(b) **Flexible cFDR results**

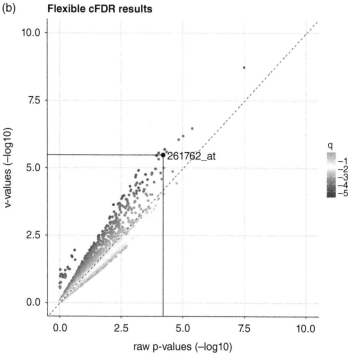

Figure 9.11 Plots of *v*-values versus 'raw' *p*-values, from the NaCl versus untreated contrast in *A. thaliana* genotypes. (a) Over the whole [0, 1] range of *v* and *p*. (b) Limited to the region near the origin, transformed to the $-\log_{10}$ scale.

most interest (small values of p and v, hence large $-\log_{10}$-transformed values), in Figure 9.11b we see that the significance of the effects on expression of many probesets has been increased (points above the diagonal line), whereas for some others the significance has been reduced (points below the line), though generally to a lesser extent. The probesets with small raw p-values, and even smaller v-values when the evidence from the auxiliary covariate is taken into account, would be the prime candidates for further investigation. In the colour version of this figure, the plotted points are colour-coded according to their value of q: deep blue for large-negative (highly significant) values, deep red for values close to zero, and pale-mauve shades for intermediate values. As expected, the tests for which v is much more significant than p are those for which q is highly significant. These can be distinguished even in the monochrome version of the figure, because in Figure 9.11b, points in the deep shades of blue and red occur well above and well below the diagonal line $v = p$, respectively, whereas points in pale shades lie close to the line. (Conversely, in Figure 9.11a, with no minus-logarithmic transformation, the deep *red* points lie well above the line, and the deep *blue* points well below.)

To further illustrate the interpretation of Figure 9.11, the results for an individual probeset, 261762_at, are now considered in more detail. The point representing this probeset is marked in Figure 9.11b with a larger black symbol, and the probeset's numerical results are presented in Table 9.2. The raw p-value for this probeset is highly significant, but the q-value is an order of magnitude smaller, and hence v is also much smaller than the raw p-value. Hence, the corresponding point on the figure is well above the diagonal line $v = p$, among the blue points.

BH-FDR values corresponding to both the raw p-values and the v-values are then obtained by the method introduced in Chapter 2, Section 2.4 and Chapter 3, Section 3.2. They are displayed graphically as described in Chapter 3, Section 3.3, by colour-coding the points on a $-\log_{10}$-transformed Q–Q plot for each set of probabilities (Figure 9.12). This method of presentation makes clear the gain in information from the auxiliary covariate. On the basis of the raw p-values, out of the $m = 5702$ tests considered, $k = 170$ (2.98% of the total) achieve the BH-FDR criterion of $q^* = 0.1$ (these tests being represented by points above the q^* line), whereas on the basis of the v-values, $k = 274$ tests (4.81% of the total) achieve this criterion. The harvest of hypotheses for further investigation has been increased by more than half ($274/170 = 1.61$), without compromising the false discovery rate. Returning to consideration of the illustrative probeset 261762_at (Table 9.2), we see that its cFDR has been substantially reduced by the contribution of information from the auxiliary covariate, relative to its FDR based on the raw p-value.

Table 9.2 cFDR results from the NaCl versus untreated contrast in *A. thaliana* genotypes, for an illustrative probeset.

Probeset	p	q	v	FDR, raw p-value	cFDR
261762_at	0.00006164	0.00000369	0.00000337	0.0207	0.0020

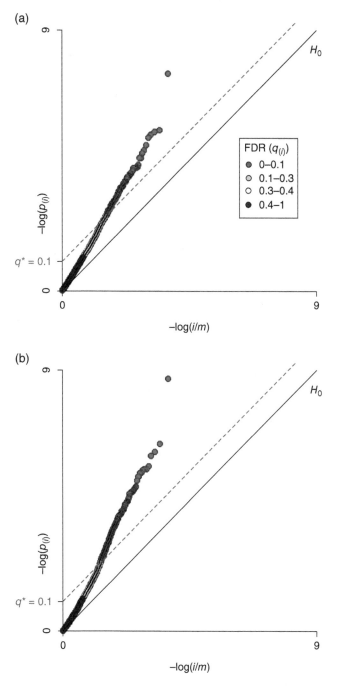

Figure 9.12 Q–Q plot, on the $-\log_{10}$ scale, of raw *p*-values and *v*-values for the NaCl versus untreated contrast in *A. thaliana* genotypes Col(gl) and Col(WT), in a representative subset of the probesets on Affymetrix array ATH1-121501. (a) Raw *p*-values. (b) *v*-values.

9.4 Summary

When multiple testing methods are applied to a set of p-values, information on 'relevant auxiliary covariates' is often also available.

A method is presented for combining the principal-trait p-values with such a parallel auxiliary variate, referred to as q, and for controlling the FDR on the basis of the combined value.

The auxiliary variate is referred to as q for consistency with the literature on this topic. N.B. This usage is not to be confused with the use of q as a symbol for the FDR itself in earlier chapters.

It is helpful to regard p-values and q-values as realisations of random variables, P and Q, respectively. The null hypothesis relating to p is then referred to as H_0^p.

The FDR based on the principal-trait p-values alone (FDR(p)) is then defined in Bayesian terms as a function of P (Equation (9.1)). The conditional FDR when the q-values are also taken into account (cFDR(p, q)) is obtained by adding the condition $Q \leq q$ to this definition (Equation (9.3)).

Methods for estimation of the cFDR, and for identifying subsets of null hypotheses for rejection on the basis of it, have been developed in the context of genetic association studies, in relation to several particular types of auxiliary covariate, including, but not limited to, a second set of p-values.

These methods are described in outline. Bayes' theorem is first applied to the formula defining the cFDR (Equation (9.3)). This leads to a function of P and Q (Equation (9.17)) corresponding to the usual conservative estimator of FDR(p) (Equation (9.7)).

In the case of the usual estimator of FDR(p), the probabilities of the observations on H_0^p (in the numerator) and the quantile ranks of these observations (in the denominator) are expressed in terms of lengths on two axes, both relating to P. However, in the case of cFDR (p, q), the observations are represented by points in the P–Q plane, and there is no single natural ordering of their values.

To deal with this situation, simplifying assumptions are made, namely, that:

- when H_0^p is true, Q is independent of P, and
- in other cases, there is a positive stochastic monotonic relationship between p and q.

The relationship between the observations that lie within the rectangle ($P \leq p$, $Q \leq q$) and the overall distribution of observations in the P–Q plane is considered.

The numerator of the estimator of cFDR(p, q) is the probability that an observation lies within the rectangle conditional on H_0^p, namely, $p \cdot P(Q \leq q | H_0^p)$. The denominator is the unconditional probability, namely, $P(P \leq p, Q \leq q)$.

Attention is focused on the case in which the auxiliary covariate comprises a second set of p-values. This is helpful because, regardless of the underlying form of the additional variable, the information it provides can often be summarised in a p-value.

The relationship between the observations within the rectangle and the overall distribution is explored using simulated data. Boundaries in the bivariate P–Q space are identified such that the probability mass within the rectangle ($P \leq p_i$, $Q \leq q_i$) is constant for all points (p_i, q_i) that lie on the boundary.

Such a region of high probability, adjacent to the P and Q axes, has been called an 'L-region', and its boundary an 'L-curve'.

A series of non-intersecting, concentric L-curves defines smaller and smaller L-regions of increasing probability density towards the origin. These regions are analogous to increasingly stringent significance criteria in the univariate distribution of P. They provide a way of combining P and Q into a single measure of the strength of evidence. But N.B. such L-curves are in practice identified on the basis of cFDR values, and not directly on the basis of the bivariate density of p- and q-values.

If the relevant auxiliary covariate Q is a p-value, it can be back-transformed to the corresponding Z-score using the function $-\Phi^{-1}(q/2)$ defined in Equation (9.23). A plot of Z-score versus p-value may then come closer to the original data. In such a plot, the region of stringent significance criteria for both variables (the angle of the L) is in the top left-hand corner.

Many datasets based on real observations conform approximately to the patterns required for the identification of L-curves and L-regions, and empirical, numerical methods for their identification have been developed.

A conservative estimator of cFDR(p, q) for a particular pair of observations (p_i, q_i) $(\widehat{\text{cFDR}}(p, q)$, Equation (9.17)) is obtained from the probability mass of the bivariate distribution that lies within the region $(P \le p_i, Q \le q_i)$, conditional on H_0^p in the numerator and unconditionally in the denominator. For this purpose, a further assumption is made, namely, that H_0^p is true for most tests.

In order to obtain a set of probabilities that combine the information from the principal-trait p-values and the q-values, and that can be used in the same way as ordinary p-values, a further step is required. The estimated cFDR values are used to define the non-intersecting boundaries of a series of concentric L-regions, the estimated cFDR being constant along each boundary. For each pair of observations (p_i, q_i), the probability density on H_0^p is then integrated over the corresponding L-region. This probability mass, called a v-value, is analogous to a p-value in the univariate case.

The rationale for defining the boundary of the L-region in relation to cFDR, and the v-value as the probability mass within the L-region on H_0^p, is clarified by relating it to the corresponding argument when only the p-values for the principal trait are considered.

Such v-values can be used to calculate BH-FDR values in the usual way. They can also be used iteratively, to incorporate additional layers of auxiliary data.

The application of these methods to non-genetic data is explored. In many non-genetic contexts, correlations between P and Q and between tests will compromise the assumptions made in the methods outlined earlier in this summary. However, it is argued that the resulting v-values and BH-FDR values are likely to be conservative, and hence may still provide useful guidance even if they cannot be taken literally.

The methods are applied to the *Arabidopsis* gene expression data introduced in Chapter 4. The NaCl versus untreated contrast for genotype Col(gl) is specified as the principal trait, and the corresponding contrast for genotype Col(WT) as the auxiliary covariate. The results from every fourth probeset on the Affymetrix array ATH1-121501 are used, as a representative subset of all probesets on the array.

There is a positive correlation between the t-statistics for the two traits, and evidence of real effects for some probesets for both traits. For both traits, there is evidence of effects in both directions: some genes are more strongly expressed in NaCl-treated plants, whereas others are more strongly expressed in untreated plants. These patterns indicate that the auxiliary covariate may be effective in supplementing the information from the principal-trait *p*-values, and that it is appropriate to base the analysis on *p*-values from two-sided tests for both traits.

The *p*-values for the auxiliary covariate are transformed to the corresponding absolute *Z*-scores, to illustrate that the analysis implementation used can cope with an arbitrary distribution of the auxiliary covariate.

L-regions corresponding to $v < 0.15$ and $v < 0.1$ are identified. The *v*-values for each probeset are obtained, and compared with the corresponding 'raw', principal-trait *p*-values. The *v*-values are shown to be smaller (more significant) than the corresponding raw *p*-values for many probesets, particularly in the region near the origin (highly significant test results), but larger (less significant) for some others, though generally to a lesser extent.

BH-FDR values are obtained from the *v*-values, and are compared with those from the raw *p*-values using Q–Q plots on the $-\log_{10}$ scale. These plots show a clear gain in information from the contribution of the auxiliary covariate to the *v*-values. While maintaining control of the false discovery rate at $q^* = 0.1$, the number of hypotheses identified for further investigation from the $m = 5702$ tests performed is increased from $k = 170$ (2.98% of the total) to $k = 274$ (4.81%).

References

Efron, B., Turnbull, B.B., and Narasimhan, B. (2015). *locfdr Vignette. Complete Help Documentation. Including Usage Tips and Simulation Example*. Stanford: Department of Statistics, Stanford University https://cran.r-project.org/web/packages/locfdr/vignettes/locfdr-example.pdf.

Hastie, T., Tibshirai, R., and Friedman, J. (2001). *The Elements of Statistical Learning. Data Mining, Inference and Prediction*. New York: Springer 533 pp.

Hutchinson, A., Liley, J., and Wallace, C. (2022). fcfdr: an R package to leverage continuous and binary functional genomic data in GWAS. *BMC Bioinformatics* 23: https://doi.org/10.1186/s12859-022-04838-0.

Hutchinson, A., Reales, G., Willis, T., and Wallace, C. (2021). Leveraging auxiliary data from arbitrary distributions to boost GWAS discovery with Flexible cFDR. *PLoS Genetics* 17 (10): e1009853. https://doi.org/10.1371/journal.pgen.1009853.

Liley, J. and Wallace, C. (2021). Accurate error control in high-dimensional association testing using conditional false discovery rates. *Biometrical Journal* 63: 1096–1130.

R Core Team (2021). *R: A Language and Environment for Statistical Computing*. Vienna, Austria: R Foundation for Statistical Computing https://www.R-project.org/.

10

An FDR-Based Analogue of the Confidence Interval:
The False Coverage Rate (FCR)

10.1 The Concept of the Coverage of a Confidence Interval

When researchers have reported a set of discoveries on the basis of the FDR, they will usually also want to report an estimate of the effect size corresponding to each discovery, in relation to a null hypothesis of 'no effect' (e.g., a difference of 0 or a ratio of 1). When a discovery is reported on the basis of an unadjusted p-value, the point estimate of the corresponding effect is usually accompanied by a confidence interval (CI), calculated on the same conceptual basis as the p-value. Researchers reporting FDRs will naturally want each of their effect estimates to be accompanied by an interval estimate that is related to the FDR in an analogous way.

In order to identify the BH-FDR-based interval that is analogous to the ordinary CI, the first step is to review the relationship between the CI and the unadjusted p-value. The CI is expressed in relation to a significance threshold α. Suppose that the true effect for the discovery in question is δ, and a point estimate of this effect, d, has been observed. A null hypothesis (H_0) concerning the true effect, $\delta = \delta_0$, is then specified. The 'exact' $(1 - \alpha)$ CI is then defined as the range of values of δ_0 that does not cause the observation d to give an extreme value, relative to the threshold α, when H_0 is tested. For example, if we specify $\alpha = 0.05$, we obtain the $(1 - 0.05)$ CI, namely, the range of values of δ_0 that do not cause a significance test on d to give $p < 0.05$.

In practice, the CI is more commonly expressed in terms of a percentage than in terms of a probability. Thus, in the present case, the $(1 - \alpha)$ CI is referred to as the

$$100 \times (1 - \alpha)\%\text{CI} = 100 \times (1 - 0.05)\%\text{CI},$$

that is, the 95% CI.

In many large-sample situations, d can be assumed to be a realisation of a normally distributed variable D with standard deviation σ_d, that is,

$$D \sim N(\delta, \sigma_d). \tag{10.1}$$

In this case, $H_0{:}\delta = \delta_0$ can be tested by calculating the corresponding Z statistic,

$$z = \frac{d - \delta_0}{\sigma_d}. \tag{10.2}$$

The False Discovery Rate: Its Meaning, Interpretation and Application in Data Science, First Edition.
N.W. Galwey.
© 2025 John Wiley & Sons Ltd. Published 2025 by John Wiley & Sons Ltd.
Companion website: www.wiley.com/go/falsediscoveryrate

On H_0, z is a realisation of a random variable Z with distribution

$$Z \sim N(0, 1).$$

So, if a two-sided test is conducted,

$$p = P((|Z| > |z|)|d, \delta_0), \tag{10.3}$$

and the $(1 - \alpha)$ CI is the range of values of δ_0 for which

$$p \geq \alpha, \tag{10.4}$$

and H_0 is not rejected.

If a test statistic other than the standard normal variable Z is used, then some measure of the discrepancy between d and δ_0 other than $(d - \delta_0)$ may be needed, and if a one-sided test is conducted, then the signed value of the test statistic, rather than its absolute value, is required in order to obtain the p-value. However, this common and simple example of a normally distributed effect and a two-sided Z-test serves to illustrate the concepts involved.

In practice, it is not necessary to explore the range of possible values of δ_0 in detail. We simply use the standard formula for calculation of the test statistic, find the values of the test statistic that correspond to $p = \alpha$, and then rearrange the formula to obtain the values of δ_0 corresponding to these boundaries of the H_0 rejection region. In the case of the two-sided Z-test, if the test result z is obtained, the corresponding p-value is

$$p = P(|Z| > |z|) = 2 \times P(Z > |z|). \tag{10.5}$$

Substituting $p = \alpha$ into Equation (10.5) and rearranging, we obtain

$$P(Z > |z|) = \alpha/2,$$

and the values of z that satisfy this criterion are designated $\pm z_{\alpha/2}$. Substituting these values into Equation (10.2), we obtain

$$\pm z_{\alpha/2} = \frac{d - \delta_0}{\sigma_d},$$

which can be rearranged to give

$$\delta_0 = d \pm z_{\alpha/2} \cdot \sigma_d. \tag{10.6}$$

These two values of δ_0 are the boundaries of the $(1 - \alpha)$ CI. The distribution of D when δ_0 is specified as each of these boundary values, and when the observed value is d in each case, is illustrated in Figure 10.1.

Before extending this approach to the FDR context, it is important to consider carefully the meaning of such a conventional CI. It is tempting to think of it as meaning that

$$P(\delta \text{ lies within the } 100(1 - \alpha)\% \text{ CI}) = 1 - \alpha, \tag{10.7}$$

but this is not quite right. In the definition of a CI, it is the estimated effect d, not true effect δ, that is specified as a realisation of a random variable, to which a probability may be attached: that is, the CI is a frequentist, not a Bayesian concept. And indeed, Equation (10.7) does not necessarily give the correct probability. This can be illustrated if, instead of considering the normally distributed variable D, we consider a variable with a binomial distribution.

Figure 10.1 (a)–(c) Distribution of the normally distributed observed effect D when the null-hypothesis value δ_0 is specified as the values at the boundaries of the CI. In panels (a) and (b), hatched areas indicate values of D that will give values of the test statistic in the rejection region.

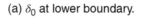

(a) δ_0 at lower boundary.

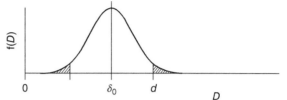

(b) δ_0 at upper boundary.

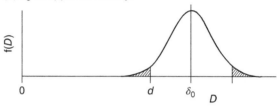

(c) CI for δ.

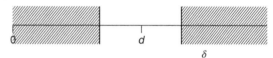

This is conventionally defined as the distribution of the number of 'successes' obtained, R, in a sample of N independent 'trials' (where, for example, a 'trial' might consist of rolling a die and a 'success' might consist of obtaining a 'six'), and is expressed symbolically as

$$R \sim \text{Binomial}(N, \pi), \tag{10.8}$$

where π is the probability of 'success' in an individual trial. The probabilities in this distribution are given by

$$P(R = r) = \frac{N!}{r!(N-r)!}\pi^r(1-\pi)^{N-r}, \tag{10.9}$$

where

$\qquad r =$ a realisation of R, that is, the observation of R from an individual sample of N trials,

and

$$N! = N \times (N-1) \times (N-2) \times ... \times 2 \times 1.$$

In this distribution, π is the unknown parameter. Of course, if the die is unbiased, then $\pi = \frac{1}{6}$, but we will not make this assumption: we will consider how π is estimated from the outcome of the sample of N trials.

Suppose that $N = 10$ trials are conducted, of which $r = 2$ gives a 'success'. We can then define the boundaries of a $100(1-\alpha)\%$ CI for π as the lowest and highest values, π_0, that would cause the null hypothesis H_0: $\pi = \pi_0$ to be rejected on this evidence when the significance threshold is specified as α. If we further specify that the rejection region for H_0 should comprise equal probability masses $\alpha/2$ in each tail of the binomial distribution, then these lower and upper boundaries are defined by

$$P(R \geq r) = \alpha/2 \tag{10.10}$$

and

$$P(R \leq r) = \alpha/2, \tag{10.11}$$

respectively, as shown for a 95% CI in Figure 10.2. (Or, equivalently to Equation (10.10), for the lower boundary,

$$P(R < r) = 1 - \alpha/2, \tag{10.12}$$

if this makes computation easier.) If the low value $\pi_0 = 0.025$ is specified, the probability of $r = 2$ or higher is $\alpha/2 = 0.025$ (Figure 10.2a), whereas if the high value $\pi_0 = 0.556$ is specified, then the probability of obtaining the observed value $r = 2$ or lower is $\alpha/2 = 0.025$ (Figure 10.2b). Putting these criteria together, we obtain the 95% CI for π, [0.025, 0.556], as shown in Figure 10.2c.

(a) π_0 at lower boundary.

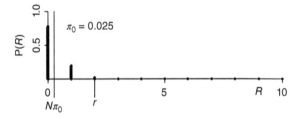

(b) π_0 at upper boundary.

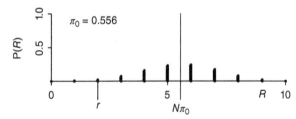

(c) CI for π.

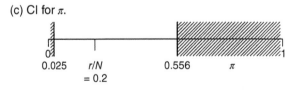

Figure 10.2 (a)–(c) Distribution of the observed binomial variable R, when the null-hypothesis value π_0 is specified as the values at the boundaries of the CI.

However, this CI is not unique. We have chosen to achieve our threshold value of $\alpha = 0.05$ in terms of equal probability masses $\alpha/2$ in each tail of the binomial distribution, but other choices could be made. Note that the present CI is not symmetrical about the unbiased point estimate of π, $r/N = 2/10$: the distance from the point estimate to the lower boundary is

$$0.2 - 0.025 = 0.175,$$

whereas the distance from the point estimate to the upper boundary is

$$0.556 - 0.2 = 0.356.$$

Nor is the probability mass for the observed outcome the same for the π_0 values at the two CI boundaries: if $\pi_0 = 0.025$, $P(R = 2) = 0.0233$, whereas if $\pi_0 = 0.556$, $P(R = 2) = 0.0210$ (a difference too small to be detectable on the plots). To obtain a symmetrical confidence interval, or one with equal probability mass at the two boundaries, we would have to allocate α unequally between the upper and lower tails of the binomial distribution.

Further exploration shows that for a binomial variable such as R, the probability that π lies within the $(1 - \alpha)$ CI is not constant even when the method for choosing the CI boundaries has been specified and the value of N has been specified: it depends on the value of π itself! The process for calculating this probability, when the CI is defined as described in the earlier text, is as follows:

- for each value of π, over the range $[0, 1]$:
  - determine whether π lies within the $(1 - \alpha)$ CI for each value $R = 0...N$. That is, determine whether the criteria $P(R \geq r|\pi) > \alpha/2$ and $P(R \leq r|\pi) > \alpha/2$ (corresponding to the boundary-value criteria in Equations (10.10) and (10.11)) are both met.
  - set the following index variable:
    $I = 1$ if π lies within the $(1 - \alpha)$ CI,
    $I = 0$ otherwise.
  - obtain $P(R = r|\pi)$,
  - perform the following calculation:

$$P(\pi \text{ lies within the } 100(1 - \alpha)\% \text{ CI}) = \sum_{r=0}^{N} P(R = r|\pi) \cdot I \qquad (10.13)$$

This probability, that the true parameter value lies within the CI, is known as the *true coverage* of the CI. The value $100(1 - \alpha)\%$ is known as the *nominal coverage*. With $\alpha = 0.05$ and sample sizes $N = 10$ and 100, this process gives the results shown in Figure 10.3. The vertical regions of the coverage function correspond to ranges where a small change in the value of π_0 causes a particular value of r to meet, or to fail to meet, one of the boundary-value criteria in Equations (10.10) and (10.11), causing a step change in the true coverage.

The main practical points to be noted concerning these CIs are as follows:

- The true coverage is always greater than the nominal value of $100(1 - 0.05)\% = 95\%$, that is, $P(\pi \text{ lies within the } 95\% \text{ CI}) > 0.95$.

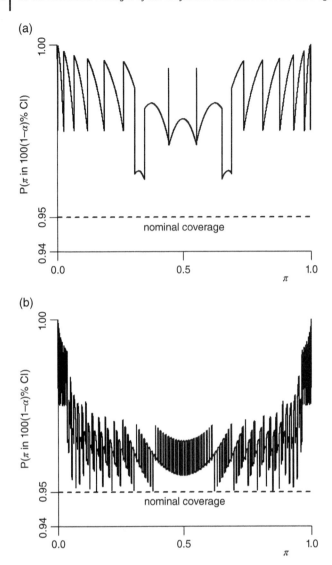

Figure 10.3 Coverage of a 95% confidence interval for an estimate of the binomial-distribution parameter π, for different values of the sample size N. (a) N = 10. (b) N = 100.

Therefore, the CI is somewhat wider than it needs to be: it is *conservative* – though because we do not know the true value π, we do not know exactly how conservative.

- Broadly speaking, the true coverage is greater for values of π close to 0 or 1, and lower (closer to its nominal value) for intermediate values of π. This pattern is particularly strong when N is large.
- A larger value of N brings the coverage of the CI closer to its nominal value. Indeed, as N approaches infinity, the binomial distribution approaches the standard normal distribution and the coverage approaches the nominal value.

The binomial CI calculated by this method is referred to as the Clopper–Pearson interval (Clopper and Pearson 1934). It is also often known as an 'exact' confidence interval, because of its exact relationship to the corresponding rejection region of the binomial distribution in relation to H_0. However, as Figure 10.3 shows, it is far from being exact with regard to the agreement between the nominal and true coverage. Other methods are available that do much better in this respect, by accepting results that will sometimes be slightly anti-conservative, that is, CIs that are somewhat narrower than they 'should' be, giving a true coverage that is slightly less than their nominal coverage. These methods are well reviewed and explained by Newcombe (1998).

Having used the binomial distribution to demonstrate the concept of the coverage of a CI, we now return to consideration of a normally distributed effect estimate, d. Because this is a realisation of a random variable D, with Distribution (10.1), the probability that the true value δ lies within the confidence interval defined by any postulated value δ_0 does not depend on δ itself (unlike the corresponding probability for an estimate of the binomial parameter π, which *does* depend on π itself): that is, the Z statistic defined in Equation (10.2) is not a function of δ. Hence, for a normally distributed effect estimate, the true coverage of the CI equals the nominal coverage. This often provides the basis for a workable approximation, even if the effect estimate is not strictly normally distributed. In particular, in the case of an observed binomial variable, if N is sufficiently large, and the estimate of π given by $\hat{\pi} = \dfrac{r}{N}$ is sufficiently far from 0 or 1, then the binomial distribution can be approximated by a normal distribution:

$$\hat{\pi} \sim N\left(\pi, \sqrt{\frac{\hat{\pi}(1-\hat{\pi})}{N}}\right). \tag{10.14}$$

If the nominal coverage of the CI can be assumed to be a reasonable approximation to its true coverage, a basis is obtained for calculating an analogue of the CI for use in multiple-testing situations, based on the FDR.

10.2 A Confidence Interval Based on the FDR-Determined Significance Threshold

If the nominal coverage and the true coverage of a CI are the same, then because of the relationship between the p-value and the CI noted in Equation (10.3) and Inequality (10.4), the meaning of the significance threshold α can be expressed in two equivalent ways:

$$P(p < \alpha \,|\, H_0) = \alpha \tag{10.15}$$

and

$$P(\delta \text{ lies outside the } 100(1-\alpha)\% \text{ CI} \,|\, H_0) = \alpha. \tag{10.16}$$

It is important to note that Equation (10.16) is not a Bayesian statement, dependent upon regarding δ as a random variable with a specified probability distribution. The Z statistic is not a function of δ (as was noted in Section 10.1), and, therefore, provided that the assumptions made are correct, Equation (10.16) is a frequentist statement about what will happen in the long run when many such CIs are calculated. (If the nominal CI is conservative, the symbol '=' in Equations (10.15) and (10.16) can be replaced by '<', that is, the probabilities on the left-hand side are *less than α*.)

Because of the relationship between the *p*-value and the CI noted in Equations (10.15) and (10.16), the FDR, which we have so far connected to the statistical test of each of a set of *m* hypotheses, can also be connected to the confidence interval for the effect associated with each hypothesis. As stated earlier (Chapter 2, Section 2.4, Inequality 2.14), the BH-FDR criterion is specified as

$$P_{(k)} \leq \frac{k}{m} q^*,$$
(10.17)

where

$$q^* = \text{the FDR to be achieved,}$$

and

$$P_{(k)} = \text{the kth-ranked } p\text{-value, that is, the largest of the ordered } p\text{-values, } p_{(i)}, i = 1...m,$$
$$\text{that satisfies Inequality (10.17).}$$

That is, the set of hypotheses that meet the FDR criterion q^* is specified by setting the significance threshold to

$$\alpha = p_{(k)}.$$

This significance threshold can then be used to construct a $100(1 - \alpha)\% = 100(1 - p_{(k)})\%$ CI for the effect estimate connected to each of the k test results announced as discoveries (Benjamini and Yekutieli 2005, Definition 1). For this purpose, the ith ordered p-value $p_{(i)}$ must be associated with:

- a true effect $\delta_{(i)}$,
- an estimate of this true effect, $d_{(i)}$, and
- a standard error of this estimate, $SE(d_{(i)})$.

The CI is calculated by adapting Equation (10.6):

$$\delta_{(i)} = d_{(i)} \pm z_{p_{(k)}/2} \cdot SE(d_{(i)}).$$
(10.18)

Note that the rank k used to obtain the appropriate threshold value $\alpha = p_{(k)}$ will not necessarily be the same as the rank i of the test under consideration.

A *False Coverage Rate* (FCR), analogous to the FDR, can then be defined in relation to the CIs for the set of k test results announced as discoveries. Its true value is

$$FCR = \frac{V}{V + S},$$

where

$$V = \text{the number of tests for which } \delta_{(i)} \text{ lies outside the } 100(1 - p_{(k)})\% \text{ CI}$$

and

$$S = \text{the number of tests for which } \delta_{(i)} \text{ lies within this interval.}$$

However, this true value is unknown, because the true value of V is unknown. Nevertheless, statements can be made that relate the FCR to q^*, corresponding to those made previously (Chapter 2, Section 2.4) about the hypothesis tests. Firstly, the criterion in Inequality (10.17) controls the FCR at

$$\mathrm{E}\left(\frac{V}{V+S}\right) = \mathrm{E}\left(\frac{V}{k}\right) \leq q^*.$$

That is, if we calculate the $100(1 - p_{(k)})\%$ CI for each of the k test results announced as discoveries, and if the true coverage of the CI is equal to its nominal coverage, then it is expected that the CI will contain the true value except in a proportion q^* of the tests or less. This is analogous to the statement that the same criterion controls the FDR at the same rate, where

$V =$ the (true, unknown) number of tests, among the k test results announced as discoveries, for which H_0 is true (Chapter 2, Section 2.4, Equation (2.9)).

Secondly, the criterion in Inequality (10.17) leads to an upper bound for the expected FCR for each test, which is the same as the upper bound for the BH-FDR, that is,

$$\mathrm{E}\left(\frac{V}{V+S}\right) \leq \frac{p_{(k)}}{k/m} = \frac{mp_{(k)}}{k},$$

as previously stated in Chapter 2, Section 2.5, Equation (2.19). Hence,

$$\widehat{\mathrm{FCR}} = \frac{mp_{(k)}}{k} \tag{10.19}$$

provides a conservative estimate of the FCR.

Like the BH-FDR, the FCR can be calculated using the value $q_{(i)}$ for each hypothesis, $i = 1...m$ (as described in Chapter 3, Section 3.2), rather than a pre-specified value q^*.

In relation to the hypothesis test, it was necessary to distinguish between two concepts: the false-positive rate, the proportion of cases in which H_0 is rejected when it is true, and the FDR, the proportion of cases in which H_0 is true when it is rejected. No such distinction is needed in relation to the FCR. The FCR relates only to the probability that the true value of the effect lies outside the CI, and no statement conditional on a particular value of the effect (such as the statement H_0) is required.

10.3 Numerical Illustration of the FCR

The calculation of the FCR can be illustrated in the context of the *Arabidopsis thaliana* data analysed in Chapter 4. In Section 4.3 (Chapter 4), p-values were obtained for the NaCl versus untreated contrast in the *A. thaliana* genotype Col(gl), for the expression level of 83 salt-related genes. Table 10.1 presents the ordered p-values for the genes giving the most significant and least significant results, together with the estimate of the contrast effect for each gene ($d_{(i)}$), the SE of the estimate ($SE(d_{(i)})$), and some other statistics. In this table (as in Chapter 2, Table 2.4), column $p_{(i)}$ gives the ordered p-values, from smallest to largest. $q_{(i)}$ gives the BH-FDR that is achieved if $p_{(i)}$ is considered significant, and k indicates the rank of the largest p-value that can be considered significant while still achieving this FDR, $\alpha = p_{(k)}$.

Table 10.1 Statistics from the analysis of the NaCl versus untreated contrast in the A. thaliana genotype Col(gl), for the expression level of 83 salt-related genes. Each gene is identified by its Probeset ID. For the relationship between Probeset ID and gene name, see Table 4.2 in Chapter 4.

i	Probeset ID	$d_{(i)}$	$SE(d_{(i)})$	t	$p_{(i)}$	$q_{(i)}$	k	$p_{(k)}$	$t_{(p_{(k)}/2),6}$	FDR-based CI boundary Lower	Upper
1	251745_at	−0.997	0.1784	−5.587	0.0014	0.116	1	0.0014	5.587	−1.993	0.000
2	249327_at	0.552	0.1249	4.423	0.0045	0.181	5	0.0109	3.632	0.099	1.006
3	246546_at	−0.371	0.0967	−3.833	0.0086	0.181	5	0.0109	3.632	−0.722	−0.019
4	253141_at	−0.489	0.1333	−3.670	0.0104	0.181	5	0.0109	3.632	−0.974	−0.005
5	260587_at	0.187	0.0515	3.632	0.0109	0.181	5	0.0109	3.632	0.000	0.374
6	245747_at	−0.497	0.1461	−3.404	0.0144	0.193	7	0.0163	3.307	−0.981	−0.014
7	258959_at	−0.343	0.1036	−3.307	0.0163	0.193	7	0.0163	3.307	−0.685	0.000
8	247650_at	0.211	0.0794	2.657	0.0377	0.391	8	0.0377	2.657	0.000	0.422
9	249884_at	−0.238	0.1080	−2.203	0.0699	0.623	41	0.3079	1.114	−0.358	−0.118
10	245868_at	0.145	0.0716	2.029	0.0888	0.623	41	0.3079	1.114	0.066	0.225
...											...
76	263469_at	−0.052	0.2225	−0.233	0.8238	0.900	76	0.8238	0.233	−0.104	0.000
77	246681_at	−0.028	0.1509	−0.183	0.8609	0.922	80	0.8891	0.146	−0.050	−0.006
78	259081_at	−0.074	0.4533	−0.163	0.8756	0.922	80	0.8891	0.146	−0.140	−0.008
79	258020_at	−0.010	0.0625	−0.154	0.8826	0.922	80	0.8891	0.146	−0.019	−0.001
80	259357_at	−0.030	0.2046	−0.146	0.8891	0.922	80	0.8891	0.146	−0.060	0.000
81	253627_at	−0.030	0.2990	−0.099	0.9243	0.945	82	0.9333	0.087	−0.056	−0.004
82	259337_at	0.016	0.1812	0.087	0.9333	0.945	82	0.9333	0.087	0.000	0.032
83	247007_at	0.001	0.1232	0.009	0.9933	0.993	83	0.9933	0.009	0.000	0.002

The values $p_{(i)}$ are presented graphically in Figure 4.8 in Chapter 4, $-\log_{10}$-transformed, and with the plotted points coded by colour or shading to indicate the corresponding FDR value.

Suppose that we want to obtain a CI for the contrast effect on the expression level of the gene with rank $i = 3$, Probeset ID '246546_at', while achieving a known FCR. We note that the BH-FDR achievable while announcing this effect as a discovery, and hence also the FCR achievable, is $q_{(3)} = 0.1815$, and that in order to achieve this value, the significance threshold that must be used to calculate the CI is $p_{(k)} = p_{(5)} = 0.010934$ (both values presented here to more places of decimals than in the table). The t statistic used to test the significance of this effect has six degrees of freedom (DF) (the residual DF in the anova of the whole experiment, Table 4.9), so the two-sided critical values of the t distribution required for calculation of the CI are

$$\pm t_{\alpha/2,\text{DF}} = \pm t_{p_{(5)}/2,6} = \pm t_{0.010934/2,6} = \pm t_{0.0054669,6} = \pm 3.63240.$$

For a CI based on the t distribution, as for the CI based on the standard normal distribution (Equation 10.6), the true coverage is equal to the nominal coverage, provided that the assumptions justifying the use of the distribution are valid. Hence, Equation (10.18) can be further adapted, with $t_{\alpha/2,\text{d.f}}$ playing the role of $z_{\alpha/2}$, as follows:

$$\text{CI} = d_{(i)} \pm t_{p_{(k)}/2,\text{d.f.}} \cdot \text{SE}(d_{(i)}) = -0.37071 \pm 3.63240 \times 0.096711 = [-0.722, -0.0194].$$

$$(10.20)$$

But we note that the value used for the threshold $\alpha = p_{(k)}$ in this calculation was $p_{(5)}$, not $p_{(3)}$, which means that we can calculate CIs using this value for all the $k = 5$ genes with ranks $i = 1...5$, and continue to achieve FCR $= 0.1815$.

We further note that the CI for Probeset ID '251745_at', the gene with rank $i = 1$, in Table 10.1 is calculated so as to achieve a lower FCR, $q_{(1)} = 0.1159$, using the lower significance threshold $\alpha = p_{(1)} = 0.0013969$. If we want to achieve the FCR $q^* = q_{(1)} = 0.1159$, then this gene is the only one for which a CI can be reported, that is, $k = 1$. But we do not have to accept this. If we are content with $q^* = q_{(3)} = q_{(5)} = 0.1815$, we can calculate an alternative CI for this gene on the basis of $\alpha = p_{(5)} = 0.010934$, by substituting appropriate values into Equation (10.20), as follows:

$$\text{CI} = -0.99653 \pm 3.63240 \times 0.178351 = [-1.6444, -0.3487].$$

We then achieve a narrower CI than that given in the table, which was $[-1.9931, 0.0000]$, and a larger harvest of genes for which we can report a CI ($k = 5$), by paying the price of a higher FCR. This illustrates the point that the FCR, like the FDR (see Chapter 3, Section 3.4), is a property of a *set* of test results, not an individual test result.

As for the CIs for the genes with the highest-ranked p-values, at first glance they do not look unreasonable. For example, the results for Probeset ID '247007_at', the gene with rank $i = m = 83$, are $d_{(83)} = 0.00108$, CI $= [0.0000, 0.0022]$. But this CI is obtained by setting the absurd threshold $\alpha = p_{(83)} = 0.9932820$, giving $q_{(83)} = 0.9933$: it is practically certain that this CI does not contain the true effect $\delta_{(83)}$.

The Benjamini–Hochberg-based FCR approach is not the only way in which CIs can be adapted to take account of multiplicity. One alternative is to use a Bonferroni-corrected significance threshold, a/m, to construct the CI. For example, in the present case, if we set $a = 0.05$, the Bonferroni-corrected critical t-values are

$$\pm t_{a/2m,DF} = \pm t_{0.05/(2 \times 83),6} = \pm t_{0.000301,6} = \pm 6.55701.$$

Applying these to Probeset ID '251745_at' $(i = 1)$ gives

$$CI = -0.99653 \pm 6.55701 \times 0.178351 = [-2.1660, 0.1729].$$

If we apply this very conservative approach to all $m = 83$ tests, we will ensure that the probability that one or more of the CIs fails to contain the true effect value is kept below 0.05, but will pay the price of extremely wide CIs.

10.4 Summary

Researchers reporting discoveries on the basis of the FDR usually wish to report the effect size associated with each discovery.

For an individual discovery, the point estimate of the effect (d) is usually accompanied by a confidence interval (CI), calculated on the same conceptual basis as the p-value. In the context of multiple testing with control of the FDR, an analogous interval related to the FDR is required.

The relationship between the CI and the unadjusted p-value is explored in detail. A null hypothesis concerning the unknown true effect (δ) is specified, namely, H_0: $\delta = \delta_0$. The 100 $(1 - a)\%$ CI is defined by the boundaries of the range of values of δ_0 that do not result in rejection of H_0 at the threshold level a.

The long-run, frequentist probability that δ lies within the $100(1 - a)\%$ CI is known as the *true coverage* of this CI, and $(1 - a)$ is known as its *nominal coverage*. If d is a realisation of a normally distributed variable, the two are equal, but this relationship is not valid for all distributions.

The discrepancy between true and nominal coverage is explored in the context of the binomial distribution.

If the nominal coverage is a reasonable approximation to the true coverage, the FDR for a set of test results reported as discoveries can be used as the basis for the calculation of an interval around each of the corresponding effect estimates. These intervals have a relationship to the FDR analogous to the relationship of a conventional CI to the p-value.

For each of the k ordered discoveries that achieve a specified FDR q^*, an estimated effect, $d_{(i)}$, is obtained. The largest p-value reported as significant, $p_{(k)}$, is specified as the significance threshold a. This value of a is substituted into the standard formula to calculate a CI for each $d_{(i)}$, $i = 1...k$. The false coverage rate (FCR) is then the proportion of tests for which the CI does not include the true effect $\delta_{(i)}$.

If the nominal coverage equals the true coverage, this procedure controls the FCR at level q^*. That is, the relationship of the FCR to the CI is analogous to the relationship of the FDR to H_0.

Like the BH-FDR, the FCR can be calculated using the value $q_{(i)}$ for each hypothesis, $i = 1...m$, where m is the total number of tests conducted, rather than a pre-specified value q^*.

The FCR is illustrated numerically in the context of the *Arabidopsis* data analysed in Chapter 4.

References

Benjamini, Y. and Yekutieli, D. (2005). False discovery rate-adjusted multiple confidence intervals for selected parameters. *Journal of the American Statistical Association* 100: 71–81. https://doi.org/10.1198/016214504000001907.

Clopper, C. and Pearson, E.S. (1934). The use of confidence or fiducial limits illustrated in the case of the binomial. *Biometrika* 26: 404–413. https://doi.org/10.1093/biomet/26.4.404.

Newcombe, R.G. (1998). Two-sided confidence intervals for the single proportion: comparison of seven methods. *Statistics in Medicine* 17: 857–872. https://doi.org/10.1002/(SICI)1097-0258 (19980430)17:8<857::AID-SIM777>3.0.CO;2-E. PMID 9595616.

11

The FDR as a Criterion for Sample Size Calculations

11.1 Review of the Standard Methods for Power and Sample Size Calculations

The conclusion from a study is often based, largely or entirely, on the significance of a particular p-value obtained from it. It is therefore prudent to ask, during the planning stage, 'How large does the study have to be, in terms of sample size, to ensure a high probability that a significant p-value will indeed be obtained, if the exposure or treatment under investigation has an effect large enough to be worth knowing about (whether for further research, for practical use, or simply as a fact of importance)?' This question is the basis of a conventional power calculation, which asks, for example,

- if the following conditions are met:
  - the study consists of a simple comparison of exposed versus unexposed (or treated versus untreated) experimental units (e.g., human individuals, samples of material or manufactured items),
  - the response in question is a normally distributed variable Y,
  - the standard deviation of Y among units at the same level of exposure (unexposed or exposed) is σ,
  - the true effect of exposure is δ,
  - the study comprises n unexposed and n exposed units,
  - the criterion for statistical significance is specified as $p < \alpha$,
- then,
  - what is the probability, β, that the study will fail to give a significant result, that is, that the outcome will be $p \geq \alpha$?

The probability that the study *will* give a significant result, $(1 - \beta)$, is then the *statistical power* of the study. If the number of units is under the control of the investigator, the calculation can be rearranged, to ask what sample size n is required to give a specified power, typically $(1 - \beta) = 0.8$ or 0.9 (80% or 90%).

Since an FDR compares the strength of evidence among a set of hypotheses all of which have actually been tested, it is a natural instrument for choosing a subset of these

The False Discovery Rate: Its Meaning, Interpretation and Application in Data Science, First Edition.
N.W. Galwey.
© 2025 John Wiley & Sons Ltd. Published 2025 by John Wiley & Sons Ltd.
Companion website: www.wiley.com/go/falsediscoveryrate

hypotheses that deserve further investigation. But if the FDR is to be used in this way, it is desirable that questions about the probability that worthwhile hypotheses will indeed be correctly identified, or how large the experiment must be to ensure that they are identified, should be expressed in terms of the FDR, instead of or as well as the *p*-value. Methods for doing so are considered in this chapter. In order to arrive at methods that are easy to understand and apply, several simplifying assumptions will be made, and these will be noted as they are introduced.

Since the false discovery rate is based on the concept of a 'discovery', announced when a 'significant' *p*-value is obtained, it is still necessary to specify a threshold significance criterion, for example, $\alpha = 0.05$. Since the *p*-value is defined in relation to a null hypothesis, H_0, this must also be specified. As usual it is assumed that H_0 is true in m_0 of the m tests conducted, and that the alternative hypothesis, H_1, is true in the remaining m_1 tests, so that $m_0 + m_1 = m$. In any given set of m tests conducted, m_0 and m_1 will be fixed, but their values cannot be known, and an assumption must be made about them. We will assume that the m hypotheses tested are randomly sampled from an infinite population of hypotheses available for test – for example, in a gene expression study, that the effect of a stimulus on the expression level of a sample of RNA transcripts is to be studied, and that the m transcripts sampled are randomly chosen from a much larger population of transcripts available for study. We will further assume that in the underlying population, H_0 is true for a proportion π_0 of the hypotheses, and H_1 is true for the remaining proportion π_1, so that $\pi_0 + \pi_1 = 1$. With such assumptions, m_0 and m_1 become random variables following a binomial distribution, such that

$$E(m_0/m) = \pi_0, E(m_1/m) = \pi_1.$$

We will further assume that m is sufficiently large that the approximations

$$m_0/m \approx \pi_0, m_1/m \approx \pi_1 \tag{11.1}$$

are acceptable.

The information required in order to control the FDR of a planned study at a specified level is similar to that required for a conventional power calculation, namely, the specification of H_0, of α, and of the statistical power to be achieved, $(1 - \beta)$, if the alternative hypothesis H_1 is true. The process of a conventional power calculation will therefore next be reviewed.

H_0 requires the specification of a particular value for the effect of the exposure or treatment under consideration, typically $\delta_0 = 0$, but H_1 covers a range of possible values of δ, namely:

- either $\delta > 0$ or $\delta < 0$, but not both, if $\delta_0 = 0$ and a one-sided test is specified, or
- $\delta \neq 0$ if a two-sided test is specified.

When calculating the statistical power of a proposed study, the whole range covered by H_1 cannot be considered simultaneously: the magnitude of a particular effect that it is desired to detect, δ_1, must be specified.

Having specified δ_0 and δ_1, δ will be estimated by

$$d = \bar{y}_E - \bar{y}_U,$$

where

$\bar{y}_E$ = mean value of Y in the exposed units;
$\bar{y}_U$ = mean value of Y in the unexposed units.

d is then a realisation of a random variable D, with distribution:

$$D \sim N\left(\delta, \sqrt{\frac{2}{n}}\sigma\right).$$
(11.2)

For simplicity, we will assume that after the study is completed, σ is effectively known, for example, because the study is large enough for it to be estimated precisely. The significance of the observed d can then be tested using the Z statistic,

$$z = \frac{d}{\sqrt{\frac{2}{n}}\sigma}.$$
(11.3)

If H_0 is true, z is a realisation of

$$Z_0 \sim N(0, 1).$$
(11.4)

If a one-sided test is to be conducted, with the alternative hypothesis $\delta > 0$, the probability of obtaining a significant result is then

$$P(Z_0 > z_\alpha) = \alpha,$$
(11.5)

where

z_α = the $(1 - \alpha)$ quantile of Z_0,

as illustrated in Figure 11.1.

To understand the basis of a power calculation related to this test statistic, we need to return to consideration of the random variable D and its realisation d. Taking the critical value of the test statistic, z_α, as defined by Distribution (11.4) and Equation (11.5), substituting it into Equation (11.3), and rearranging, it follows that the test statistic Z will be significant in cases where

$$d > \sqrt{\frac{2}{n}}\sigma z_\alpha.$$
(11.6)

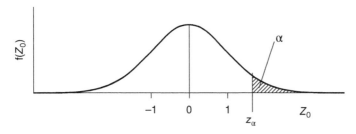

Figure 11.1 The standard normal distribution, showing the significance threshold probability α and the corresponding value of Z.

If H_0 is true, the probability that this will be the case is, of course,

$$P\left(D_0 > \sqrt{\frac{2}{n}}\sigma z_\alpha\right) = \alpha,$$

where

$$D_0 = D|H_0,$$

that is, the symbol D_0 represents the variable D, conditional on H_0 being true. The distribution of D_0 and the region of this distribution that corresponds to a significant result are illustrated in Figure 11.2a. However, if H_1 is true and, specifically, if $\delta = \delta_1$, then d is a realisation of

$$D_1 \sim N\left(\delta_1, \sqrt{\frac{2}{n}}\sigma\right), \tag{11.7}$$

where

$$D_1 = D \mid (\delta = \delta_1).$$

Comparing the significance threshold from Inequality (11.6) with Distribution (11.7), the probability of obtaining a significant result is then

$$1 - \beta = P\left(D_1 > \sqrt{\frac{2}{n}}\sigma z_\alpha\right), \tag{11.8}$$

(a) for $n = 3$

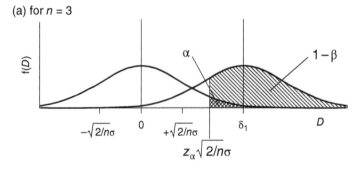

(b) for $n = 5$

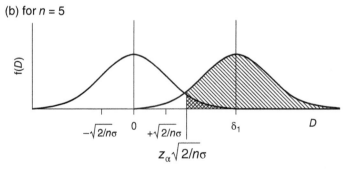

Figure 11.2 (a) and (b) The distribution of D on H_0 and H_1, showing the region corresponding to a significant test result on each hypothesis.

and this is the power of the significance test. From the relationship between Distribution (11.7) and the standard normal distribution (11.4), this probability can also be expressed as

$$P\left(D_1 > \sqrt{\tfrac{2}{n}}\sigma z_\alpha\right) = P\left(Z_0 > \frac{\sqrt{\tfrac{2}{n}}\sigma z_\alpha - \delta_1}{\sqrt{\tfrac{2}{n}}\sigma}\right) = P\left(Z_0 > z_\alpha - \frac{\delta_1}{\sqrt{\tfrac{2}{n}}\sigma}\right). \tag{11.9}$$

The distribution of D_1, and the region of it that corresponds to a significant result, are also illustrated in Figure 11.2a.

Equivalently, it follows from Distribution (11.7) that when $\delta = \delta_1$, z is a realisation of

$$Z_1 \sim N\left(\frac{\delta_1}{\sqrt{\tfrac{2}{n}}\sigma}, 1\right). \tag{11.10}$$

The probability of obtaining a significant result is then naturally expressed as

$$1 - \beta = P(Z_1 > z_\alpha), \tag{11.11}$$

and from the relationship between Distribution (11.10) and the standard normal distribution (11.4),

$$P(Z_1 > z_\alpha) = P\left(Z_0 > z_\alpha - \frac{\delta_1}{\sqrt{\tfrac{2}{n}}\sigma}\right).$$

In summary, the probability of obtaining a significant result is

$$1 - \beta = P\left(D_1 > \sqrt{\tfrac{2}{n}}\sigma z_\alpha\right) = P(Z_1 > z_\alpha) = P\left(Z_0 > z_\alpha - \frac{\delta_1}{\sqrt{\tfrac{2}{n}}\sigma}\right).$$

Visual comparison of the distribution of D_1 in Figure 11.2a with the standard normal distribution in Figure 11.1 confirms the equivalence of these representations. The form

$$1 - \beta = P\left(Z_0 > z_\alpha - \frac{\delta_1}{\sqrt{\tfrac{2}{n}}\sigma}\right) \tag{11.12}$$

is the most useful for practical purposes.

A numerical example will illustrate how increasing the sample size of a study can increase the power of its hypothesis test. Figure 11.2a was produced on the assumption that:

- the significance threshold is $\alpha = 0.05$, whence for a one-sided test, $z_\alpha = 1.645$;
- the standard deviation of Y is assumed (e.g., on the basis of previous knowledge) to be $\sigma = 2$;
- the investigator is interested in detecting an effect of magnitude $\delta_1 = 4$;
- it is proposed that the sample size at each exposure level should be $n = 3$.

The power of the study will then be

$$1 - \beta = P\left(Z_0 > 1.645 - \frac{4}{\sqrt{\frac{2}{3}} \times 2} \right) = P(Z_0 > -0.805) = 0.789.$$

However, if $n = 5$, we obtain Figure 11.2b, and

$$1 - \beta = P\left(Z_0 > 1.645 - \frac{4}{\sqrt{\frac{2}{5}} \times 2} \right) = P(Z_0 > -1.517) = 0.935.$$

Comparison on the scale of D shows how the increase in n narrows the distributions and increases the power of the test. However, the test will of course be conducted on the scale of Z, not D, and presenting the distributions on this scale is also revealing (Figure 11.3). It allows the power of the tests, $(1 - \beta)$, to be compared more clearly, on a single plot. The narrowing of both distributions when n is increased is no longer represented, but the increase in separation of the null and alternative distributions that is achieved is now clearer.

If the value of n cannot be controlled by the investigator, the procedure described in this section so far can provide a valuable indication of whether the proposed study is worth doing. But if n is within the investigator's control, further steps can be taken to determine what sample size will produce a study that *is* worth doing. By analogy with Equation (11.5), we specify

$$P\left(Z_0 > z_{(1-\beta)}\right) = 1 - \beta. \tag{11.13}$$

Then combining Equations (11.13) and (11.12),

$$P\left(Z_0 > z_{(1-\beta)}\right) = P\left(Z_0 > z_\alpha - \frac{\delta_1}{\sqrt{\frac{2}{n}}\sigma} \right),$$

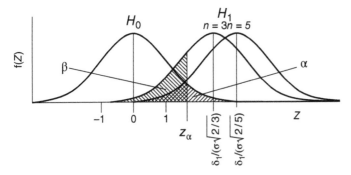

Figure 11.3   The distribution of Z on H_0 and H_1, for different values of n. Total hatched area to left of z_α represents β when $n = 3$. Cross-hatched area represents β when $n = 5$.

whence

$$z_{(1-\beta)} = z_\alpha - \frac{\delta_1}{\sqrt{\frac{2}{n}\sigma}}. \tag{11.14}$$

We also note that, from the symmetry of the standard normal distribution about 0,

$$z_{(1-\beta)} = -z_\beta. \tag{11.15}$$

Substituting Equation (11.15) into Equation (11.14) and rearranging, we obtain

$$n = 2\left[(z_\alpha + z_\beta)\frac{\sigma}{\delta_1}\right]^2. \tag{11.16}$$

Thus, if we are able to specify:

- the significance threshold α that we propose to use,
- the statistical power $(1 - \beta)$ that we seek to achieve,
- a value of the standard deviation of Y that we believe is realistic, namely, σ, and
- a value of the effect size if H_1 is true, sufficiently large that we would be sorry if we failed to detect it, namely, δ_1,

then we can then specify a sample size, n, at each exposure level that is likely to achieve our goal.

For example, suppose we specify that we seek to design a study with power

$$1 - \beta = 0.8,$$

often expressed as '80%', whence

$$\beta = 1 - 0.8 = 0.2,$$

then keeping the values $\alpha = 0.05$, $\sigma = 2$ and $\delta_1 = 4$ specified previously, we obtain

$$n = 2 \times \left[(z_{0.05} + z_{0.2}) \times \frac{2}{4}\right]^2 = 2 \times \left[(1.645 + 0.842) \times \frac{2}{4}\right]^2 = 3.091.$$

That is, since the sample size must be a whole number, we require $n = 4$ units per exposure level.

11.2 Connection of Statistical-Power-Related Concepts to FDR-Related Concepts

The next step is to connect the concepts of the significance threshold α (sometimes rather mysteriously called the 'size' of the significance test) and the statistical power $(1 - \beta)$ to the other concepts related to the FDR. If all the variables in Equation (11.12) except α are held constant, then the probability of obtaining a significant result when H_1 is true – the power of the test – can be expressed as a function of α:

$$F_1(\alpha) = 1 - \beta = P\left(Z_0 > z_\alpha - \frac{\delta_1}{\sqrt{\frac{2}{n}\sigma}}\right). \tag{11.17}$$

The probability of obtaining a significant result when H_0 is true is also a function of α – the simplest possible one, namely, α itself:

$$F_0(\alpha) = \alpha. \tag{11.18}$$

These probabilities, together with the proportions of the tests for which H_1 and H_0 are true, namely, π_1 and $\pi_0 = (1 - \pi_1)$, respectively, can be used to populate the confusion matrix with the expected proportion of tests in each cell, as shown in Table 11.1.

Using the relationship between the confusion matrix and the FDR introduced in Chapter 2, Section 2.3, the expected value of the FDR (referred to as pFDR) is then seen to be

$$\text{pFDR} = \frac{\pi_0 F_0(\alpha)}{\pi_0 F_0(\alpha) + \pi_1 F_1(\alpha)} = \frac{\pi_0 \alpha}{\pi_0 \alpha + \pi_1 F_1(\alpha)}. \tag{11.19}$$

This approach was presented and explored by Cai et al. (2010): Equation (11.19) in this section is Equation (3) in their foundational paper. Expressing the power of the test solely as a function of α has the merit of permitting further exploration and argument concerning pFDR to be pursued without reference to a particular test statistic: the conclusions will be relevant to t, F and χ^2 tests, etc., as well as to the Z test. However, there are two contexts in which the underlying variables that determine the power must be kept in mind:

- δ_1 is a particular value of assumed effect size, whereas in practice the effect size will usually vary among the cases in which H_1 is true. A common approach to this problem is to specify an assumed probability distribution of the effect sizes, then specify the mean value of this distribution as δ_1, and make the further assumption that the results of power calculations based on this value will be a reasonable approximation to those that would be obtained from the whole distribution.
- If achievement of a specified pFDR is to be used as the criterion to determine an appropriate sample size, the value of n must be brought back into consideration. The process for doing this will now be considered.

The level at which pFDR is to be controlled is designated η: that is, we desire

$$\text{pFDR} \leq \eta. \tag{11.20}$$

Table 11.1 The confusion matrix expressed in terms of expected proportions.

	Conclusion from evidence		
True hypothesis	H_0	H_1	Total
H_0	$\pi_0(1 - F_0(\alpha))$	$\pi_0 F_0(\alpha)$	π_0
H_1	$\pi_1(1 - F_1(\alpha))$	$\pi_1 F_1(\alpha)$	π_1
Total			1

(The symbol η is used here for consistency with the notation of Cai et al. It is equivalent to the symbol q^* used by Benjamini and Hochberg (1995) and introduced in Chapter 2, Section 2.4.) Combining Equation (11.19) and Inequality (11.20), we obtain

$$\frac{\pi_0 \alpha}{\pi_0 \alpha + \pi_1 F_1(\alpha)} \leq \eta,$$

which can be rearranged to give

$$\frac{\pi_0}{\pi_1} \cdot \frac{\alpha}{F_1(\alpha)} \leq \frac{\eta}{1 - \eta}. \tag{11.21}$$

This may seem an unnecessarily elaborate way in which to specify the relationship between the FDR and the significance threshold. However, Inequality (11.21) can be re-expressed in a way that makes it consistent with intuition, as follows. On the left-hand side,

$$\frac{\pi_0}{\pi_1} \cdot \frac{\alpha}{F_1(\alpha)} = \frac{\pi_0 \alpha / (\pi_0 \alpha + \pi_1 F_1(\alpha))}{\pi_1 F_1(\alpha) / (\pi_0 \alpha + \pi_1 F_1(\alpha))} = \frac{E(FDR)}{E(\text{true discovery rate})}. \tag{11.22}$$

On the right-hand side,

$$\frac{\eta}{1 - \eta} = \frac{\max(\text{acceptable FDR})}{\min(\text{acceptable true discovery rate})}. \tag{11.23}$$

Then, substituting Equations (11.22) and (11.23) into Inequality (11.21),

$$\frac{E(FDR)}{E(\text{true discovery rate})} \leq \frac{\max(\text{acceptable FDR})}{\min(\text{acceptable true discovery rate})}, \tag{11.24}$$

which is as it should be. Inequality (11.21) can be further rearranged as

$$\frac{\alpha}{F_1(\alpha)} \leq \frac{\pi_1}{\pi_0} \cdot \frac{\eta}{1 - \eta}, \tag{11.25}$$

so that the left-hand side is a function only of α.

11.3 Sample Size Required to Achieve a Specified FDR

The left-hand side of Inequality (11.25) can then be evaluated for different values of n, to identify those that meet the criterion. For example, with the assumptions and specifications about α, σ and δ_1 made earlier, we have seen that if $n = 3$, then

$$\text{power} = 1 - \beta = F_1(\alpha) = 0.789.$$

If we further assume that $\pi_1 = 0.1$, and specify that we wish to control the FDR at the rate $\eta = 0.1$, we find that

$$\frac{\pi_1}{\pi_0} \cdot \frac{\eta}{1 - \eta} = \frac{0.1}{0.9} \times \frac{0.1}{1 - 0.1} = 0.01234, \tag{11.26}$$

and we can substitute these values into Inequality (11.25) to obtain

$$\frac{0.05}{0.789} \le 0.01234 \tag{11.27}$$

$$0.0633 \le 0.01234.$$

This statement is false: that is, the condition is not met, and pFDR is not controlled at the desired rate. Trying $n = 5$, we obtain

$$F_1(\alpha) = 0.935$$

and

$$\frac{0.05}{0.935} \le 0.01234,$$

$$0.0535 \le 0.01234,$$

and the condition is still not met. Increasing n from 3 to 5 has reduced the ratio $\alpha/F_1(\alpha)$, but not by very much.

In fact, there is no value of n that will enable us to control the FDR with the choices of α, π_1 and η specified here. To understand this, note that because $F_1(\alpha)$ is a probability,

$$0 \le F_1(\alpha) \le 1,$$

and therefore,

$$\alpha \le \frac{\alpha}{F_1(\alpha)}. \tag{11.28}$$

Combining Inequalities (11.25) and (11.28), we obtain

$$\alpha \le \frac{\pi_1}{\pi_0} \cdot \frac{\eta}{1-\eta}. \tag{11.29}$$

Neither π_1 nor $\pi_0 = (1 - \pi_1)$ nor η is a function of n, which therefore influences Inequality (11.25) only through its effect on $F_1(\alpha)$. Hence, n has no influence on Inequality (11.29), and this inequality indicates the maximum value of α that can be specified when the desired values of π_1 and η have been chosen, regardless of the value of n.

Overall, the key to controlling the FDR is to reduce the ratio $\alpha/F_1(\alpha)$. Inspection of Figure 11.3 shows that if α is reduced, and hence z_α is increased, the value $F_1(\alpha) = (1 - \beta)$ is unfortunately also reduced. However, the proportional reduction of $F_1(\alpha)$ is small compared with the proportional reduction of α, so the value of $\alpha/F_1(\alpha)$ is reduced, as intended. We conclude that in order to control the FDR at a worthwhile level, we must specify a stringent (i.e., low) value of α.

From Equation (11.26) and Inequality (11.29), we see that, with the present specifications of π_1 and η, we must specify $\alpha \le 0.01234$. If we therefore lower the specified significance threshold to $\alpha = 0.01$, we can proceed to explore how, as n is increased, $F_1(\alpha)$ increases and hence $\alpha/F_1(\alpha)$ decreases (Table 11.2).

Table 11.2 Value of n required to achieve a specified FDR (η), given specifications $\delta_1 = 4$, $\sigma = 2$, $\pi_1 = 0.1$ and $\alpha = 0.01$.

n	$F_1(\alpha)$	$\alpha/F_1(\alpha)$	$\dfrac{\alpha}{F_1(\alpha)} \leq \dfrac{\pi_1}{\pi_0} \cdot \dfrac{\eta}{1-\eta} = 0.01234$
1	0.18085	0.05529	False
2	0.37208	0.02688	False
3	0.54900	0.01821	False
4	0.69219	0.01445	False
5	0.79840	0.01253	False
6	0.87239	0.01146	True
7	0.92151	0.01085	True
8	0.95290	0.01049	True
9	0.97234	0.01028	True
10	0.98406	0.01016	True
11	0.99096	0.01009	True

This table shows that if $n \geq 6$, $\eta \leq 0.1$ is achieved. In more detail, substituting numerical values into Equation (11.17), $z_\alpha = z_{0.01} = 2.326$, so when $n = 6$, the power is

$$1 - \beta = F_1(\alpha) = P\left(Z_0 > 2.326 - \frac{4}{\sqrt{\frac{2}{6}} \times 2}\right) = P(Z_0 > -1.138) = 0.872,$$

whence

$$\frac{\alpha}{F_1(\alpha)} \leq \frac{0.01}{0.872} = 0.01146,$$

and

$$0.01146 \leq 0.01234$$

is true.

There is one further consideration that must be explored, in order to establish the credentials of this method for specification sample size on the basis of control of the FDR. We have established that n greater than a particular value will control the FDR at rate η when a particular significance threshold α is specified – but is it possible that some more liberal threshold (i.e., a *larger* value of α) would control the FDR at the same or a lower rate, for the same or a smaller value of n? If so, this would allow more hypotheses to be retained for further investigation, without increasing the FDR and without expending additional resources, and this would surely be a superior outcome. The idea seems implausible, but it needs to be evaluated more rigorously.

In order for a larger value of α to permit control of the FDR at a lower rate η, it would have to permit a lower value of $\eta/(1-\eta)$, and Inequality (11.25) shows that to achieve this it would have to reduce the ratio $\alpha/F_1(\alpha)$: that is, the increase in α would have to produce a more-than-proportional increase in $F_1(\alpha)$. In the preceding example, the opposite was the case: increasing α from 0.01 to 0.05 produced only a relatively slight proportional increase in $F_1(\alpha)$. We will now explore the relationship between α and $\alpha/F_1(\alpha)$ more generally.

We continue to consider the case of a Z test for the significance of an effect estimate d, which is a realisation of a random variable D with Distribution (11.2). For the true effect δ, we consider the hypotheses $H_0{:}\delta = 0$ and $H_1{:}\delta > 0$, specifying the particular value $\delta = \delta_1$ for the purpose of power calculations. Then,

$$F_0(\alpha) = P(Z > z_\alpha \mid \delta = 0) = \alpha,$$
$$F_1(\alpha) = P(Z > z_\alpha \mid \delta = \delta_1) = 1-\beta,$$

as illustrated in Figure 11.3. We note also that $F_1(\alpha)$ can be conveniently calculated from Equation (11.17), where Z_0 has the standard normal distribution (11.4). The next step is to consider the values of $F_0(\alpha) = \alpha$ and $F_1(\alpha)$ over the whole range of possible critical values for the test statistic, $-\infty \le z_\alpha \le +\infty$ (Figure 11.4). When $z_\alpha \to -\infty$, all test results obtained are counted as significant, whether $\delta = 0$ or $\delta = \delta_1$, and when $z_\alpha \to +\infty$, all test results are counted as non-significant. In between, for any value of z_α, the proportion of significant results is always smaller if $\delta = 0$ than if $\delta = \delta_1$. This is consistent with intuition – we expect to get more significant results when a real effect is present – but it is also important to note that the ratio between these two conditional probabilities, $F_0(\alpha)/F_1(\alpha)$, becomes smaller and smaller as the critical value of the test statistic, z_α, is increased. The more stringent the significance criterion, the smaller the proportion of significant test results that will be false-positives.

Finally, we move from the scale of Z to the scale of α, and consider the relationship between the ratio $F_0(\alpha)/F_1(\alpha) = \alpha/F_1(\alpha)$ and α (Figure 11.5). This is seen to be monotonically increasing: the larger the value of α, the larger the value of $\alpha/F_1(\alpha)$. No larger value of α will give a lower FDR with the same value of n. It follows that a stringent significance threshold α must be specified if the FDR is to be controlled at a low rate η with a realistic sample size n – or perhaps no matter how large the sample. And this is surely consistent with intuition.

This monotonic relationship between $F_0(\alpha)/F_1(\alpha)$ and α is an instance of a *monotone likelihood ratio* (MLR), though this concept is formally defined in terms of the probability densities of Z_0 and Z_1 (given by Distributions 11.4 and 11.10, respectively), not their cumulative distributions (Lehmann 1986, Chapter 3, Section 3, Distributions with monotone likelihood ratio). Such a monotonic positive relationship between $F_0(\alpha)/F_1(\alpha)$ and α is a feature of

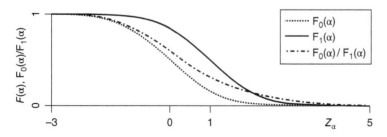

Figure 11.4 The relationship between $F_0(\alpha)$, $F_1(\alpha)$ and z_α. The functions are plotted with the specifications $\delta_1 = 1$ and $\sqrt{\dfrac{2}{n}}\sigma = 1$.

Figure 11.5 The relationship between $\alpha/F_1(\alpha)$ and α.

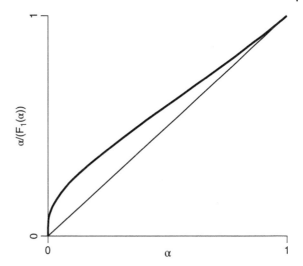

many other test statistics as well as the Z test. Cai et al. (2010) have noted that a test will have this feature if it meets all the following criteria (which they state more formally):

- Its probability density function has the MLR property.
- It is right-tailed, that is, values to the right of (larger than) the critical value are considered significant.
- The distribution is shifted to the right when H_1 is true, relative to its position on H_0.

Cai et al. state that 'Many commonly used distributions, such as normal, noncentral t, non-central chi-square and non-central F distributions, belong to this family of distributions'. The *noncentrality parameter* of a probability distribution is a value that specifies how far it is shifted left or right, relative to its position on H_0. For example, the noncentrality parameter of Z_1 is $\dfrac{\delta_1}{\sqrt{\dfrac{2}{n}\sigma}}$. For a more formal presentation of this concept, see Dodge (2003), or https://en.wikipedia.org/wiki/Noncentral_distribution, accessed 17 May 2024. Note that symmetrical two-sided significance tests, such as the two sided t- and Z-tests, can be expressed as right-tailed if the significance threshold is expressed in terms of the absolute value of the test statistic, stripped of its plus or minus sign: that is, in the case of the Z-test, if the significance threshold is expressed as $|Z| > z_{\alpha/2}$. Indeed, it is difficult to imagine a useful significance test that does *not* meet the criteria of Cai et al.

11.4 Significance Threshold (α) Required to Achieve a Specified FDR When Sample Size Is Fixed

If the sample size n cannot be controlled by the investigator, the monotonic relationship between $F_0(\alpha)/F_1(\alpha)$ and α can be used in combination with Inequality (11.25) to find the largest value of α that will control the FDR at a specified rate. For example, suppose that we are planning a study in which, once again, it seems reasonable to assume that $\sigma = 2$ and $\pi_1 = 0.1$, to specify $\delta_1 = 4$, and to control the FDR at $\eta = 0.1$, but in which we are limited by circumstances beyond our control to $n = 3$. To achieve this FDR, we search for the largest value of α that satisfies

$$\frac{\alpha}{F_1(\alpha)} < \frac{\pi_1}{\pi_0} \cdot \frac{\eta}{1-\eta} = \frac{0.1}{0.9} \cdot \frac{0.1}{1-0.1} = 0.01235.$$

Starting with $\alpha = 0.0001$, we obtain $z_\alpha = 3.719016$, and, hence, from Equation (11.17),

$$F_1(\alpha) = P\left(Z_0 > 3.719016 - \frac{4}{\sqrt{\frac{2}{3}} \times 2}\right) = P(Z_0 > 1.26953) = 0.10213,$$

whence

$$\frac{\alpha}{F_1(\alpha)} = \frac{0.0001}{0.10213} = 0.00098,$$

indicating that the FDR is controlled at the specified rate. Continuing to explore values of α over the range from 0 to 1, we obtain the results presented in Table 11.3. To the level of precision explored, $\alpha = 0.0058$ is the largest significance threshold that satisfies $\frac{\alpha}{F_1(\alpha)} < 0.01235$, and hence controls the FDR at $\eta < 0.1$.

In their more formal presentation of the ideas in this chapter, Cai et al. (2010) consider the case where the approximations concerning m, m_0 and m_1 (Display (11.1)) are not acceptable, because the total number of tests, m, is so small that:

- there is a non-negligible probability that $m_1 = 0$, that is, there are no tests for which H_1 is true, and/or

Table 11.3 Values of α for which it is possible to control the FDR at a specified level ($\eta = 0.1$, whence $\alpha/F_1(\alpha) \leq 0.01235$), given the specifications $\delta_1 = 4$, $\sigma = 2$ and $\pi_1 = 0.1$.

α	$F_1(\alpha)$	$\alpha/F_1(\alpha)$	FDR controlled?
0	0.00000	Undefined	Undefined
0.0001	0.10213	0.00098	True
0.0002	0.13773	0.00145	True
0.0003	0.16302	0.00184	True
⋮			⋮
0.0056	0.46537	0.01203	True
0.0057	0.46784	0.01218	True
0.0058	0.47027	0.01233	True
0.0059	0.47266	0.01248	False
0.0060	0.47502	0.01263	False
⋮			⋮

- there is a non-negligible probability that $R = 0$, that is, H_0 is not rejected for any test, so that the standard specification of the expected FDR, $E(V/(V + S)) = E(V/R)$ in the notation of the confusion matrix (Chapter 5, Section 5.5, Table 5.14), requires division by zero.

The first of these situations requires a rather elaborate refinement to the function $F_1(\alpha)$, the power of each test (Equation 8 of Cai et al.). The second requires a similarly elaborate refinement of the formula for the FDR (Equation 4 of Cai et al.). However, in most of the situations in which FDR should be taken into account in the planning of a study, it seems unlikely that these issues will make a practical difference, in which case the formulae presented here, using π_0 and π_1 in place of m_0/m and m_1/m, can be applied.

The formulae and arguments in this chapter are based on the assumption that the significance tests are independent in the m_0 cases in which H_0 is true. However, as noted in Chapter 2, Section 2.8, if there are positive correlations among these tests, the BH-FDR criterion is conservative. Cai et al. considered the implications of this for sample size calculations, and noted that

> our simulation result shows that even when the hypotheses are correlated, the sample size derived from our procedure can still achieve the desired average power in most of the cases. In only a few cases with common correlation structure, the achieved average power could be less than the desired value... And the loss of power in such cases is relatively small (<5%).

The need for a multiple-testing significance threshold that is fairly stringent, yet not as severe as a Bonferroni-corrected threshold, has sometimes been recognised more informally, without explicit reference to control of the FDR. For example, Simon et al. (2004, Chapter 3, Section 3.8, Number of biological replicates needed) presented an approach to the design of genetic and gene-expression microarray experiments (in which thousands of hypotheses are typically tested), on the basis of a fairly stringent significance threshold of $\alpha = 0.001$, combined with a relatively conventional power criterion of $(1 - \beta) = 0.95$. Cai et al. explored how this proposal performs with regard to control of the FDR, and their conclusions are summarised here. Substituting these values of α and $(1 - \beta) = F_1(\alpha)$ into Inequality (11.25), we obtain

$$\frac{0.001}{0.95} \leq \frac{\pi_1}{\pi_0} \cdot \frac{\eta}{1 - \eta}.$$

Remembering that $\pi_1 = 1 - \pi_0$, this can be rearranged to give

$$\pi_0 \leq \frac{950\eta}{1 + 949\eta}.$$

So, for example, control of pFDR at $\eta = 0.10$ can be achieved provided that

$$\pi_0 \leq \frac{950 \times 0.10}{1 + 949 \times 0.10} = 0.9906,$$

that is, $\pi_1 \geq 0.0094$, and H_1 is true for more than about 1% of the tests. If H_1 is true for a larger proportion of tests, this criterion becomes conservative: it will overestimate the pFDR. Overall, the approach advocated by Simon et al. gives reasonable results in terms of the FDR.

11.5 Summary

If the outcome of a study is to be assessed on the basis of a *p*-value, then at the planning stage, it is conventional to perform power and sample size calculations. These are intended to ensure that if a real effect, large enough to be of interest, is present, there is a high probability that it will be detected by the proposed significance test.

By analogy, if the outcome of a multiple-testing study is to be assessed on the basis of the FDR, it is advisable to perform calculations at the planning stage, to ensure detection of a large proportion of the cases in which H_1 is true, while maintaining a low FDR level.

To achieve this while retaining simplicity, it is necessary to specify a significance criterion (α), a common null and a common alternative hypothesis (H_0 and H_1) over the *m* tests, a proportion of the tests for which H_1 is true ($\pi_1 = 1 - \pi_0$), an effect of treatment or exposure on H_0 (typically $\delta_0 = 0$) and a constant effect size on H_1 (δ_1).

For simplicity, it is further assumed that the observed effect (*d*) is a realisation of a random variable (*D*) with known standard deviation after the study is completed, so that its significance can be tested with the *Z* statistic.

The calculations for a conventional power calculation are reviewed. The power of the significance test $(1 - \beta)$ is the probability of obtaining a significant result when H_1 is true and $\delta = \delta_1$. It is shown to increase as the sample size at each exposure level (*n*) is increased.

The concepts used in a conventional power calculation are related to those used to achieve a specified FDR. The probability of obtaining a significant result when H_0 is true and when H_1 is true are expressed as functions of α, namely, $F_0(\alpha) = \alpha$ and $F_1(\alpha) = (1 - \beta)$, respectively. The expected FDR (pFDR) is expressed as a function of $F_0(\alpha)$, $F_1(\alpha)$, π_0 and π_1. The level at which pFDR is controlled (η) is then expressed as a function of these variables, namely,

$$\frac{\pi_0}{\pi_1} \cdot \frac{\alpha}{F_1(\alpha)} \leq \frac{\eta}{1-\eta} \qquad \text{(Inequality 11.21)}$$

This inequality can be re-expressed in a way that is consistent with intuition, namely,

$$\frac{E(\text{FDR})}{E(\text{true discovery rate})} \leq \frac{\max(\text{acceptable FDR})}{\min(\text{acceptable true discovery rate})} \qquad \text{(Inequality 11.24)}$$

Inequality (11.21) can also be rearranged as $\dfrac{\alpha}{F_1(\alpha)} \leq \dfrac{\pi_1}{\pi_0} \cdot \dfrac{\eta}{1-\eta}$ (Inequality 11.25). Because $F_1(\alpha)$ is a probability $(0 \leq F_1(\alpha) \leq 1)$, in all cases, $\dfrac{\alpha}{F_1(\alpha)} \leq \alpha$, and $\alpha \leq \dfrac{\pi_1}{\pi_0} \cdot \dfrac{\eta}{1-\eta}$ (Inequality 11.29).

None of the terms in Inequality (11.29) is a function of *n*, which affects the achievable value of η only through its effect on $F_1(\alpha)$.

Hence, the FDR cannot be controlled solely by specifying a large value of *n* for any desired value of α. It is also necessary to specify a sufficiently low value of α.

A numerical method is illustrated for identifying the required value of *n*, after α has been specified, so as to achieve the required value of $\dfrac{\alpha}{F_1(\alpha)}$.

The possibility that a larger value of α might give a lower value of η, permitting a smaller value of n, seems implausible, but is formally explored. It would require that the ratio $F_0(\alpha)/F_1(\alpha)$ should decrease as α is increased, whereas in fact this relationship is monotonically increasing for the Z test, and for many other standard significance test statistics, for example, t, χ^2 and F.

A numerical method is demonstrated for identifying the maximum value of α that can be specified when n is fixed by external circumstances.

The method for control of the FDR presented here is used to evaluate a proposed design of genetic and gene-expression microarray experiments (Simon et al. 2004), in which the need for a fairly stringent multiple-testing significance threshold was recognised without explicit reference to control of the FDR.

This proposal recommended a significance threshold of $\alpha = 0.001$, combined with a relatively conventional power criterion of $(1 - \beta) = 0.95$. The performance of these criteria in terms of the FDR is shown to be satisfactory, provided that H_1 is true for more than about 1% of the tests.

References

Benjamini, Y. and Hochberg, Y. (1995). Controlling the false discovery rate: a practical and powerful approach to multiple testing. *Journal of the Royal Statistical Society B* 57: 289–300.

Cai, G., Lin, X., and Lee, K. (2010). Sample size determination with false discovery rate adjustment for experiments with high-dimensional data. *Statistics in Biopharmaceutical Research* 2: 165–174. https://doi.org/10.1198/sbr.2009.0058.

Dodge, Y. (2003). *The Oxford Dictionary of Statistical Terms*. Oxford, UK: Oxford University Press ISBN 0-19-920613-9.

Lehmann, E.L. (1986). *Testing Statistical Hypotheses*. New York: Wiley, 604 pp.

Simon, R.M., Korn, E.L., McShane, L.M. et al. (2004). *Design and Analysis of DNA Microarray Investigations*. New York: Springer, 199 pp.

Index

Note: *Italic* page numbers refer to *figure* and **Bold** page numbers refer to **tables**

The False Discovery Rate: Its Meaning, Interpretation and Application in Data Science, First Edition.
N.W. Galwey.
© 2025 John Wiley & Sons Ltd. Published 2025 by John Wiley & Sons Ltd.
Companion website: www.wiley.com/go/falsediscoveryrate